The Pleasures of Statistics

Frederick Mosteller (1916-2006)

Editors
Stephen E. Fienberg
Department of Statistics
Carnegie Mellon University
5000 Forbes Avenue
Pittsburgh PA 15213-3891
USA
fienberg@stat.cmu.edu

David C. Hoaglin
Abt Bio-Pharma Solutions, Inc.
181 Spring Street
Lexington MA 02421-8030
USA
david.hoaglin@abtbiopharma.com

Judith M. Tanur
Department of Sociology
State University of New York,
Stony Brook, 11794
USA
jtanur@notes.cc.sunysb.edu

ISBN 978-0-387-77955-3   e-ISBN 978-0-387-77956-0
DOI 10.1007/978-0-387-77956-0
Springer New York Dordrecht Heidelberg London

Library of Congress Control Number: 2009942419

Printed on acid-free paper

Springer is part of Springer Science+Business Media (www.springer.com)

Frederick Mosteller

The Pleasures of Statistics

The Autobiography of Frederick Mosteller

Edited by Stephen E. Fienberg, David C. Hoaglin, and Judith M. Tanur

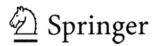 Springer

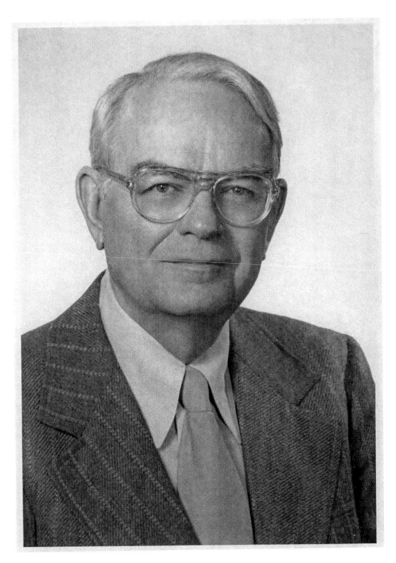

Fred Mosteller, 1980.

Preface

In the summer of 2003, as Steve Fienberg was traveling through New England, he stopped to visit with Fred Mosteller and Dave Hoaglin, in part to discuss progress on the preparation of a volume of Fred's papers. That work had inched along over an extended period of time, and we were trying to get the effort back on track. (The volume appeared the week after Fred passed away in the summer of 2006.) During the visit, Fred brought out a typewritten manuscript. It was an autobiography that he had prepared in the late 1980s. The latest draft was dated in 1990, and the manuscript was still not complete. Apparently this was one of the few occasions when Fred had not followed through on his own dictum, "Finish the job that's nearest done," and he had missed the deadline for a series of autobiographies being published by a major private foundation. Cleo Youtz, Fred's longtime assistant and collaborator, had retrieved the manuscript and was encouraging him to work on it. He felt that he was no longer able to do so and asked us to arrange for its publication. We agreed to take charge of the manuscript and secured the collaboration of Judy Tanur.

We chose to retain Fred's voice and organizational schema, and have worked mainly to clean up details and put the manuscript into publishable form. Fred's manuscript ended around 1990, even though he continued to work and publish throughout the following decade and a half. In a few places we have added footnotes, references, and brief commentaries (especially at the end of each of the opening six chapters) for completeness or explanation. We made no attempt to use Fred's style to extend the chronology for the further decade and a half of his life, but with the help of John C. Bailar III, Graham A. Colditz, John D. Emerson, John Hedley-Whyte, Howard H. Hiatt, Debra Milamed, and James H. Ware we prepared an epilogue to supplement the material on Fred during his time at the Harvard School of Public Health and bring the text to a graceful finish.

The manuscript that we inherited had no title. After considering a number of possibilities, we chose *The Pleasures of Statistics*. We hope Fred would have approved.

Very late in the editorial process we discovered another bit of Fred's manuscript, a short piece labeled "Introduction." We were uncertain whether Fred intended this material to be an introduction to the whole book or to the first section. We decided to use it to introduce the first section, but the reader should be aware that this was our decision and not necessarily Fred's.

Fred's original text describing many of his projects was interspersed with lists of members of the various working groups in which he had participated. This was in his usual spirit of giving credit to all members of his team, but it also interrupted the text and, we believed, would distract the reader. We have retained all such lists but moved them into a "Notes" section at the end of the chapter.

For most of his chapters Fred had collected lists of references. His text mentions them, explicitly or implicitly, but contains few citations in the form usually found in a technical paper or monograph. If a chapter has references, we have placed them in a "References" section at the end of the chapter, where interested readers can readily find them. Those sections also contain the references cited in our commentaries.

We thank John Kimmel, our editor at Springer-Verlag, for agreeing to publish this volume. Springer has previously republished Fred's book with David Wallace on the Federalist Papers, as well as *A Statistical Model* in 1990 and Fred's *Selected Papers* in 2006. These related volumes offer other glimpses of Fred's life and his contributions to statistics. In particular, *Selected Papers of Frederick Mosteller* contains a brief biography and full bibliography.

Among the three editors only Dave Hoaglin had seen parts of the manuscript before 2003. Even so, after we secured the commitment to publish it, the task of putting it in final form has taken far too long. We know that many people commented on drafts during the 1980s. If Fred were writing this preface, he would acknowledge them all with his customary care. Alas, we received no information on their contributions. We do know that Marge Olson did most of the original typing; much of the manuscript was not in electronic form. Also, Cleo Youtz had helped throughout; and after we took charge of the manuscript, she typed most of it into Word Perfect, though she was in her 90s!

Bill and Gale Mosteller, Fred's children, provided most of the photographs from family files and helped to identify the people depicted and when and where the photos taken. They also contributed to a series of editorial decisions and helped with proofreading.

At Carnegie Mellon, where we prepared the final manuscript, several people contributed to the effort: Heather Wainer, Caroline Sheedy, Heidi Sestrich, Ximena Marinero, and most of all Kira Bokalders, who worked with us to insert the photographs and add captions, as well as to clean up the LATEX files for the final published version.

We are grateful to Graham A. Colditz, John D. Emerson, Mark Glickman, Sidney Klawansky, and especially Michael A. Stoto for help with references for Chapters 21, 22, and 23.

Also, we extend our thanks to Sally Thurston, Martha Stewart, Harvard University, and the Ford Foundation for granting us permission to use various photos and stills of Fred throughout the years, which so appropriately capture many of the special moments in his life and career.

Fred's papers are archived at Harvard University Library Archives, the American Philosophical Society Library, and Iowa State University Library's Special Collections Department (MS 610). The American Statistical Association has archived digital copies of the tapes from *Continental Classroom* as well as the 1987 lecture "Broadening the Scope of Statistics and Statistical Education" (DS019) and a related conversation with Fred and John Tukey (DS020) as part of its ongoing project, *Filming of Distinguished Statisticians*.

We feel especially privileged to be able to share with others the personal details of the life of a great scientist, someone who was both a friend and mentor to us and a long-time collaborator, and who has positively affected the lives of countless statisticians, scientists, and ordinary citizens.

Pittsburgh, PA	Stephen E. Fienberg
Lexington, MA	David C. Hoaglin
Montauk, NY	Judith M. Tanur

July 4, 2009

References

Fienberg, S. E., Hoaglin, D. C., Kruskal, W. H., and Tanur, J. M., editors (1990). *A Statistical Model: Frederick Mosteller's Contributions to Statistics, Science, and Public Policy.* New York: Springer-Verlag.

Fienberg, S. E. and Hoaglin, D. C., editors (2006). *Selected Papers of Frederick Mosteller.* New York: Springer-Verlag.

Mosteller, F. and Wallace, D. L. (1984). *Applied Bayesian and Classical Inference: The Case of The Federalist Papers.* (2nd edition of *Inference and Disputed Authorship: The Federalist*). New York: Springer-Verlag.

Contents

List of Figures

Part I

Examples of Quantitative Studies

Introduction

I suppose that, beyond family life, professors mainly teach, administer education, carry out scholarly work, and participate in public work for the advancement of their profession and of society. The first part of the book deals mainly with my scholarly and public work through discussions of six examples.

When readers unfamiliar with a scientific field begin to learn about it, they need examples that illustrate modes of inquiry, objectives, and its variety. To provide this, I start with examples of studies that show statistics in practice—informing the public about politics, evaluating research on human sexual behavior, producing mathematical theory that describes outcomes of human and animal psychological experiments, resolving a humanistic historical question through modeling, assessing a potential public health hazard in medicine, and evaluating equality of educational opportunity. These examples give me a chance occasionally to express some personal opinions and perspectives.

I illustrate many methods and principles in these real studies where statistics plays a major role. In many studies, statistics plays a critical but minor role, and later chapters take up such topics.

My engagement in all these projects came after I had become a faculty member at Harvard University, first in the Department of Social Relations and later also in the Department of Statistics. Later parts of the book deal with my education and scientific development, teaching, administrative activities, and collections of scholarly activities.

So much of my work has been carried out with groups of people that it would be misleading not to mention them, but it is often not feasible to treat them individually. Consequently I often include lists of names that readers may find helpful in understanding the composition of the group.

1

Why Did Dewey Beat Truman in the Pre-election Polls of 1948?

On election night in 1948, like many other people, I attended to the media later and later, and finally about 1:30 a.m. I abandoned hope of a decision and went to bed. Next morning we found that Harry Truman had defeated Thomas Dewey for the presidency of the United States, contrary to all the media wisdom. More important from a statistical point of view, the media had been continuously and confidently informed by the various polling organizations (such as Crossley, Gallup, and Roper) that Dewey would be the winner. These events led to my participation in a large social science study of pre-election polling.

For a short time, it seemed all right to me that experts should be taken down a peg or two, but that view did not last. Samuel A. Stouffer, the sociologist who encouraged bringing me to Harvard, regarded sample surveys as a pre-eminent tool of the social sciences, comparable in value if not in precision to the microscope for the biologist or the telescope for the astronomer. Consequently he felt that a major mistaken forecast using sample surveys was not merely a joke for newspaper columnists but a catastrophe requiring careful scientific investigation and, unlike most research, that an investigation had to be made immediately if useful information was to be recovered. Sam kept saying, "Fred, I wish you could come and help with this, but I suppose you have classes." He well knew what classes I had. Sam met at once with James B. Conant, formerly a chemist, then president of Harvard University, who said, "This reminds me of an explosion in a chemical laboratory. It doesn't stop research, but it makes a terrible mess and takes a long time to clean up."

Although the *Literary Digest* had made a grave error in forecasting the outcome of the Roosevelt-Landon election in 1936, the nation had come to believe that pre-election forecasting now had a sound scientific basis and could be expected to be correct. By 1948, opinion polling was widely used for marketing work, and at the Bureau of the Census, researchers such as Morris Hansen, William Hurwitz, and William Madow had impressively advanced the theory and practice of sample surveys. Although opinion polling was a research field and the problems of sampling and interviewing were being studied, most

F. Mosteller, *The Pleasures of Statistics: The Autobiography of Frederick Mosteller*,
DOI 10.1007/978-0-387-77956-0_1,
© Springer Science + Business Media, LLC 2010

people were not aware of the difficulties of opinion and pre-election polling, over and above those encountered in making unambiguous measurements from members of samples drawn from a well-defined population of objects, like the population of buildings over 20 stories tall.

Organizing

Among the problems were: some people would not respond; others would, but incorrectly; the interviewer could influence the answer; some people had no opinion; and people changed their minds. (Gallup read aloud a letter sent to him by a regretful respondent to his poll, apologizing for having changed his mind in the voting booth after reporting his intention to the Gallup interviewer. The respondent sincerely regretted that he personally had caused the error in forecasting.) Rensis Likert at the Survey Research Center at Michigan, Hadley Cantril at Princeton University, and Paul Lazarsfeld in the Bureau of Applied Social Research at Columbia University were among those who were trying to carry out research in opinion polling in addition to groups in the government, especially the Bureau of the Census.

Rumors flew that many groups of social scientists were planning to inquire into the reasons for the 1948 error in forecasting. A key organization whose purpose was to plan and promote research in social fields was the Social Science Research Council (SSRC), consisting then of seven associated social science organizations.[1]

In 1948, each associated organization had 3 members on the Board of Directors; some additional Board members were chosen at large, and some members of the staff such as the president were also Board members. Most of SSRC's research work was carried out by committees with the aid of a small staff. When social scientists saw clear needs for innovation, especially of an interdisciplinary sort, they often turned to SSRC for aid in developing the new topic. Foundations cooperated with SSRC in supporting such developments. Often foundations liked to have SSRC handle fellowship and educational programs that they funded. Thus SSRC was a facilitator and catalyst without substantial funds of its own. At this time, the president was Pendleton Herring, a political scientist.

The Social Science Research Council and the National Research Council had a joint Committee on Measurement of Opinion, Attitudes and Consumer Wants (chaired by Samuel A. Stouffer). This Committee had been carrying out research on sampling, on the effect of interviewers on expression of attitudes and opinions, and studies of panel methods of interviewing (the same people serve as respondents in several successive surveys). One concern about the election forecasting error was that, unless some authoritative group launched a serious study of what had happened in the 1948 surveys, all studies of opinions and attitudes would fall into disrepute.

The exact order of activities would be hard to establish from any record. Stouffer always used the long-distance phone incessantly and wrote letters only when his secretary or a colleague drafted, typed, and put a completed letter in front of him to sign. It wasn't that Sam found it hard to write, quite the opposite. As a young man, he had been a journalist and a student of English literature before turning to quantitative sociology. Instead, he had a driving urge to get things done, and he couldn't stand to wait for letters or write letters when simple "yeses" or "noes" on the phone would settle matters. I never did have a letter about my academic appointment before I went to Harvard, even after many requests. Sam's suits were always covered with cigarette ashes, and he paced the floor incessantly wherever he was working, in a class, an office, or a hotel room.

In trying to develop an effort such as this pre-election poll investigation, he would plan carefully all the people to call to get an organization to do what he thought was needed. It seemed like simple planning, but Sam always made it sound like a conspiracy. Perhaps that was part of his fun. Donald Young, then president of the Russell Sage Foundation, once said to me, "We know Sam thinks he's scheming, but we like the plan and we like the product, so what does it matter?"

To return to the plan for the investigation, with Stouffer's leadership the Social Science Research Council decided to set up a Committee on Analysis of Pre-election Polls and Forecasts[2] under the chairmanship of S.S. Wilks, my thesis professor at Princeton.

The membership was most impressive, including leading figures from mathematical statistics, applied statistics, history, demography, psychology, political science, economics, business, and sociology. This panel would be hard to beat as representatives of the top quantitative social scientists in the country, nearly all of whom used survey data in their professional work. This group was appointed eight days after the election, unheard-of speed. The SSRC at that time tended to think for a year or so about establishing a committee and what its appropriate membership should be, an approach that has its benefits when funding is hard to come by and more ideas are available than good people to carry them out.

Three days after its appointment this new Committee met, together with most of the people who ultimately formed the staff.[3] These people were still scrambling to rearrange their lives because, whether teachers, government employees, or members of other organizations, projects or classes had to be set aside or new personnel found. Ivy League schools did not take their teaching commitment lightly. Leo Goodman was a beginning graduate student in mathematics at Princeton, and Duncan MacRae reminds me that Leo helped us by running decks of IBM cards through sorters.

Even before the Committee was appointed, the American Association for Public Opinion Research acted to support the appointment of a committee, agreed to cooperate with its investigation, and urged others to as well. Such a move was most helpful, and the list of contributors of polling information [4] might have been much shorter without this support.

Although at first it seemed hopeless for me to break loose and help with this work, the two Sams—Stouffer and Wilks—wanted me to be chief of staff, and by now I was enthusiastic too. With the help of Dean Paul Buck and the Department of Mathematics at Harvard, the statistician John Gurland, who was visiting Harvard at the time, was kind enough to take over my course in mathematical statistics. My wife, Virginia, and I were in the process of supervising the building of our house, and regular inspections would have to be omitted for a while because I had to move to Princeton for several weeks.

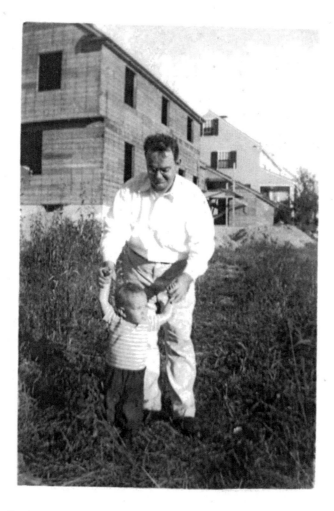

Fig. 1.1. Fred at the Belmont house construction site with his son, Bill, in 1948.

At Princeton, Fred Stephan, sociologist and statistician, whom I had known through SSRC and the American Statistical Association and at a conference at Lake Junaluska in North Carolina, not only made all the local arrangements for space and other support, but hurled himself into the intellectual work, acting as part of the staff. Fred and his wife served the staff a marvelous Thanksgiving dinner in Princeton. Philip J. McCarthy was a statistics student in the same graduate class with me and Wilfrid Dixon in Wilks's statistics program, and I knew him well. I had gotten acquainted with Eli S. Marks, an expert in sampling, in my Washington, D.C., work during World War II; and I knew David B. Truman, a political scientist, from other work with the SSRC. Among the staff, then, only Herbert Hyman was a totally new acquaintance. Sam Stouffer and Duncan MacRae, Jr., then a graduate student in Social Relations at Harvard, volunteered to do a chapter on the last-minute swing to Truman. Forty years later maybe I can say that so many people volunteered to do this chapter that they had to be fought off—it was regarded as the plum job of the investigation. From far and near many fine researchers wrote asking to be the authors of that chapter. I was too inexperienced to be good at declining, and some of the staff would have liked a shot at this chapter as well.

Leonard Doob, editor of the *Public Opinion Quarterly*, generously produced a chapter on the public presentation of polling results.

With a staff consisting of people who by the age of 30 have already shown that they will be stars in their fields, and that has been assembled by the top people in their disciplines with an eye to what was needed in the report, one meeting can accomplish a great deal.

I was used to meeting during WWII with John Williams at the New York branch of the Statistics Research Group of Princeton with the leader outlining the problem, and then staff trying to take it apart. Here we all seemed to know the problem and why we were here, and so in response to the question, "What shall we do?" the experts present indicated what they thought we should do and what they hoped to contribute. We soon had a list of chapters laid out with authorship ready to hand. I've never been involved in a book that shaped up more rapidly—not that some chunks weren't added later, but the main plan of the work was developed in a meeting that lasted less than two hours, even though there was a suitable amount of moaning about the difficulty of the task and how much had to be done in a short time. Of the 11 chapters, need for and authorship of 9 were settled at this first meeting, including the subject of the chapter by Doob, though we did not then know who would be its author. One of the other two chapters was an obligatory chapter by Wilks as chairman of the Committee we were staffing.

Naturally, the primary focus of our work was on the big three polling agencies: Crossley, Gallup, and Roper. At the beginning, the staff visited each polling organization and got its views of the problem. And they were not entirely alike. Roper alone, though, had the problem of explaining his published view that pre-election polling and forecasting was so easy that polling organizations should give it up.

In some ways the hardest task was Hyman's, because he had to check up on the questionnaire design and on control of error in editing, coding, and tabulation. This required repeated visits and interviews at the polling organizations, one in Princeton where we were based and the others in New York City where we weren't.

Without much more ado than this, we all trotted off to write our chapters. The polling organizations willingly supplied data as appropriate. Much of the data we needed were available from the Princeton University Library. Some came from post-election follow-up surveys. As fast as the drafts came in from the authors, I edited the manuscripts—they were being written very rapidly—and discussed them with Stephan and with the authors. When they had time, authors read one another's manuscripts, but just getting one's own chunks finished was a heroic task. My chapter was prepared fairly quickly because it was based primarily on readily available historical material. That gave me more time to read the chapters others wrote and to look for omissions in them. More important was to guard against being excessively knowledgeable after the fact.

I am always amused to hear the evening business report tell the cause of every move in the stock market all day long, even though the same people did not know on the day before whether specific events would send the market up or down. In criticizing the work of others a similar hazard arises. One has a tendency to say that people could have known or that they had methods of investigation they could have used, when the methods may not have been tried in cold blood forecasting, but seem very promising to researchers in the forefront of the field. Often what people might have done would merely have offered an additional vector pointing in a direction somewhat different from a confusing profusion of pointers already available. Integrating these signals is still a problem. I had time to think about claims we wanted to make about what could or should have been done, and after discussion with the team we were able to avoid several instances of claiming more after-the-fact knowledge than we had.

Can you use a method just proved to be defective to find out what is wrong with it? To some extent. These things are largely a matter of degree.

Through the years since 1948, dozens of people have personally explained to me their considered view of what went wrong with the pre-election polls of 1948, some knowing I had served on the staff of the Committee and others oblivious. I have enjoyed this information least at dinner, because responding to the firm statement, "The thing that went wrong with the pre-election polls of 1948 was..." requires great restraint and forbearance. Do you say, "Oh, really?" or "I'm glad to know how that was"?

Allen Wallis, then editor of the *Journal of the American Statistical Association*, once summed the findings up very well: "If there is one thing the SSRC report shows, it is that no one thing caused the errors in the forecasts of the 1948 pre-election polls." As he knew, it was even worse; many things produced the errors.

In a view from the perspective of today, we should have been worried about the possibility of fraud by the polling agencies. I doubt if non-auditors, non-detectives, non-prosecutors would have been very effective at searches for fraud. Some kinds of peculiarities could have started us on a hunt for such behavior, but none were found. (All polling organizations have to guard against interviewers who cheat and have various ways of checking for that kind of fraud. It is so much easier to fill out the forms at home than to go out and locate and talk to respondents that the temptation to cheat must always be present. Fortunately many interviewers enjoy the work itself.)

George Gallup, in a poor-country-boy kind of presentation at the annual meeting of the American Statistical Association in 1949, claimed that the report said that he was honest but stupid, or words to that effect. The report had not attacked the honesty nor played down the intelligence of any of the leaders of polling agencies. Anyone who knew Gallup's professional history regarded him as brilliant. He had gone from a midwestern professor of journalism to an entrepreneur with columns in an enormous number of newspapers, even if we don't bother to count other commercial contracts of great value. I respected him too much to accept this "I'm so dumb and innocent" mien, though the humor went over well at the meeting.

Findings

Just what was the error in the 1948 forecasts? I wrote a chapter on measuring the error and tried to put it into the perspective of the sizes of errors made in many other election forecasts based on opinion surveys.

An important problem in predicting the presidential election in the U.S.A. emerges from the process of awarding state electoral votes. Each state has its own election, and the outcome for the total comes from adding up the 48 (now 50) state electoral votes for each candidate. Thus, instead of estimating which candidate has a majority of the popular vote, the problem is to decide for each state which candidate will receive the electoral vote. I note, regretfully, in retrospect, that the staff did not consider what would be the best way to make an estimate of the winner in these circumstances. It did note the problem as distinctly harder than that of predicting the candidate with the higher national percentage. Not all features of the electoral college approach are negative for forecasting, because some states currently and traditionally prefer a particular party, so that its candidate is likely to carry the state's electoral vote. Even so, plenty of states will be left in a border capacity. Thus the problem was not quite as hard as that of predicting 48 separate elections, but not nearly as easy as predicting one majority vote for the nation. Just where the degree of difficulty falls in between would vary from election to election.

From the research of the staff and other contributors to the report, the Committee concluded that the pollsters had overestimated their predictive ability and neglected the difficulties in predicting a close election. One way of putting it was that the election was too close to call, even without biases in the measuring process that I mention below. The Committee thought the pollsters should have paid attention to their past errors and the implications of those errors for this election. (Of course, they had been right in the 1936, 1940, and 1944 elections, though Crossley made no forecast in 1940.) In saying that they had been right, it should be noted that Crossley and Gallup were about seven percent low in 1936. The errors in the past in estimating the percentages were often substantial. Having only three previous presidential elections limits the amount of data.

We concluded that the 1948 errors were not much out of line with previous errors, and that the polls in presidential elections had not shown yet an ability to improve on persistence forecasting. In trying to forecast weather, one measure of accuracy is to see how much better the forecaster is than someone who always makes as the next prediction whatever the weather is now. Similarly, one could always predict the percentage Republican vote in the next election to be the same as it was in the previous election. I found the magnitude of persistence forecasting errors comparable to those of Crossley and Gallup (smaller in 1936 and 1948, the same in 1944, and larger in 1940). We said that the polls had gotten more than their due in credit for their previous successes and now were reaping a similar unfair amount of blame for errors of much the same magnitude.

We also criticized them for not adequately educating the public about the magnitudes of their errors. After years of teaching, radio listening, and TV viewing, I conclude that we may not know how to do this. Indeed, the whole problem of risk communication, in this case risk of error, is still open for major improvements.

The reader should understand that during the period of the investigation the staff had a hard time finding out what the actual vote and electoral vote were. When we spoke of the outcome as of a given date, we were still uncertain about the vote in the Cleveland area, where 200,000 votes were waving in the breeze, as I recall, enough to change Ohio's vote. I no longer recall why the fact that we couldn't settle the Ohio vote was not discussed in the report. The Committee Report recommends better reporting of the official vote.

Roper's situation was unusual. He had developed a doubly-biased sample that was intended to balance its biases. Such an approach turns out to invite trouble, because one never knows how the extent of the biases will work out in the next election.

The Committee said two major causes of errors were (a) errors of sampling and interviewing and (b) errors of forecasting, including assessing future behavior of undecided voters and not allowing for shifts in voting intentions near the end of the campaign. (Fair enough criticism, but such allowances had not been used much in previous elections.)

Two forms of selection of respondents were in principal use at the time: quota sampling and probability sampling, with quota sampling more common.

In quota sampling, the central office assigned the interviewer in the field a part of the quota information about the distribution of the respondents—so many in each age group, so many in each socioeconomic class, and so many of each sex, for example. Then it was up to the interviewer to fill the quota as nearly as she or he (most interviewers were women) could manage.

In the probability samples, the attempt was usually made to assign a specific person to be interviewed: go to a specific household and in that household interview a specific person (the oldest male, the oldest female, or other choices settled in advance, usually by listing the household in an order together with choices).

Everyone—staff and Committee—was concerned about the use of quota sampling versus probability sampling. Although we all "knew" that probability sampling was preferable, the evidence was not present in the data. As McCarthy pointed out, since neither the quota samples nor the probability samples were carried out as they were planned, we cannot tell whether *in practice* one was better than the other. (Today I feel I still don't know, even though my prejudice is still for the probability sample.)

Let us return to the popular questions. What about a last-minute swing to Truman? Stouffer and MacRae offer us a cautious "yes, there was." In postelection surveys about one-seventh of those who said they voted claimed they made up their mind in the last two weeks, and three-quarters of these said they voted for Truman.

In discussing the undecided votes, Marks noted that Gallup had found the percent undecided in 1948 nearly twice that in 1944: 15.8 percent versus 8.9 percent. Marks says that we need not ask whether 1948 was an abnormal election, because from the point of view of the pollsters what was abnormal was having a presidential election without Franklin Roosevelt as a candidate.

In our work we frequently had to remind ourselves that, although many people might have excellent ideas about how to go about allocating the undecided responses, the research verifying that such ideas actually worked had not been done. Such a care must be especially appreciated, because some of the polling organizations had tried to develop special sets of filters to find out whether people were likely to vote and how they leaned; and although these methods were studied and tested in earlier elections, they did not save Crossley, for example, from error in 1948. It is easy to have good ideas, but verified methods require much more.

What the Committee accomplished through its research effort was to get a clear statement of the procedures used by Crossley, by Gallup, and by Roper. It emphasized how difficult presidential election polling was and outlined research needs. Because of its strong auspices, cooperation from many other polling organizations gave an opportunity to assess some of the causes of error and estimate the sizes of their effects. They found the sources of error to be large in number and difficult to evaluate—that is, to sort out. The pollsters seemed to have reached their errors by somewhat different routes, with Crossley and Gallup more nearly alike while Roper was different.

What was the size of the error in predicting the national percentage vote for president (rather than the electoral vote)? Crossley underestimated the Democratic percentage by 4.6 percentage points, Roper by 12.3. Gallup understated the Democratic percentage of the two-party vote by 5.3 percent. The errors of Crossley and Gallup were more than double their errors in 1944; and Roper had errors of no more than 1.5 percent in 1936, 1940, and 1944, so the 12.3 was shocking. The debacle and the report stimulated new interest in the methodology of opinion polling, and research has continued. The care and speed to publication of the Committee's report—8 weeks after the election— probably helped avoid a congressional investigation, and that greatly relieved the polling industry. The industry did take a hard look at itself and cooperated with our work.

Turning now to 1988, Irving Crespi has written *Pre-election Polling: Sources of Accuracy and Error*, a modern analysis of performance in election predictions based on sample surveys. He says that the four major sources of error identified by our study in 1948 were "(1) the use of flawed sample designs, (2) failure to screen nonvoters out of the sample, (3) inadequate methods for treating 'undecided' responses, and (4) failure to measure late changes in voting preference." He concludes that these problems are still present and important but offers hope from research, past and future.

Editors' Postscript

In the years since 1948 polling has become a standard part of campaigns in the US and around the world. It is worthwhile distinguishing between three kinds of election forecasting: pre-election polling of the sort described in this chapter, use of early election results to predict the final result, and exit polling. Most polling organizations now use some form of probability sampling, albeit with very substantial rates of non-response, and most have developed proprietary methods to help them decide which respondents are likely to vote. Eliminating or de-emphasizing the responses of those unlikely to vote improves the accuracy of predicting the results of the election, but pre-election polls appear to be plagued by many of the other problems that Fred describes from 1948.

Since television began to report election returns on a national scale in 1952, the public's interest in prompt knowledge of the results has given rise to elaborate mechanisms for using early election returns (Link, 1972; Fienberg, 2007) and then, later, exit polls of samples of voters right after they have cast their ballots. Exit polls typically use systematic samples of early voters, and statistical models project their results to provide forecasts of winners and to supply newscasters with analytic details for on-air reporting. Controversy arose in the 1970s about the possibility that declaring winners of elections on the east coast of the United States before the polls closed on the west coast might affect turnout on the west coast and thus even the outcome of the election.

In the 2004 national election, early results of exit polls were leaked to the public, creating the impression that John Kerry had a large lead over George W. Bush. When those early impressions turned out to be false, both the exit polls and the election itself underwent careful scrutiny, including by the Social Science Research Council (Traugott, Highton, and Brady, 2005), the organization that sponsored the 1948 exploration which Fred participated in. Conclusions seem to indicate that both the exit polls and the election itself were somewhat flawed. In fact, because both pre-election polls and exit polls have high levels of nonresponse, in part because of the difficulty of implementing timely followup, as well as response biases, both pollsters and critics would do well to revisit the discussion in the 1948 SSRC report (Edison Media Research/Mitofsky International, 2005; Baiman et al., 2005).

Notes

1. Social Science Research Council Associated Organizations
    American Anthropological Association
    American Economic Association
    American Historical Association
    American Political Science Association
    American Psychological Association
    American Sociological Society
    American Statistical Association

2. Committee on Analysis of Pre-election Polls and Forecasts
    S.S. Wilks, *Chairman*, Princeton University
    Frederick F. Stephan, *Executive Secretary*, Princeton University
    James Phinney Baxter, 3rd, Williams College
    Phillip M. Hauser, University of Chicago
    Carl I. Hovland, Yale University
    V.O. Key, Johns Hopkins University
    Isador Lubin, New York City
    Frank Stanton, Columbia Broadcasting System
    Samuel A. Stouffer, Harvard University

3. Technical Staff
    Frederick Mosteller *(chief of staff)*, Harvard University
    Herbert Hyman, National Opinion Research Center
    Philip J. McCarthy, Cornell University
    Eli S. Marks, U.S. Census Bureau
    David B. Truman, Williams College

4. Contributors of Polling Information

Boston Globe Poll of Massachusetts Opinion
    Robert L.M. Ahern, Research Director
The California Poll (Field & Peacock Associates)
    Thomas Peacock
The Sun-Times Straw Poll (Chicago)
    Karin Walsh, City Editor
    Richard J. Finnegan, Editor
Colorado Poll (*Denver Post* and Research Services, Inc.)
    W.N. McPhee, Vice-President
The 1948 Election Study (Elmira, New York)
    Elmo Wilson
    Helen Dinerman
The *Bulletin* Poll (The *Evening Bulletin* and the *Sunday Bulletin*, Philadephia)
    Paul Trescott
    P.L. Snyder
Illinois Poll (Ben Gaffin & Associates)
    Ben H. Gaffin
The Iowa Poll
    Henry J. Kroeger, Director of Research
    Norman C. Meier, Consultant
The Iowa Public Opinion Panel (Central Surveys, Inc.)
    Charles E. Parker
    W. M. Longman
The Minnesota Poll
    Sidney Goldish, Editor
The New Jersey Poll
    Kenneth Fink, Director
    Robert G. Lutz
The Texas Poll (Joe Belden & Associates)
    Joe Belden, Director
The Trenton Poll
    Carroll S. Moore, Jr.
The *Washington Post* Poll
    John J. Corson
    Brandon Marsh
Election Poll of Washington Public Opinion Laboratory
(Washington State College and University of Washington)
    J.N. Bachelder, Co-Director
    Stuart C. Dodd, Co-Director

References

Baiman, R., Dodge, D., and Doop, K. (2005). The 2004 Presidential Election: Exit Poll Error or Vote Miscount? U.S. Count Votes' National Election Data Archive Project. http://www.electionmathematics.org/em-exitpolls/USCV_exit_poll_analysis.pdf.

Crespi, I. (1988). *Pre-election Polling: Sources of Accuracy and Error*. New York: Russell Sage Foundation.

Edison Media Research/Mitofsky International (2005). Evaluation of Edison/Mitofsky Election System 2004. http://www.electionmathematics.org/em-exitpolls/EvaluationJan192005.pdf.

Fienberg, S. E. (2007). Memories of election night predictions past: Psephologists and statisticians at work. *Chance*, 20(4):8–17.

Link, R. F. (1972). Election night on television. In J. M. Tanur, F. Mosteller, W. H. Kruskal, R. F. Link, R. S. Pieters, and G. R. Rising, editors, *Statistics: A Guide to the Unknown*. San Francisco: Holden-Day. 137–145. (Also appears in the 2nd edition [1979] and the 3rd edition [1989].)

Mosteller, F., Hyman, H., McCarthy, P. J., Marks, E. S., and Truman, D. B., with the collaboration of L. W. Doob, D. MacRae, Jr., F. F. Stephan, S. A. Stouffer, and S. S. Wilks (1949). *The Pre-election Polls of 1948*. New York: Social Science Research Council Bulletin 60.

Traugott, M., Highton, B., and Brady, H. (2005). A Review of Recent Controversies Concerning the 2004 Presidential Election Exit Polls. National Research Commission on Elections and Voting, Social Science Research Council. http://elections.ssrc.org/research/ExitPollReport031005.pdf.

Sexual Behavior in the United States: The Kinsey Report

Sex talk titillated the public in the 1950s the way the national deficit, drugs, AIDS, and malfeasance in government excite us today; but in the 1950s we had more fun, feeling very devilish when discussing bedroom topics in the open. In this milieu, the book *Sexual Behavior in the Human Male*, generally called the Kinsey Report, filled a niche in 1948. It fitted with the changing attitudes and sexual behavior of the whole of society in the United States, a trend that ultimately peaked following the introduction of oral contraceptives and changed again with the AIDS epidemic. The Kinsey Report got enormous publicity from radio talk shows of the time and from interest generated when nearly every comic based jokes on it. Nevertheless, I doubt that many people actually read it, because it was a serious scholarly work based on about nine years of field work by Alfred C. Kinsey and his colleagues Wardell B. Pomeroy and Clyde E. Martin. It was lush with tables and methodological descriptions, and so it took an avid and diligent reader to find out that more people seemed to be engaged in more diverse sexual activities than the general public had appreciated. The reported extent and variety of these behaviors shocked the U.S. population.

Organizing for Evaluation

When such a serious book on such a socially inviting topic comes out, reviewers study it very carefully and give it thorough criticism. "The more serious the book, the more serious the criticism" is not a rule; but a serious book is a challenge to the reviewer. Although this book was by no means the first scientific work published on sexual behavior, it was more extensive in its coverage, and its methods differed from those of most other investigators. Furthermore, the research leader was a biologist rather than a physician or a social scientist, disciplines that had more traditionally produced books on research in human sexual behavior.

Support for the research carried out by Kinsey and his associates at the Institute for Sex Research at Indiana University came partly from the National

F. Mosteller, *The Pleasures of Statistics: The Autobiography of Frederick Mosteller*,
DOI 10.1007/978-0-387-77956-0_2,
© Springer Science + Business Media, LLC 2010

Research Council's Committee for Research in Problems of Sex. Although in late 1950 that Committee continued to support the research, the avalanche of criticisms of the statistical methods used in the research persuaded the Committee through George Corner to write to Isador Lubin, in his capacity as chair of the Commission on Statistical Standards of the American Statistical Association, to "provide counsel regarding the research methods of the Institute for Sex Research."

Corner's letter emphasized problems of statistical analysis and expressed hope that work on the companion volume on the human female, then in preparation, could take advantage of this counsel. Kinsey in his turn offered full cooperation with a committee that might be set up by the American Statistical Association and outlined a number of tasks that he hoped such a committee would undertake, including a review of the statistical criticisms of the book already published about the male, as well as a comparison of methods of research used by other researchers in similar fields with those used by his group. He also made it clear that the book on the human female was far along and that the impact of a committee on its content would be limited.

As president of the American Statistical Association at this time, Samuel S. Wilks appointed a special committee of the Commission on Statistical Standards, no doubt with the advice of the Commission's members, to make the review. The members of the Committee were William G. Cochran, chairman, then the chair of the Department of Biostatistics in the School of Hygiene and Public Health at the Johns Hopkins University and a well-known researcher in the field of sampling of human populations, as well as a scholar in the statistics of health and medicine; John W. Tukey of the Department of Mathematics at Princeton University and of Bell Telephone Laboratories; and me from the Department of Social Relations at Harvard University.

By now I had a well-established teaching load, carried on a good deal of statistical advising for students and faculty at Harvard, mostly in Social Relations, was helping Henry Beecher at Massachusetts General Hospital, and had various University and professional committee tasks as well as my own research work. So this appointment was not altogether a welcome one, even though the study of human sexual behavior sounded like an exciting new field for me. Throughout the effort, more than usual I found myself very hard-pressed for time. No doubt the other Committee members had similar problems. The famous financier Bernard Baruch is said to have advised doing two fewer things than you can, and I had overshot. We were induced because of a feeling of responsibility as professional statisticians.

Kinsey cannot have been very pleased either. His group, which we conveniently abbreviate as KPM, was so far along with their book on the human female that we jointly decided not to treat that new work, even though Corner had specifically mentioned it in the preliminary correspondence. Our committee was already finding the work related to the book on the human male a challenge. For KPM, inevitably an extra study committee not responsible for production makes demands on time and resources and at best is something of a nuisance.

Neither the Commission on Statistical Standards nor Wilks gave our committee a specific charge. They simply handed us the correspondence from George Corner to Lubin and Kinsey's letter to Wilks that made several suggestions about the potential composition of the Committee and the tasks it should undertake.

Doing the Evaluation

Soon we went to Bloomington, Indiana, met with KPM, discussed some plans for our work, and learned firsthand about the interviewing methods being used. Like special research centers at many institutions, Kinsey's group had quarters in a rather low-ceiling basement. Much of the space was used for a library devoted entirely to books on sex.

It turned out that Kinsey was a collector. For example, some of his biological work had been devoted to gall wasps, and he had collected every book and article on this topic that he could find. I was astonished that so much had been written about these wasps. It was a very substantial separate library from that on sexual topics.

Similarly, he had a large record collection of classical music. For some parties in his home, he laid out formal concerts based on this collection. Before each piece was played, he introduced it in scholarly fashion, explaining who composed it and where it was first performed, along with other historical notes.

We did not get off to a good start with our study. I had just learned the words to a song in a Gilbert and Sullivan opera, and it turned out that both Cochran and Tukey were Gilbert and Sullivan buffs. Cochran was also frequently involved in singing groups. And so, as we walked in the rain from our accommodations to the offices of the Institute for Sex Research, we sang a couple of stanzas from H.M.S. Pinafore about becoming Ruler of the Queen's Navee; but, it being my first such experience, I was not very good at it. When we got to the offices, we were shown to a room that we could have "all to ourselves." We had about an hour before our first meeting with the Kinsey group, and so we shut the door and I suggested instead of buckling down to work that we try another stanza of the song to straighten me out. We hadn't gotten very far into it when there was a noisy pounding on the door. Kinsey and some of the staff were there to admonish us. Like so many quarters, including mine at Harvard, sound traveled perfectly from one room to all the others, and so we were distracting the work of the whole Institute, as well as appearing rather light-hearted about what was surely a serious matter to the local organization. I was always a one-note singer anyway, so not much has been lost by restricting my training.

Table 2.1. Age and Sexual Outlet Marital Intercourse: Average Frequency Per Week.

Age	U.S. Population Average Frequency
16–20	3.92
21–25	3.34
26–30	2.89
31–35	2.45
36–40	2.05
41–45	1.74
46–50	1.80
51–55	1.33

Sample has been corrected for age, marital status, and educational level for the U.S. Census, 1940 (Source: Kinsey, Pomeroy, and Martin, 1948, Table 56, p. 252).

The reader might appreciate a few examples of KPM's findings. I give a few excerpts from their vastly more extensive tables and figures. Table 2.1 gives the average frequency per week of marital intercourse as estimated for the U.S. white male population by five-year intervals for ages 16 to 55. The rates show a fairly steady decline from nearly 4 times per week for late teen ages to about 1.3 times per week in the early fifties. Beyond these ages, KPM did not project.

KPM wanted to compare the behavior of people in different generations. To do this, they broke their sample about evenly into those under age 33 and those over age 33. Some critics would have preferred that the generations be defined according to birth date rather than age. Table 2.2 gives the accumulative incidence curve for intercourse for U.S. white males who have completed no more than the eighth grade of schooling. The percentages estimate the portion of the U.S. population that have had some form of intercourse by the age given. Few of either generation have had intercourse of any form by age 10; but by age 15 in the older generation 34.3 percent report at least one experience, and in the younger generation 51.5 report such an experience. Thus the rate seemed to be going up.

The reader may wish to know about better educated groups. I do not give a table, but by age 15 both generations with education level 13+ had almost exactly the same experience of intercourse in any form: 9.4 percent for the older and 9.5 percent for the younger.[1]

To get an idea of the distribution of sources of outlets for U.S. white males, I have read results from the graph for age group 31–35 (Table 2.3). The 82 total in the second panel differs from the 81 in the first panel because of reading and rounding errors. As before, the U.S. population estimates come

Table 2.2. Accumulative Incidence Curve: Education Level 0–8, Total Intercourse

Age	Older generation		Younger generation	
	Cases	Percent	Cases*	Percent
10	324	0.3	476	0.0
15	324	34.3	466	51.5
20	324	84.9	299	89.6
25	324	96.0	173	95.4
30	324	98.5	80	95.0

* The numbers of cases decrease with increasing age because they depend on the age at date of interview (Source: Kinsey, Pomeroy, and Martin, 1948, Table 101, p. 404).

from adjusting the sample values for age, marital status, and education. KPM give similar results for other age groups.

Kinsey had requested that we examine the statistical criticisms of his work as they appeared in the reviews. A. Kimball Romney, then a graduate student in the Department of Social Relations at Harvard and now a very well-known quantitative anthropologist, helped us with this. After we had selected six papers for review, with Kinsey's cooperation, Romney broke them up according to their criticisms. Then each criticism was typed on a sheet of paper, and these were sorted into categories. The slips of paper were of various lengths and

Table 2.3. Distribution of Sources of Outlets for U.S. White Males. (From Kinsey, Pomeroy, and Martin, 1948, Figure 126, p. 488)

Source of outlet	Percent
animal contact	near 0
homosexual outlet	6
intercourse	81
petting to climax	2
nocturnal emissions	3
masturbation	8
	$\overline{100}$

The third line for heterosexual coitus can be categorized further as

Source	Percent
post-marital with companions	2
extra-marital with companions	3
intercourse with prostitutes	3
marital intercourse	67
pre-marital intercourse	7
	$\overline{82}$

rather inconvenient to handle. Cochran, Mosteller, and Tukey then divided up the topics and prepared comments on the remarks of the original reviewers. All this is reproduced in the 110-page Appendix A of the Committee's published book *Statistical Problems of the Kinsey Report*. As might be expected, we often agreed and often disagreed with the critics.

When one is involved with lots of slips of paper, some trouble can be expected to arise. One trouble that happened to us was inadvertent plagiarism. A slip from one critic's paper was accidentally edited slightly by us and converted into our own remarks without attribution. The critic, our friend W. Allen Wallis, pointed this out to us, his main complaint being that the comment had been better stated before our editing. I hope that slip was the only one we so converted.

A second task Kinsey requested was a comparison of the statistical work of his group with that of others who had written books on sex. William O. Jenkins, a faculty member in the Department of Social Relations and an experimental psychologist, reviewed nine books on results of sex research and the Kinsey Report itself from the point of view of samples and sampling methods, interviewing methods, statistical methods, checks (internal and external to the work), and results; he produced the 67-page Appendix B for our report. He ranked the works separately for their handling of samples, interviewing, statistical methods, and checks, and then summed the ranks to get a final ranking. He concluded that KPM should be ranked first and that "the KPM study is a monumental endeavor."[2]

We also produced a 39-page appendix on further work, a 40-page appendix on probability sampling, and another of 23 pages on principles of sampling.

We had one major disappointment. We had hoped to get some idea of what sort of accuracy in sexual information might be needed by people such as marriage counselors or physicians, who counseled on sexual matters. I know now from experience in several fields that it was naive of us to suppose we could get anywhere with that sort of question without mounting a major research project of our own. Unless professionals have been studying the accuracy of the methods used in their work, they have no very good way to think about the value of knowing things more accurately.

The kinds of questions we could not get answered by physicians were: [3]

1. What information is it that is regarded as pertinent for these physicians?
2. Why do the physicians need this information?
3. How can the physician use the information?
4. If we reduce all rates and incidences in the book by a factor of 2 or 10, will it make any difference in the physician's therapeutic behavior? What if we raise them?
5. Are the tables in KPM of much assistance, or is it the verbal material describing the patterns of behavior of certain groups that is of most value?
6. If it is the verbal material, would it make any difference whether the patterns described represented only one or two outstanding individuals

or whether they represented rather well 90 percent of the persons in the group described?

7. Is the knowledge of the existence of extreme cases really of most value, setting as they can bounds below which the upper limit cannot fall and above which the lower limit cannot fall?

By and large the tendency among investigators had been to standardize interviewing for each respondent, using exactly the same questions in exactly the same order. KPM used a different approach. Their interviewers memorized all their questions and were able to gather and record their answers in the order received. Thus when a respondent's narrative answered questions not yet asked, they could record responses without waste of time. KPM preferred interviewing to filling out questionnaires, because often explanations were required and because they intended to represent the whole U.S. white male population including the illiterate. Although KPM's interviewing style was out of step with the prevalent methodology, the critics did not have a well-grounded basis for objection. No one knew what methods were more accurate. KPM used several kinds of checks on their interviewing, more than other investigators.

A more vulnerable point was the sampling. No attempt was made to get a probability sample of the U.S. males. Our committee regarded a probability sample as an unattainable goal, at least when KPM began their interviewing. They interviewed groups of people wherever they could find them, working especially hard on groups such as students, church classes, clubs, and other organizations. It is hard to describe the population actually sampled. Perhaps it would be fair to say that in trying to develop the U.S. white male population they strove for what William Kruskal and I call coverage as a form of representativeness—an attempt to get some of each kind of group, even if one cannot get properly weighted samples. Even today, many people would not be willing to be interviewed about their sexual behavior, and in the late 1940s the reluctance would have been much stronger. The basic question always is whether the people who are not interviewed differ much in their behavior and responses from those who are interviewed.

When in election polling pollsters report the percentage favoring a party, they are likely to include a statement about the margin of error associated with the poll. For example, they may say that the margin is plus or minus 3 percent. This margin is usually based on an assumption of a random sample plus a further assumption that those not responding will split about like those who have responded. If I were to tell you that the margin of error was 3 percent but that 10 percent of the sample had not responded, you might shrewdly note that the missing 10 percent could all vote for one party or all for the other party and thus create a 10-percent swing and thus about a 5-percent error. For example, if the actual response were 50 percent Democrat, 40 percent Republican, and 10 percent non-response, the pollsters would be likely to report among those responding 56 percent Democrat and a margin of error of 3 percent. But the 10 percent non-responders could produce 60 percent Democrat if all voted Democrat or 50 percent Democrat if none voted Democrat, and so the margin of error of 3 percent based on simple sampling theory would be dominated by the larger possible error that could be produced by the unknown behavior of the non-responders.

We do not expect such extreme swings as this, but even today we do not have very extensive evidence about the behavior of non-responders, and their behavior may be seriously related to the kind of subject being studied. Although the illustration above shows what extremes can occur with a 10 percent non-response rate, the actual situation in the 1940s may have been much worse: perhaps more than 50 percent would not respond, and the potential swings in the percentages could be huge. This feature is not special to inquiries about sexual behavior, but to any sensitive behavior that respondents may not care to divulge—for example, interviews about occasions when the person being interviewed has broken the law or has behaved in some other way society disapproves.

To try to investigate the effect of non-response, KPM declared some groups to be 100 percent groups, meaning that they would get all members of the group. They then could compare the 100 percent reports with those from partial groups. If the groups are comparable to begin with, this would help get at the bias from non-responders or resistant responders. For this approach

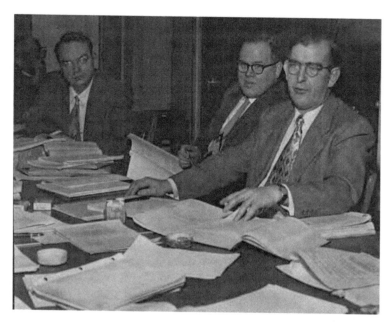

Fig. 2.1. Fred Mosteller, John Tukey, and Bill Cochran, circa 1950, in a meeting with Alfred Kinsey in Bloomington, Indiana.

to give its full value, the 100 percent groups should be chosen in advance. KPM chose to name a group as a 100 percent group after they found substantial success with that group; consequently the choice already has some bias toward readiness to respond. Whether the 100 percent groups so named actually had all members interviewed, I do not know. In 1989, someone suggested to me that not all were. Deciding to try hard for 100 percent and succeeding are not quite the same.

KPM liked to do their own methodology, and so they did a variety of sampling experiments to find out what sample sizes were needed for a given accuracy. Such sampling was based on the simple theory of random sampling, which was already well worked out. Nevertheless they, like me, may have learned a good deal about sampling fluctuations from such investigations. In new problems even if theory has been worked out, I often find simulations very instructive.

The kinds of problems KPM dealt with were much more complicated than simple random sampling because they were sampling from clusters with variable amounts of non-response of unknown effect.

To represent the national population, they needed to adjust the measures for the groups to match up to the national counts. For example, they might adjust for geographical region and education. Although their interviews came from many parts of the country, the greatest number came from Indiana, their base state; also they were heavy on youth. Consequently adjustments were required to try to project from the sample to the nation. Critics complained about the U.S. corrections partly because they were unable to check them. KPM had not given enough detail to make this possible, because they based their weights on finer breakdowns than the reader had available.

Because KPM started their work in wartime and because Indiana University was not a center of statistical activity like the University of Iowa or Iowa State University, they did not have ready access to statistical groups working on sampling problems. Even if they had had such access, they needed advice from someone at the very cutting edge of work in sampling design and analysis if they were to cope with the deeper difficulties of their work. Given these circumstances, we could scarcely criticize them for not having more statistical support.

Without going into further details, our summary remark for the whole report was:

> Our own opinion is that KPM are engaged in a complex program of research involving many problems of measurement and sampling, for some of which there appear at the present to be no satisfactory solutions. While much remains to be done, our overall impression of their work to date is favorable.[4]

Once our work was over, I saw no more of Kinsey nor, as far as I know, of Martin. But Pomeroy and I have crossed paths in airports and airplanes several times and have discussed mutual interests. Pomeroy has written a book,

Kinsey and the Institute for Sex Research, published by the Yale University Press in 1972, second edition in 1982.

The Institute continues, and I believe it has carried out a probability sample. Among its many studies, one has been informative of practices that bear upon research in the prevention of AIDS.

Editors' Postscript

In the years since the Kinsey report quite a few surveys have studied sexual behavior, many of them using random sampling and achieving very respectable response rates. Perhaps the earliest was a study of college students carried out by William Simon and John Gagnon (Simon and Gagnon, 1970), based at the Institute for Sex Research at Indiana University. Using a scheme designed by Seymour Sudman, the study randomly sampled 12 colleges and from each college randomly chose 25 students at each year in school. Their response rate was over 70%. The earliest probability sample covering the full U.S. population seems to be the one carried out by Albert Klassen and Eugene Levitt somewhat later than the Gagnon and Simon study but not published until 1989 (Klassen, Williams, and Levitt, 1989). This study concentrated on attitudes toward homosexuality, but contained some questions about sexual behavior. Much more recently, and in part in response to the AIDS epidemic, a major national probability survey of sexual behavior attained a 78% response rate (Michael, Gagnon, Laumann, and Kolata, 1994; Laumann, Gagnon, Michael, and Michaels, 1994).

The debate about whether interviewing should be standardized or more conversational continues. Suchman and Jordan (1990) raise some of the issues and expose them to discussion. Conrad and Schober (2000) provide some empirical evidence that suggests that standardized interviewing is most efficient when the respondent's situation is uncomplicated but conversational interviewing yields more accurate results when the situation is unusual.

Notes

1. See Kinsey (1948), Table 99, p. 400.
2. Cochran, Mosteller, and Tukey (1954), p. 219.
3. Cochran, Mosteller, and Tukey (1954), pp. 306–307.
4. See Cochran, Mosteller, and Tukey (1954), p. 2.

References

Cochran, W. G., Mosteller, F., and Tukey, J. W., with the assistance of W. O. Jenkins (1954). *Statistical Problems of the Kinsey Report on Sexual Behavior in the Human Male*. Washington, D.C.: The American Statistical Association.

Conrad, F. G. and Schober, M. F. (2000). Clarifying question meaning in a household telephone survey. *Public Opinion Quarterly*, 64:1–28.

Jenkins, W. O. (1954). Comparison with other studies. Appendix B in W. G. Cochran, F. Mosteller, and J. W. Tukey, with the assistance of W. O. Jenkins, *Statistical Problems of the Kinsey Report on Sexual Behavior in the Human Male*. Washington, D.C.: The American Statistical Association.

Kinsey, A. C., Pomeroy, W. B., and Martin, C. E. (1948). *Sexual Behavior in the Human Male*. Philadelphia: W. B. Saunders Co.

Kinsey, A. C., Pomeroy, W. B., Martin, C. E., and Gebhard, P. H., Research Associates; Staff of the Institute for Sex Research, Indiana University (1953). *Sexual Behavior in the Human Female*. Philadelphia: W. B. Saunders.

Klassen, A. D., Williams, C. J., and Levitt, E. E. (1989). *Sex and Morality in the U.S.: An Empirical Enquiry Under the Auspices of the Kinsey Institute*. Middleton, CT: Wesleyan University Press.

Kruskal, W. H. and Mosteller, F. (1980). Representative sampling, IV: The history of the concept in statistics. *International Statistical Review*, 48:169–195.

Laumann, E. O., Gagnon, J. H., Michael, R. T., and Michaels, S. (1994). *The Social Organization of Sexuality*. Chicago: University of Chicago Press.

Michael, R. T., Gagnon, J. H., Laumann, E. O., and Kolata, G. (1994). *Sex in America: A Definitive Survey*. Boston: Little, Brown and Company.

Pomeroy, W. B. (1972, 1982). *Dr. Kinsey and the Institute for Sex Research*. New Haven, CT: Yale University Press.

Simon, W. and Gagnon, J. H. (1970). *The End of Adolescence: The College Experience*. New York: Harper & Row.

Suchman, L. and Jordan, B. (1990). Interactional troubles in face-to-face survey interviews (with discussion). *Journal of the American Statistical Association*, 85:232–253.

3

Learning Theory: Founding Mathematical Psychology

Accidental happenings—coincidences—have a way of influencing large segments of one's life. Knowing William Cochran through the Kinsey work probably led to our later association at Harvard. My work in the field of mathematical learning theory also developed through an entirely unexpected and unanticipated route.

In the large and varied Department of Social Relations, we had many visitors. Rubbing shoulders with the many scholars visiting here was one frequent source of accidental happenings for me in the early years. Often academicians advance their work by visiting another university where a somewhat different scholarly atmosphere will redirect their imaginations, and breaking with a normal schedule helps free up the imagination, too. Visits can be as short as a few days, but usually last a quarter, a semester, or a year. The degree of association with the host department may be loose or strong. Sometimes visiting scholars merely want a supportive atmosphere to carry forward work they have long wanted to complete but lacked the uncluttered time for. Other times they want to interact directly and intensely with researchers at the institution they are visiting.

My research association with Robert R. Bush was of the latter sort. He wanted to be in a lively social science environment, and because of his natural science background and Princeton connections rather naturally gravitated toward me when he came to Harvard. He came jointly sponsored by the National Research Council (NRC) (the operating arm of the National Academy of Sciences) and the Social Science Research Council (SSRC), in 1949. At that time these organizations jointly gave postdoctoral fellowships for social scientists who wanted to get some training in the natural sciences or for natural scientists who wanted training in the social sciences. Bush was in the latter category. (My understanding is that few people applied from the physical sciences for training in the social sciences.)

As the reader may know, by the close of World War II, many physicists were in personal turmoil over the military uses of scientific research, especially research linked to the atomic bomb. To air these concerns, a group of natural

F. Mosteller, *The Pleasures of Statistics: The Autobiography of Frederick Mosteller,*
DOI 10.1007/978-0-387-77956-0_3,
© Springer Science + Business Media, LLC 2010

scientists at Princeton organized a regular seminar held at the Institute for Advanced Study on the topic, "Are the methods of physical sciences applicable to the social sciences?" Such social science stars as Margaret Mead, Gregory Bateson, and Abraham Kardiner addressed the seminar. Among the organizers of the seminar was Bush, who at that time was a young nuclear physicist and a friend of J. Robert Oppenheimer. Oppenheimer, in turn, was a member of the NRC-SSRC crossover fellowship committee.

An outgrowth of these interdisciplinary meetings was that Bush applied for one of the NRC-SSRC fellowships, initially for a two-year stint, and chose to spend the fellowship time at Harvard's three-year-old Department and Laboratory of Social Relations. With hundreds of undergraduates, over 150 graduate students, and nearly a hundred professional staff people, this Lab/Department was an exciting and stimulating place. It was divided into four distinct disciplines: clinical psychology, social psychology, sociology, and social anthropology. The scholars in these four disciplines shared department space and interacted vigorously and productively among themselves, as well as with other branches of social science, such as the Laboratory of Human Development, the Psychology Department, and the Education Department, all lively enterprises. Social Relations research ran from entirely non-quantitative, non-empirical social philosophy and wide-open anthropological field studies, to the tightest of laboratory experiments on animals; from completely empirical studies to totally theoretical mathematical ones. Sites for this research included nursery schools, hospitals, mental institutions, work camps, even the stage for work on psychodrama. Bush found it easy to join the various groups, whether in seminars and courses with graduate students or in discussions with faculty. By participating in many of the informal student-faculty study groups, he learned a lot of psychology and social science quickly, making a reputation for himself that ultimately led to his appointment to the staff.

In those days, preliminaries for placement of a special visitor included making sure that someone at the host institution would be responsible for making the visitor welcome and facilitating his work. In some cases the possibility of explicit collaboration was raised. As a recent Princeton Ph.D. in mathematics myself and as a member of the new Department of Social Relations who had some direct ties to the Social Science Research Council, it was natural that Bush and I would fall in step.

Bob was already a productive researcher, having coauthored four articles in physics. He wanted to start research as soon as he arrived, and his arrival turned out to be the start of our eight years of extensive and congenial collaboration.

Thinking that we might work together on one of them, I suggested three possible research areas: (1) investigating problem solving in small groups (related to departmental work then in progress by R. Freed Bales, earlier my office-mate), (2) discovering the links between various psychological scaling methods through theory and experiment (based on a course I had given in psychometric methods), and (3) developing mathematical models for learning. (The third topic was suggested by some data on the relief of pain in postoperative patients from successive doses of analgesics brought to my attention by Henry K. Beecher of Massachusetts General Hospital. Whether patients received medication or placebo, their relief from pain improved with the passage of time, though more from the medication. In analyzing these data, I found considerable improvement in relief over time that, when plotted up, was reminiscent of improvements in task performance that accompanied practice [learning]. Presumably the healing process was causing the increased relief, but the data reminded me very much of a slow learning process, even though it was merely an analogy. I wanted to develop some mathematical models to describe this behavior.)

As soon as Bob came, we spent a few days looking into these three problem areas. As for the first, we could not see at that time how to get a sharp mathematical wedge into small-group problem solving. For the second area, in the light of his later sustained and fundamental work on scales of measurement and their relationships that has become a classic in the field, it may amuse the psychological reader to learn that S.S. Stevens advised us that the field was settled and so there was nothing left to do. We were not put off by this advice, but Bob did not care for research on scaling even though the major question looked tractable both mathematically and experimentally—he said he wanted something more social, more directly involving human beings. This is amusing too because Stevens's later work was directed exactly to the social, or at least societal, uses of scaling. It all belongs to the *New Yorker*'s "Department of the Clouded Crystal Ball."

Before Bob came—actually about a year before, when Clyde Coombs, a psychologist from the University of Michigan deep in using mathematical methods for psychological studies, Paul Lazarsfeld, a leader in quantitative sociology, especially in the sample-survey field, Sam Stouffer, another quantitative sociologist, and I were working on a large scaling project—Doris Entwisle had become my mathematical assistant. With her double major in mathematics and psychology as well as a master's degree in psychology from Brown University, she had a good background for the learning project that we chose. (By 1967, she was an associate professor in both the Departments of Social Relations and Electrical Engineering at the Johns Hopkins University. Bob pointed out to her as she launched her own independent research career that it was going to be hard for her to get the strong assistance that she had provided for us.)

Models for Learning

Turning to the third area, we both saw ways to start on probabilistic models for learning. And so in a matter of three days, we chose and began to work on a problem that turned into years of effort. The vast store of empirical work and tidy experiments made this area particularly attractive to Bob because we had at hand a reliable base of solid information to use in informing our theoretical efforts. While inevitably these empirical data proved to be less useful than we had hoped, they nevertheless probably represented the largest body of solid work in social science at that time.

To get the notion of a mathematical or statistical model, let me describe a very crude model for learning a short list of words. We will build the model by assuming that, each time you are shown a word on the list, you increase the probability that you remember it next time by 0.2. If you do ever remember it, you always remember it after that. Let the list have 10 words. Initially you know nothing about the list and so each word has probability 0 of being recalled. After running through the list once, each word moves up to a probability of 0.2 of being recalled. Next time through the list you are likely to remember a few and these few will move up to probability 1, the others to 0.4.

After 5 times through the list, you have it memorized, for sure, but you might get all correct sooner.

On the second round, the average number correct is $10 \times 0.2 = 2$. The remembered ones now have probability 1 and the rest have 0.4 (because we saw them before). The average number correct on the third round is now $2(1) + 8(0.4) = 5.2$.

We can answer such questions as, what is the probability that you get all correct after the third round. The probability that a specific word has reached 1 after the third round can be computed as 0.808. The probability that all 10 words reach 1 by this round is $(0.808)^{10} = 0.118608$ or about 0.12.

You will ask, how do I know people behave in such a manner, but that is a matter for empirical investigation. The kinds of models described in this chapter have been used to describe very well the learning of a list of words, but those models are a little more complicated than the model I just described. Still, it is adequate to give the idea of a dynamic model—one that changes the probabilities on successive trials depending on what happens.

The speed with which we launched our eight-year collaboration was rather characteristic of Bob's "Let's do something, and let's do it now" attitude toward work and play. Wherever possible, he preferred to try various approaches out and see what worked, rather than to argue or even to think very hard about which alternative was preferable. Being quick, well organized, and so well focused on the relevant issues, he made this approach work, where others might not have been able to. Also, he was versatile and had a broad enough view of the world so that almost any problem he chose to work on might have been worth some time. In the instance under discussion, if the learning research had not been productive, we could readily have turned to one of the other two areas. For both of them we had more extensive preparation than for the learning project, and there were plenty of other promising problems as well.

Bob's work style was efficient. When I knew him, he started the day with a "shopping list" of the things to be accomplished that day, more or less in the order he planned to do them. These lists were a heterogeneous mixture of academic and housekeeping tasks. For example, on a given day, he might plan to revise a research paper, prepare an examination, deliver a typewriter for repair, give two lectures, and attend a committee meeting. He expected to complete his list each day (many of us do not), and if he finished before bedtime, which was fairly often, he felt entirely free to play. He planned ahead for this play as well, but he did not feel comfortable to start to play until everything on the work list was checked off. More than once I remember his working very late at a party previously scheduled at his own house, long after the guests arrived, because he found it hard to start to play when his work list for the day was not complete.

He had an especially good deep voice and had had some training in operatic singing. He also had a great sense of humor. These together with very legible handwriting and well-organized blackboard technique helped a lot in all aspects of our work. We usually met in Emerson Hall, either in my office or in a room the laboratory used for meetings and speakers. In both these places, the acoustics, blackboards, and other facilities were pitifully inadequate for research of any kind, let alone research involving mathematical explorations that might go on for a week at a time. There was one ditto machine capable of making at most 80 good copies from one master, and in those days modern copying was far over the horizon. To emphasize how meager the facilities were in those days, the reader should know that there were about half a dozen phone lines for a faculty, most of them senior, numbering over two dozen. My phone extension, for example, served five offices, some with more than one person, with no way except shouting down the hall to transfer calls from office to office. For a long time Bob had no extension that he even shared.

With his fellowship, Bob's time was his own. We were frequently able to spend half a day at a time together on research and then half a day apart. Memoranda were written very rapidly. Often he worked at home, and long phone calls were frequent.

As Bob learned about animal experiments on conditioning and reinforcement, from time to time he would try out some of the relevant principles on a human being. Small wonder that my son William, who was 2 at the time, upon seeing Bob used to race up to him shouting, "subset, subset." This was Bill's first serious word, painstakingly inserted in Bill's verbal repertoire by Bob.

The learning models Bush and I were developing took on a mathematical form exactly like that of some models being independently developed by William Estes at Indiana University, so correspondence with Estes and his group quickly sprang up. These models are termed "linear" because they define relationships where the outcome is some multiplicative and/or additive combination of the explanatory concepts. For example, in a T-maze when a rat is running down the stem, it comes to the bar of the T and has a choice of turning right or left. On one side, say the left, a bit of food may reward the rat, while on the right side there is no food. The basic idea underlying the model is that initially the rat has some specific non-zero probability of turning left, but if the rat turns left and gets the food, the probability of turning left next time it runs the T-maze will be increased because of the reinforcement produced by the food. If, instead, the rat turns right and gets no food, the rat may now be more likely to turn right again just to go with the habit of doing what has been done, or the rat may now be less likely to turn right because of lack of reward. The linearity in the model comes from the fact that the likelihood of turning left (or right) increases or decreases by some multiplicative function related to each event, and the changes can be added up as event after event occurs.

Although first-hand experience with rats might have something to say about the actual likelihood of these various acts, the formal model does not. In our model, then, it was not necessary to decide which choice the animal would make. Rather the model enabled one to assess the effect of any set of choices on future choices. Thus the models could, in principle, describe the details of some kinds of laboratory experiments then in common use both for animals and for humans: two-choice situations with various schedules of reward (usually food) or non-reward.

The models had the feature that a subject had two or more possible choices, and at a given moment one of the choices was sure to be taken. Accordingly the probabilities assigned to the various choices totaled 1. (The rat was not allowed to stop, paralyzed by indecision, at the top of the maze.) After any particular choice was made, the outcome (reward, punishment, etc.), together with the choice itself, prompted a change in the probabilities of future choices. For example, suppose the initial likelihood that the rat would turn left is 50-50, but after finding food when turning left the likelihood goes up to 0.55. This implies that the likelihood of a choice to the right goes down from 0.50 to 0.45.

Changes in probabilities of choices take on a specific mathematical form, easiest to describe with just two choices, as for the T-maze example, but generalizable to more than two choices. If in the T-maze the rat was always rewarded on the left and never rewarded on the right, it is reasonable that after repeated trials, the rat will go left nearly all the time, that is, with probability practically 1. The model we devised changed the probability of going left, say, according to the intensity or strength of the reward or reinforcement, and according to how far the probability of turning left was from its limiting value, in this instance 1. For example, we assumed that the effect of a reward on the first trial, when chances are 50-50, is some fixed fraction of the total probability available $(1 - .50)$. In the case of a 0.05 increment, the fraction is one-tenth. The next round, though, the probability of turning left is 0.55, so the fraction too is less, $.1(1 - .55) = .045$. This has the sensible outcome that when the rat has had considerable experience and turned left many times, the probability is nearly 1, perhaps .95, of turning left. At that point the reward does not much increase the probability of turning left, compared to what it would do if the initial probability were low. Thus, if the rat started at 0.5 for going left and had a learning rate of 0.1, then going left once and being rewarded would move the probability from 0.5 to 0.55 (one-tenth of the way to 1). But if the rat started at 0.9, one rewarded left turn would move the probability only to 0.91, one-tenth of the way from the starting probability (0.90) to the limit of 1.

Each possible treatment (reward or punishment together with choice) leads to a possibly different change in the probabilities depending upon when the rat starts and what the specific set of choices is. To evaluate the actual parameters describing the amount of change in any organism prompted by a set of learning experiences requires some information from data procured when an actual experiment of this variety was carried out.

Such models, although discussed so far in terms of animals, could be adapted to human learning as well. Essentially we devised a probability vector (set of probabilities) giving the probabilities associated with various choices, together with a set of mathematical operators that changed the numerical values of the components of the vector. Each operator was associated with a choice by the subject in the experiment and the outcome of the choice. Although many other forms of operators were possible, we thought it would be wise to stick to one form and explore it extensively, trying it out on as many different experimental situations as we could. We wanted to see how far we could go using only a few tools. Ultimately we wanted to explore other possible forms of operators, and both Bob and I did this later.

In our first paper, "A Mathematical Model for Simple Learning," we explained the relation between our approach and that of Estes; we emphasized reinforcement concepts, he emphasized association theory. We were both trying to describe instrumental conditioning or operant conditioning, behavior that changes because of experience with the environment, and not Pavlovian conditioning, which depends on internal physiological mechanisms.

Our strong emphasis was on the discrete trial-by-trial approach. However, when we need to relate probabilities, latent times, and rates, we are led naturally to differential equations and "continuous" rather than discrete results.

The paper discusses free-responding situations as in bar-pressing in Skinner boxes under extinction, fixed ratio, and random ratio reinforcement conditions, as well as aperiodic and periodic reinforcement. Most of these interpretations required us to go to differential equations, but we never emphasized them so heavily again. We wanted to describe the learning in fine detail. The differential equations were describing situations where we had little data available for verifying assumptions. When a pigeon ballistically put on a burst of pecks at a key, we could not believe that the individual pecks were independent actions in the sense of the model. True, one might still be able to fit the actual learning curves because a model with several parameters can fit a complicated shape. But we wanted the model to describe the detailed process, not just fit means, and this idea of studying fine (detailed) structure was new to mathematical learning theory. Prior to this, most learning curves came from averaging performance of individuals without much attention to the details leading up to the averages.

To describe experiments in stimulus generalization and discrimination,[1] we need to measure similarity of stimuli. We generalized and adapted Estes's set theoretic approach to treat these problems and applied the results to several experiments.

One of our most important analytical devices was the idea of a mythical "statistical" subject. We called them stat-rats, so christened, I believe, by Doris Entwisle. In the kinds of learning experiments we studied, a sequence of trials could have many properties, and we could rarely measure the actual probability in the animal, except perhaps when it was near 0 or 1. Consequently it was desirable to simulate an experiment by running stat-rats trial by trial to imitate the behavior of the real subjects. But in those days before computers, simulations were not often used because they were so tedious to calculate by hand. Nevertheless, we applied the same mathematical model to describe each stat-rat's behavior as the model being fitted to the experimental data. Such simulations, now called Monte Carlo methods, made it possible to get at many theoretical properties of the data without analytically describing extremely complex distributions. We exploited this idea repeatedly in *Stochastic Models for Learning*, especially in the Solomon-Wynne experiment (Chapter 11) and in the eight models paper.

In the Solomon-Wynne experiment dogs learned to avoid an electric shock by jumping over a bar when a light flashed. Dogs with unimpaired nervous systems learned in relatively few trials to do this without fail. Initially they had a probability of nearly 0 of jumping over the bar but soon raised their probabilities of jumping following the light to 1. A paradoxical feature of this laboratory experiment was that the behavior did not extinguish even when on trial after trial dogs were never shocked again.

Bush put together a model for what might be called insight or one-trial learning. When he presented it orally to a group of psychologists, they complained that he already had a model, the linear operator model, and that one model was enough. This attitude, although perhaps given partly in fun, distressed us both, and so we thought it would be instructive to try to prepare a set of alternative models for the same learning situation, essentially the Solomon-Wynne experiment. We thought that it would be helpful to see what variety there would be in mathematical models that attempted to describe various theories of learning. This work led to our paper on eight models mentioned earlier.

In this paper we used the dog data to explore how various psychological theories could be translated into mathematical models that would account for these same data. Our general idea was that if a model was correct, then it should match any statistical feature of the data. For example, in the Solomon-Wynne experiment, the model should be able to reproduce the mean and standard deviation of the number of failures of the dogs to jump, it should reproduce the average number of runs of successes and failures to avoid the shock, it should tell what fraction of dogs succeed on, say, trial six. In other words, the successful model would be virtually perfect from a statistical point of view in all respects. By considering departures from perfection, we could find out what features various mathematical models would find difficult to imitate. Our notion here was not to determine the "best" models, but rather the features that specific formulations did not reproduce very well. For example, one of the theories did not change the probabilities as fast as the real dogs changed theirs. It turned out that both our model and one developed by Frank Restle fitted the data well, though this was not the point of the exercise.

An aspect of the work on mathematical learning fits well with the axiomatic ideal. One sets down conditions and from these flow the legitimate operations. Our feeling was that what we were doing was empirical and ad hoc—choosing the particular operators and following them where they led, ordinarily from one set of experimental data or learning theory phenomenon to another. In one set of studies, we took a somewhat different tack and asked whether there were essential properties that learning operators for probability models should have, and if so, what classes of operators would be admissible under these properties.

We came up with what we called the "combining classes" criterion: the probability vector should have the property that, if some distinct classes of behavior were actually treated by the organism and by the system of reinforcements in the "same" way, then it should not matter to the model whether these categories had their probabilities combined before applying the operators or after applying them. (To see how we could be sure that different outcomes were treated the same way, imagine in the T-maze experiment that, when the rat turns left, someone on the other side of the world tosses a coin and it comes up heads or tails, and we now define the choice by the rat as left turn-heads or left turn-tails to create two categories of choices instead of just "left turn." Barring ESP, the rat is not influenced by this artificial dichotomy, and so the learning model ought to produce the same total new probability of turning left if it ignores the flip of the coin to begin with or if it carries out the adjustment of the probabilities for the two artificially created choices separately and then adds the probabilities at the end.)

In mathematical language, the criterion asks that the operation of combining categories be commutative with the operation we call the learning operator. Initially we were pleased with this idea and after using up a great many paper napkins at the Midget Restaurant developing it, we made some progress. It was easy to find that the learning operators we had been using had this property. It was harder to settle what other models had the property. First, L.J. Savage, of whom you will read more later, and then later Gerald Thompson, a mathematician, helped us with this work, and we finally proved that, when there were 3 or more choices, there were no probability models other than the linear operators we were using that had the requested property.

Far from pleasing us, this chilled our enthusiasm for the axiomatic approach. We realized that this exercise revealed the tremendous power of a seemingly small axiomatic request. We knew very well that we wanted to be able to use other models than those having the form of operators that ours had. We also knew that, by insisting on being prepared to combine classes making irrelevant distinctions, we were also imposing the form of operator on classes where the distinctions were relevant to learning. Mathematics can be very sneaky that way.

Many real-world problems have surprising features when one tries to impose axioms on them. Essentially what happens is that a few seemingly reasonable requirements are laid out, but they come into some subtle conflict that makes solution impossible.

Other areas where it is easy to overload the conditions are those of justice or fairness or preferences. Kenneth Arrow has a famous book *Social Choice and Individual Values* showing the impossibility of satisfying simultaneously several very acceptable rules for making choices in a voting paradigm. Because so much debate has flourished in the field of justice and fairness, Arrow's work, making clear mathematically that we can think of more ideas of fairness than we can systematically accommodate, shows that society has a never-ending problem. Our "combining classes" idea is an illustration of the concept of "the irrelevance of irrelevant alternatives," which comes up in Arrow's book and often in other modeling situations.

About two years after Bush came to Harvard, the John and Mary K. Markle Foundation gave money to the SSRC for some interuniversity summer research seminars in social science research. We applied for funds to run such a summer seminar. George A. Miller, then in psychology at Harvard, and I organized it, though he insisted that I be chairman. In the summer of 1951 at Tufts University, Cletus J. Burke, William Estes, then both of Indiana University, George A. Miller, David Zeaman, then of the University of Connecticut, Bush and I, together with then graduate student William McGill, later president of Columbia University, Katherine Safford Harris, and Jane E. Beggs, worked on learning models. Someone talked about current research progress nearly every day for about an hour and a half, but the rest of the time was spent on research. We lunched together at the faculty club, sometimes with the psychologist Leonard C. Mead, who arranged for our quarters, and sometimes with the psychologist Leonard Carmichael, then president of Tufts. It was the period when Bush and I made our greatest and fastest progress. Toward the close of that summer Bush and I decided to write a book. But it is a long way from deciding to write a book to completion of the task, in this case three years.

In addition to the mathematical material, *Stochastic Models for Learning* treated experimental data on free-recall verbal learning, avoidance training, imitation, T-maze experiments, three-choice experiments, and runway experiments. The runway experiments dealt with running times and required special developments to adapt our discrete approach to continuous distributions. We had especially to face up to the individual difference problem in a rather virulent form—subjects are definitely not all alike in their performances.

In writing the book, we had help from a number of research assistants: Lotte Lazarsfeld Bailyn, Doris Entwisle, David G. Hays, Solomon Weinstock, Joseph Weizenbaum, Thurlow R. Wilson, and Cleo Youtz.

Around 1953 Doris Entwisle's physician husband George completed his duties in the Korean War, and soon after they moved to Baltimore. She then completed her doctorate at The Johns Hopkins University and launched her own extensive research career, mainly studying problems related to social structure and elementary school children's cognitive and affective development.

Cleo Youtz came as research mathematician and through the years has supported the preparation of my research papers and books. Often she has had to double as department secretary or administrator. She helped with the completion of the learning book and has contributed to the lion's share of my research and writing since then.

When Bob moved to Columbia in 1956, he continued his work on learning, and he and I occasionally did things together. Maurice Tatsuoka, at first a student in the Graduate School of Education at Harvard and later a professor at the University of Illinois, and I did some work on situations with two attractive goals. We wanted to see how our stat-rats or stat-asses would do in the Buridan's ass situation where two attractive goals are available. Buridan's ass starved to death between two piles of hay. We found instead that, using our models, the subject would ultimately become totally attracted by one of the goals, even though both were attractive.

In those days of sexist writing, we called it the blond-brunette problem, but feared to use such a name then, lest Senator Proxmire produce a golden fleece award for the work. Again, the idea is that a young man has two (and only two) equally attractive lady friends—labeled for our convenience, blond and brunette—whom he dates. Perhaps initially he has a 50-50 chance of dating the blond, and whichever young woman he dates, he finds attractive and that increases his probability of dating her next time. But there will likely still be a substantial chance that he will date the other one next. The question is, does he just wander back and forth from one to the other, or does he ultimately become captured by one of the women? The model we developed has the feature that, although he may wander for a while, ultimately his probability of dating one of them becomes so high that from then on he dates only her. In some physical science problems where particles or processes wander, sometimes according to random walks, as does the probability of dating the blond, the probability extremes of 1 (blond) or 0 (brunette) are called absorbing barriers. Of course, the results delivered by the model do not prove anything about the real world, but we do learn what such models will and will not do.

The development of these learning models by Bush and me and by Estes, Burke, Miller, Frank Restle and others produced a modeling literature for psychologists very different from the data analysis literature of statistics and offered the advantage to social scientists of training in modeling in a field whose results had some interest for them.

When I worked on the Committee on the Mathematical Training of Social Scientists for the SSRC, I felt that it was going to be difficult to teach mathematical modeling to scholars who started their advanced mathematical studies as late as graduate school. Students would ask, "How do you get started building a mathematical model?" When I reflected on this, I realized that those of us who were trained through the physical sciences route had been practicing building these models, starting as early as our senior year in secondary school. My many college mathematics, physics, and mechanics courses were full of modeling, although unfortunately the generality across various applications was not made as clear then as it actually was. How was it possible to make up for the practice these courses gave physical science students? Part of the answer lay in giving social science students materials that fit well with their concerns. It is perplexing but nevertheless true that manipulations of familiar concepts are easier to comprehend than the same manipulations performed on unfamiliar concepts.

Although Persi Diaconis tells me that currently interest has renewed in the kinds of models that Bush and I worked on, probably as Eugene Galanter and R. Duncan Luce have said, the big value of the book *Stochastic Models for Learning* was to start "a new area: mathematical psychology."

Although Bush and I continued working on models, my last original publication was in 1960 with Tatsuoka on the "Ultimate choice between two attractive goals." But this paper had been over a year in the refereeing process before the delinquent reader reported that the manuscript was lost as well, and so I must not have been doing much in this field by 1959.

When Bush and I quit working on such models, we had been turning to "attention" in learning. In learning lists of words for example, what seemed to matter was whether you could keep your mind on a particular word or nonsense syllable long enough to store it. Without Bob there to keep us fresh, though, I turned to other things.

Aside from our work on learning models, Bob and I wrote a very long didactic piece on statistical methods useful in social sciences for the first edition of Gardner Lindzey's *Handbook of Social Psychology*. I pulled the topics together and wrote a draft. Bush saw the value of making the effort more systematic in two ways: (a) by providing an example of the application of each method; and (b) by providing tables of approximations in order to use the methods. These additions made the difference between an assembly of ideas and a practical article ready for the research worker to use. They also doubled the length of the article. In this instance Bush was not comfortable with our usual Bush and Mosteller (alphabetical) authorship and insisted that we reverse the order.

Bush left Harvard in 1956 to join the faculty at Columbia. Later he chaired two Departments of Psychology, first at the University of Pennsylvania and then at Columbia University.

Editors' Postscript

The Bush-Mosteller work on learning theory was an integral part of the beginnings of mathematical psychology, yet decades later this particular topic in psychology tends to be mainly of historical interest, although there are exceptions (e.g., Heit, 1995). But other areas of science appear to draw upon it in the study of game theory and reinforcement learning that has emerged in economics (Evev and Roth, 1998), network analysis (Pemantle and Skyrms, 2004; Skyrms and Pemantle, 2000), and computer science (Unsal, Kachroo, and Bay, 1999).

A search via Google Scholar *in the summer of 2006 showed 620 URLs for* Statistical Models for Learning, *attesting to its enduring influence.*

Notes

1. Bush and Mosteller (1951b).

References

Arrow, K. (1970). *Social Choice and Individual Values.* 2nd edition. New Haven, CT: Yale University Press.

Brunswick, E. (1939). Probability as a determiner of rat behavior. *Journal of Experimental Psychology*, 25:175–197.

Brush, F. S., Bush, R. R., Jenkins, W. O., John, W. F., and Whiting, J. W. M. (1952). Stimulus generalization after extinction and punishment: An experimental study of displacement. *Journal of Abnormal and Social Psychology*, 47:633–640.

Bush, R. R. (1959). Sequential properties of linear models. In R. R. Bush and W. K. Estes, editors, *Studies in Mathematical Learning Theory.* Stanford, CA: Stanford University Press. 215–227.

Bush, R. R. and Mosteller, F. (1951a). A mathematical model for simple learning. *Psychological Review*, 58:313–323. (Reprinted in R. D. Luce, R. R. Bush, and E. Galanter, editors, *Readings in Mathematical Psychology*, Vol. I, 1963. New York: Wiley. 278–288.)

Bush, R. R. and Mosteller, F. (1951b). A model for stimulus generalization and discrimination. *Psychological Review*, 58:413–423. (Reprinted in R. D. Luce, R. R. Bush, and E. Galanter, editors, *Readings in Mathematical Psychology*, Vol. I, 1963. New York: Wiley. 289–299.)

Bush, R. R. and Mosteller, F. (1955). *Stochastic Models for Learning.* New York: Wiley.

Bush, R. R. and Mosteller, F. (1959). A comparison of eight models. In R. R. Bush and W. K. Estes, editors, *Studies in Mathematical Learning Theory.* Stanford, CA: Stanford University Press. 293–307.

Bush, R. R., Mosteller, F., and Thompson, G. L. (1954). A formal structure for multiple-choice situations. In R. M. Thrall, C. H. Coombs, and R. L. Davis, editors, *Decision Processes*. New York: Wiley. 99–126.

Bush, R. R. and Sternberg, S. (1959). Single operator model. In R. R. Bush and W. K. Estes, editors, *Studies in Mathematical Learning Theory*. Stanford: Stanford University Press. 204–214.

Bush, R. R. and Whiting, J. W. M. (1953). On the theory of psychoanalytic displacement. *Journal of Abnormal and Social Psychology*, 48:261–272.

Bush, R. R. and Wilson, T. R. (1956). Two-choice behavior of paradise fish. *Journal of Experimental Psychology*, 51:315–322.

Evev, I. and Roth, A. E. (1998). Predicting how people play games: Reinforcement learning in experimental games with unique, mixed strategy equilibria. *American Economic Review*, 88:838–881.

Goodnow, R. E., Beecher, H. K., Brazier, M. A. B., Mosteller, F., and Tagiuri, R. (1951). Physiological performance following a hypnotic dose of a barbiturate. *Journal of Pharmacology and Experimental Therapeutics*, 102:55–61.

Hays, D. G. and Bush, R. R. (1954). A study of group action. *American Sociological Review*, 19:693–701.

Heit, E. (1995). Belief revision in models of category learning. In J. D. Moore and J. F. Lehman, editors, *Proceedings of the Seventeenth Annual Conference of the Cognitive Science Society*. Hillsdale, NJ: Erlbaum. 176–181.

Humphreys, L. G. (1939). Acquisition and extinction of verbal expectations in a situation analogous to conditioning. *Journal of Experimental Psychology*, 25:294–301.

Miller, N. E. (1948). Theory and experiment relating psychoanalytic displacement to stimulus-response generalization. *Journal of Abnormal and Social Psychology*, 42:155–178.

Miller, N. E. and Kraeling, D. (1951). Displacement: Greater generalization of approach than avoidance in a generalized approach-avoidance conflict. Paper read at Eastern Psychological Association, Brooklyn, New York.

Mosteller, F. and Bush, R. R. (1954). Selected quantitative techniques. Chapter 8 in G. Lindzey, editor, *Handbook for Social Psychology*. Cambridge, MA: Addison-Wesley. 289–334.

Mosteller, F. (1974). Robert R. Bush: Early career. *Journal of Mathematical Psychology*, 11:163–178.

Mosteller, F. and Tatsuoka, M. (1960). Ultimate choice between two attractive goals: Predictions from a model. *Psychometrika*, 25:1–17. (Reprinted in R. D. Luce, R. R. Bush, and E. Galanter, editors, *Readings in Mathematical Psychology*, Vol. I, 1963. New York: Wiley. 498-514.)

Pemantle, R. and Skyrms, B. (2004). Network formation by reinforcement learning: The long and the medium run. *Mathematical Social Sciences*, 48:315–327.

Skyrms, B. and Pemantle, R. (2000). A dynamic model of social network formation. *Proceedings of the National Academy of Sciences*, 97:9340–9346.

Unsal, C., Kachroo, P., and Bay, J. S. (1999). Multiple stochastic learning automata for vehicle path control in an automated highway system. *IEEE Transactions on Systems, Man and Cybernetics, Part A*, 29:120–128.

Whiting, J. W. M. and Child, I. L. (1953). *Child Training and Personality.* New Haven, CT: Yale University Press.

4

Who Wrote the Disputed Federalist Papers, Hamilton or Madison?

When I worked at the Office of Public Opinion Research with the social psychologist Hadley Cantril, beginning in 1940, I got to know Frederick Williams, a political scientist. He and I collaborated on some articles in the study of public opinion that appeared in a book edited by Hadley Cantril. One day in 1941, Fred said, "Have you thought about the problem of the authorship of the disputed *Federalist* papers?" I didn't know there were *Federalist* papers, much less that both Hamilton and Madison had claimed authorship of some of them. I had attended an engineering school where very little classical literature was taught at the time. I had, however, been reading in the statistical journal *Biometrika* articles by G. Udny Yule and by C. B. Williams (a different Williams) on the resolution of some disputes about authorship.

Yule used the properties of the distribution of sentence length measured by number of words. Yule asked whether *De Imitatione Christi* might have been written by Thomas à Kempis or by Jean Charlier de Gerson, recognizing that still others might be contenders. Both Yule and C. B. Williams used properties of the distribution of the number of words in a sentence to distinguish authorship. More specifically, Yule used the mean and the standard deviation. Comparing the distribution of sentence lengths in known writings of these two authors with those in the *Imitatio*, Yule concluded that the "results are completely consonant with the view that Thomas à Kempis was, and Jean Charlier de Gerson was not, the author of the *Imitatio*."

Yule (1871–1951) was among the first statisticians to work in the field of statistical stylistics. (Of course, many have worked on codes and ciphers.) I have been told that he worked hard on this subject after the authorities refused, because of a physical defect, to give him a license to fly airplanes, a hobby he would have much preferred in his seventies.

C. B. Williams had suggested in an article that analysts might be able to distinguish authors according to the shape of the distribution of the logarithm of their sentence lengths. I was therefore "set up" for studying *The Federalist* papers. Being young, I knew little enough that it seemed to me that Fred Williams and I might have no difficulty distinguishing the authorship of *The*

F. Mosteller, *The Pleasures of Statistics: The Autobiography of Frederick Mosteller*,
DOI 10.1007/978-0-387-77956-0_4,
© Springer Science + Business Media, LLC 2010

Federalist papers. By gathering sentence lengths, we might solve a problem that had troubled historians for over a hundred years.

David Wallace and I, after working together for a long time on this authorship problem, wrote a brief description of the *Federalist* controversy which I repeat here with minor revisions.

> The *Federalist* papers were published anonymously in 1787–88 by Alexander Hamilton, John Jay, and James Madison to persuade the citizens of the State of New York to ratify the Constitution. Seventy-seven papers appeared as letters in New York newspapers over the pseudonym "Publius." Together with eight more essays, they were published in book form in 1788 and have been republished repeatedly both in the U.S. and abroad. The *Federalist* remains today an important work in political philosophy. It is also the leading source of information for studying the intent of the framers of the Constitution, as, for example, in decisions on congressional reapportionment, because Madison had taken copious notes at the Constitutional Convention.

> It was generally known who had written *The Federalist*, but no public assignment of specific papers to authors occurred until 1807, three years after Hamilton's death as a result of his duel with Aaron Burr. Madison made his listing of authors only in 1818, after he had retired from the presidency. A variety of lists with conflicting claims have been disputed for a century and a half. There is general agreement on the authorship of 70 papers—5 by Jay, 14 by Madison, and 51 by Hamilton. Of the remaining 15, 12 are in dispute between Hamilton and Madison, and 3 are joint works to a disputed extent. No doubt the primary reason the dispute existed is that Madison and Hamilton did not hurry to enter their claims. Within a few years after writing the essays, they had become bitter political enemies and each occasionally took positions opposing some of his own *Federalist* writings.

> The political content of the essays has never provided convincing evidence for authorship. Since Hamilton and Madison were writing a brief in favor of ratification, they were like lawyers working for a client; they did not need to believe or endorse every argument they put forward favoring the new Constitution. While this does not mean that they would go out of their way to misrepresent their personal positions, it does mean that we cannot argue, "Hamilton wouldn't have said that because he believed otherwise." And, as we have often seen, personal political positions change. Thus the political content of a disputed essay cannot give strong evidence in favor of Hamilton's or of Madison's having written it.

The acceptance of the various claims by historians has tended to change with political climate. Hamilton's claims were favored during the last half of the nineteenth century, Madison's since then. While the thorough historical studies of the historian Douglass Adair over several decades support the Madison claims, the total historical evidence is today not much different from that which historians like the elder Henry Cabot Lodge interpreted as favoring Hamilton. New evidence was needed to obtain definite attributions, and internal statistical stylistic evidence provides one possibility; developing that evidence and the methodology for interpreting it was the heart of our work.

The writings of Hamilton and Madison are difficult to tell apart because both authors were masters of the popular *Spectator* style of writing—complicated and oratorical. [1]

Perhaps an extreme example of a sentence drawn from *The Federalist* will give an idea of the complexity of the writing: "Had no important step been taken by the leaders of the Revolution for which a precedent could not be discovered, no government established of which an exact model did not present itself, the people of the United States might, at this moment, have been numbered among the melancholy victims of misguided councils, must at best have been laboring under the weight of some of those forms which have crushed the liberties of the rest of mankind." [2]

Early Attempts with Fred Williams

Returning now to 1941, Fred Williams and I decided to approach the problem using sentence lengths. We bought duplicate copies of the book and began counting words in each sentence. We got our wives to help with the counting, though with modified rapture, for both were already fully employed. Soon we found that we couldn't count correctly, even though it seemed an easy task. It was not that we couldn't decide what to do with a date like February, 1786, or that the treatment of hyphenated words caused difficulties. It was just that we could not count words reliably in the agreed-on manner. Consequently checks had to be created. This was a very educational experience for a statistician. Much later the psychologist George Miller proved after considerable research that people weren't very good at counting, especially beyond 7.

After a time, we had counted all sentence lengths for the book. When we assembled the results for the known papers the average lengths for Hamilton and Madison were 34.55 and 34.59, respectively—a complete disaster because these averages are practically identical and so could not distinguish authors. We looked at the variability of sentence lengths too, but without much hope, and rightly. The standard deviations were 19 for Hamilton and 20 for Madison. And so sentence length gave us absolutely nothing. That's not quite fair; it told us that we were up against a much harder problem than other literary disputes I had read about. It also gave us word counts of the papers to use in further work. Talk about discouraged!

As a result of reading some stylistic work by psychologists, Hadley Cantril suggested that we look at the noun-adjective ratio. Consequently, we soon learned a lot more about English grammar: in complicated writing it is not as easy as you might think to tell whether a word is a noun. I recall that deciding about "own" led to lengthy discussions. In later years a small revolution took place: grammarians decided that the grammar we had learned in school was based on Latin and that Latin grammar was not identical with English grammar after all. Thus the rules today may be slightly different from those we were following. At any rate, with the help of dictionaries and grammars and special rules, we produced counts of nouns for Hamilton and for Madison. There were modest differences between Hamilton's and Madison's performance, but not enough to be compelling. A similar plunge into adjectives was expensive and gave only a small payoff.

This experience chastened us further, and so we cast about for some variables that were easily detected and counted, for example, one- and two-letter words, and the number of *the*'s. Naturally we computed the rates of use of each. The standard method for distinguishing between two categories is called Fisher's discriminant function. When we applied Fisher's discriminant function to the unknown papers, we found that, if the question were whether Hamilton or Madison had written all the disputed papers (as a group), then Madison was the author. But this was not the question. Instead, the task was to decide the author for each paper separately, and the discriminant we had was too weak to settle this with reasonable confidence. World War II separated Fred Williams and me, and we were never able to return to the problem together.

In later years, I used our *Federalist* experiences in elementary statistics classes at Harvard University to illustrate the difficulty of getting reliability in such simple matters as counts and the importance of operational definitions for such hard problems as deciding whether a word is a noun. In more advanced classes, that research illustrated a use of the discriminant function in a situation everyone could understand, though it also illustrated well that the method might not be as effective as a researcher could desire. Disappointments are very common.

The historian Douglass Adair heard of my discussions in statistics classes and was stimulated to write suggesting that I (or more generally, statisticians) should get back to this problem. He pointed out that words might be the key, because he had noticed that Hamilton nearly always used the form *while* and Madison the form *whilst*. The only trouble was that many papers contained neither of them.

Working with David Wallace

Meanwhile, starting in 1955, David Wallace, of the University of Chicago, and I had been puzzling about why Bayesian inference was not more widely used in real statistical problems, as opposed to another approach called the frequency theory, which had been popularized by Jerzy Neyman, Egon Pearson, and, though he might not have agreed on the name, R. A. Fisher. Wallace and I had been educated through the same route—attended Carnegie Institute of Technology (now Carnegie Mellon University), captured by E.G. Olds, a mathematics professor with strong interests in probability and statistics and their applications to quality control and other engineering problems. Olds managed to get us both admitted to Princeton to study with Samuel S. Wilks; we even have the same birthday, December 24, though we were not born the same year. I had not gotten to know Wallace when he taught for a year at Massachusetts Institute of Technology, but when I spent a sabbatical year (1954–55) at the University of Chicago with the support of the Fund for the Advancement of Education created by the Ford Foundation, we became much better acquainted.

Dave loved to work on complicated theoretical problems, and he had a memory for lengthy formulas that dazzled both me and his students. From the beginning of the computer revolution he saw its importance both for statistical and for mathematical calculation and hurled himself into it. Daily teas at the Committee on Statistics (later Department of Statistics) led to intense discussions of many statistical topics with faculty members K.A.(Alec) Brownlee, L.J. (Jimmie) Savage (an ardent Bayesian), William Kruskal, Murray Rosenblatt, Raj Bahadur, and occasionally Harry Roberts and W. Allen Wallis, the chairman, and several graduate students including Herbert T. David, Morris DeGroot, John Gilbert, Albert Madansky, and Jack Nadler, and visitors Willem van der Byl, Dennis Lindley, and Irving Schweiger.

One productive result of this visit and my acquaintance with the faculty was that the yet-unborn Department of Statistics at Harvard University profited from visits by Kruskal, Paul Meier (who joined the Chicago department after my visit), and Wallace coming to Cambridge to teach the summer courses. Some of these visits helped Dave and me to do some of our later work together in Cambridge.

In ideal circumstances, Bayesian inference provides the investigator with a systematic way to handle uncertainty and use new information. Formulas guide the investigator in adjoining information about previous beliefs—called priors—to new data, and thus revise the previous beliefs by taking proper account of the additional information. This calculation yields posterior information, which in turn becomes the prior information for the future. If enough information is added, we come close to certainty.

During the summer of 1959, David Wallace came down from New Hampshire twice to discuss our plans. We were coming to believe that we could understand more about Bayesian inference by choosing a substantial problem involving data and working it out carefully using Bayesian statistics. We had had many talks with Jimmie Savage about this field. During 1960 Jimmie was pressing colleagues at Chicago to adopt the Bayesian approach. He was just back from a year with Bruno de Finetti in Italy. Jimmie was trying to revolutionize statistics by turning it to Bayesian thinking, and he spoke ardently about this at many meetings and wrote about it in papers and books, though with only a few applications. Later he wrote an applied Bayesian paper for psychologists with one of my doctoral students, Ward Edwards, a psychologist, as a coauthor.

Earlier Harold Jeffreys had written a book on Bayesian inference to encourage its use in physical science. Although the book was impressive in its scholarship, it did not move many statisticians away from the more standard frequency approach. In talking with me, S.S. Wilks expressed concern that the Bayesian approach would reduce the collection of original data and thus, by implication, lead to decisions by guesswork and authority. Of course, there is something to this, and it is not all bad. The field of operations research has a rule that if you don't know a needed number, you should guess it. The Bayesian approach is usually mixed in with decision theory. It often turns out in decision situations that the same decision will be made for a broad variety of situations. When this is true, we may not need to know the actual situation very accurately to make the preferable decision. In a sense, then, we may need less data to make a satisfactory decision.

Most of the resistance to Bayesian inference at this time, nevertheless, came from the need to choose a prior in the first instance—seemingly an act

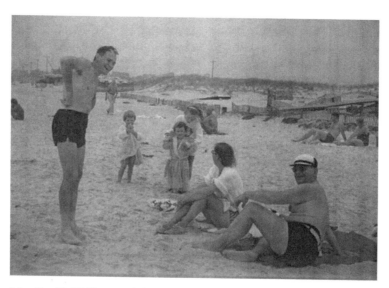

Fig. 4.1. David Wallace and his two daughters, with Gale, Virginia, and Fred Mosteller at the beach in West Falmouth, circa 1960.

of faith a scientist might not want to make. All the same in many parts of theoretical statistics and probabilistic arguments, Bayesian moves were made by all statisticians. What one saw little of was actual Bayesian analysis in problems dealing with practical data as opposed to the coins and dice and card problems in textbooks on probability.

When Adair's letter suggesting the use of particular words to distinguish authorship of the Federalist papers came in the middle of our discussions, we were spurred to action. Here was a problem we already knew to be hard. In principle we could get lots of data on style, and we could have full control of it, gathering what we needed. And best of all, unlike other problems that we had considered, we had no time bind. True, Adair was in a hurry to know, but history is good at waiting. We decided to make a serious project of it. I suppose we had a modest research paper in mind originally, but before we got very far along, the issues, methods, and information began to mount up. We did not initially realize how large the task would become, and we were unprepared for that from the point of view both of personnel and funding. In the end, the work was funded over several years from several small grants from different sources.

Cleo Youtz, our mathematical assistant, took a serious hand in the work and made sure that the efforts were documented and recorded systematically. She also did much of the original computing and managed the personnel when we employed several people.

We took Adair's basic suggestion and began to think about kinds of words that might be used to discriminate. The idea of contrasting forms of words was attractive, and in the end it did supply some information, though we didn't find it through this route. For example, the pair *toward* and *towards* did not give us much help. Indeed, the more we tried to think of paired words, the more discouraging it seemed. We picked up two other ideas.

One was, why not use all the words and weight them according to their ability to discriminate? (Bayesian theory would tell us how.) We knew why, of course: the rate of use of some words would be heavily determined by context. For example, no matter who the author was, if he wrote about the Army and the Navy or the War Department, then military words must be used at a higher rate than when discussing, say the Supreme Court. Therefore words whose usage varied a lot according to topic needed to be given low weight, because the topic rather than the author largely determined differential rates of use.

Our other idea was that "function" words might be useful. These are all the little essentially meaningless words like conjunctions, prepositions, and articles. Our thought was that their rates of use would depend more on the author than on the topic. This was an excellent idea, and it included most of the paired marker words like *while* and *whilst*.

We needed counts for all these words. At first we did it all by hand. The words in an article were typed one word per line on a long paper tape, like adding machine tape. Then with scissors the tape was cut into slips, one word per slip. These then were alphabetized by hand. We had many helpers with this. That was in 1959–60; it all seems primitive, even laughable now. When the counting was going on, if someone opened a door, slips of paper would fly about the room. You might think we would have been using high-speed computers, but their use in processing English text was just beginning at Harvard, and it took a long time to write a program for a concordance.

We asked Albert Beaton, who was in charge of the Statistical Laboratory of Harvard University, to write a concordance program. After many months, this program worked. We could then type the material onto cards that the computer used. The program would then not only alphabetize the words and count their uses, but also give the line and position in the line of text for each use. The program did this beautifully up to some indeterminate point around 3000 words, and then it would go crazy, destroying everything it had done so far. David Wallace says that I exaggerate when I say that 1500 words of *The Federalist* was as much as anyone (even a computer) could stand, however important these political writings may be. We never found out the full story as to why it did this, but we did learn to stop the machine before the trouble started and take off the information, and then start over with a clean slate at the next word. That way we were able to merge the pieces and get the results for full papers.

We also used computers for heavier calculations. Miles Davis developed the programs and ran them at Harvard, and David Wallace carried out computing for the Bayesian mathematics at the University of Chicago as he developed some of the theory needed for our work.

When Dave and I were apart, we made many phone calls to keep the work moving, and, of course, big packages of mail went both ways. The phone has the advantage of maintaining the research project on everyone's agenda. The mail was very effective at this time. For example, in 1964 Cleo often sent an air-mail package from Cambridge, Massachusetts one morning, and it would arrive at the Center for Advanced Study in the Behavioral Sciences in Stanford the next morning. One can get such service today, but it costs the better part of $10 (for a small package). In working with people at a distance, reliable mail plays a most important role. When a mailing is slow to arrive, one fears that the precious package has gone astray. In the end, for peace of mind, today one pays the extra premium for the overnight delivery.

Markers—words used almost exclusively by one author—contribute a lot to discrimination when they can be found, but they also present difficulties. We have noted that *while* or *whilst* occurs in less than half of the papers. They are absent from the other half and hence give little evidence for either author. We might hope to surmount this by finding enough different marker words or constructions so that one or more will always be present.

A second and more serious difficulty is that from the evidence in 14 essays by Madison, we cannot be sure that he would never use *while*. Other writings of Madison were examined and, indeed, he did lapse on two occasions. The presence of *while* then is a good but not sure indication of Hamilton's

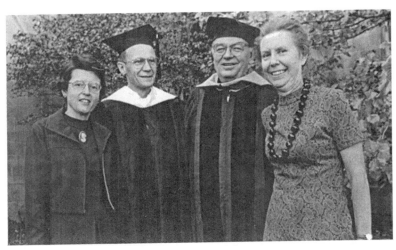

Fig. 4.2. The Wallaces, Anna Mary and David, with the Mostellers at the University of Chicago commencement ceremony in which Fred received an honorary degree in 1973.

authorship; the presence of *whilst* is a better, but still imperfect, indicator of Madison's authorship, for Hamilton too might lapse.

A central task of statistics is making inferences in the presence of uncertainty. Giving up the notion of perfect markers leads us to a statistical problem. We must find evidence, assess its strength, and combine it into a composite conclusion. Although the theoretical and practical problems may be difficult, the opportunity exists to assemble far more compelling evidence than even a few nearly perfect markers could provide.

Instead of thinking of a word as a marker whose presence or absence settles the authorship of an essay, we can take the rate or relative frequency of use of each word as a measure pointing toward one or the other author. Of course, most words won't help because they were used at about the same rate by both authors. But since we have thousands of words available, some may help. Words form a huge pool of possible discriminators. From a systematic exploration of this pool of words, we found no more pairs like *while-whilst*, but we did find single words used by one author regularly but rarely by the other. The best single word we found was *upon*, much used by Hamilton and rarely by Madison; similarly, *enough* was much more often used by Hamilton than Madison.

As I noted earlier, for the statistical arguments to be valid, information from meaningful, contextual words must be largely discarded. Such a study of authorship will not then contribute directly to any understanding of the greatness of the papers, but the evidence of authorship can be both strengthened and made independent of evidence provided by historical analysis.

Avoidance of judgments about meaningfulness or importance is common in classification and identification procedures. When art critics try to authenticate a picture, in addition to the historical record, they consider little things: how fingernails and ears are painted and what kind of paint and canvas were used. Relatively little of the final judgment is based upon the painting's artistic excellence. In the same way, police often identify people by their fingerprints, dental records, and scars, without reference to their personality, occupation, or position in society. For literary identification, we need not necessarily be clever about the appraisal of literary style, although it helps in some problems. To identify an object, we need not appreciate its full value or meaning. We may deal with the analogs of fingernails and ears—lowly words like *by* and *from*.

What non-contextual words are good candidates for discriminating between authors? In addition to prepositions, conjunctions, and articles, many other more meaningful words also seem relatively free from context: adverbs such as *commonly, consequently, particularly,* or even abstract nouns like *vigor* or *innovation*. We want words whose use is unrelated to the topic and may be regarded as reflecting minor or perhaps unconscious preferences of the author.

Consider what can be done with filler words. Some of these are the most used words in the language: *the, and, of, to,* and so on. No one writes without them, but we may find that their rates of use differ from author to author.

Table 4.1. Frequency Distribution of Rate per Thousand Words for the 48 Hamilton and 50 Madison Papers for *by, from,* and *to*.

by Rate per 1000 words	H	M	*from* Rate per 1000 words	H	M	*to* Rate per 1000 words	H	M
1-3	2		1-3	3	3	20-25		3
3-5	7		3-5	15	19	25-30	2	5
5-7	12	5	5-7	21	17	30-35	6	19
7-9	18	7	7-9	9	6	35-40	14	12
9-11	4	8	9-11		1	40-45	15	9
11-13	5	16	11-13		3	45-50	8	2
13-15	6		13-15		1	50-55	2	
15-17	5		Totals	48	50	55-60	1	
17-19	3					Totals	48	50
Totals	48	50						

*From Mosteller and Wallace (1972).

Table 4.1 shows the distribution of rates for three prepositions—*by, from,* and *to*. First, note the variation from paper to paper. Madison uses *by* typically about 12 times per 1000 words, but sometimes has rates as high as 18 or as low as 6. Even on inspection, though, the variation does not obscure Madison's systematic tendency to use *by* more often than Hamilton does. Thus low rates for *by* suggest Hamilton's authorship, and high rates Madison's. Rates for *to* run in the opposite direction. Very high rates for *from* point to Madison, but low rates give practically no information. The more widely the distributions of rates of the two authors are separated, the stronger the discriminating power of the word. Here, *by* discriminates better than *to*, which in turn is better than *from*.

To apply any of the theory of statistical inference to evidence from word rates, we must construct an acceptable probability model to represent the variability in word rate from paper to paper. Setting up a complete model for the occurrence of even a single word would be a hopeless task, for the fine structure within a sentence is determined in large measure by nonrandom elements of grammar, meaning, and style. But if our interest is restricted to the rates of use of one or more words in blocks of text of at least 100 or 200 words, we expect that detailed structure of phrases and sentences ought not to be very important. The simplest model can be described in the language of balls in an urn, so common in classical probability. To represent Madison's usage of the word *by*, we suppose there is a typical Madison rate, which would be somewhere near 12 per 1000, and we imagine an urn filled with many thousands of red and black balls, with the red occurring in the proportion 12 per 1000. Our probability model for the occurrence of *by* is the same as the probability model for successive draws from the urn, with a red ball corresponding to *by*, a black ball corresponding to all other words. To extend the model to simultaneous study two or more words, we would need balls of three or more colors. No grammatical structure or meaning is a part of this model, and it is not intended to represent behavior within sentences. What is desired is that it explain the variation in rates—in counts of occurrences in long blocks of words, corresponding to the essays.

We tested the model by comparing its predictions with actual counts of word frequencies in the papers. We found that, although this urn scheme reproduced variability well for many words, other words showed additional variability. The random variation of the urn scheme represented most of the variation in counts from one essay to another, but in some essays authors change their basic rates a bit. We had to complicate the theoretical model to allow for this, and the model we used is called the negative binomial distribution.

The test showed also that for Hamilton and Madison pronouns like *his* and *her* are exceedingly unreliable authorship indicators, worse even than words like *war*.

Each possible route from construction of models to quantitative assessment of, say, Madison's authorship of some disputed paper, required solutions of serious theoretical statistical problems, and new mathematics had to be developed, most of it by Wallace. A chief motivation for us was to use *The Federalist* problem as a case study for comparing different statistical approaches, with special attention to the Bayesian method that expresses its final results in terms of probabilities, or odds, of authorship.

By whatever methods are used, the results are the same: overwhelming evidence for Madison's authorship of the disputed papers. Our data independently supplement the evidence of the historians. Madison is extremely likely, in the sense of degree of belief, to have written the disputed *Federalist* papers, with the possible exception of paper number 55, and there our evidence yields odds of 80 to 1 for Madison—strong, but not overwhelming. Paper 56, next weakest, is a very strong 800 to 1 for Madison. The data are overwhelming for all the rest, including the two papers historians feel least certain about, papers 62 and 63.

Of course, combining and assessing the total evidence is a large statistical and computational task. High-speed computers worked many hours in making the calculations, both mathematical calculations for the theory and empirical ones for the data.

High-speed computers at this time had much less power than today's personal computers, and the machines were slow. Furthermore, software such as can be purchased today for many purposes had to be written through painfully slow and frustrating processes. We had no interactive computer.

You may have wondered about John Jay. Might he not have taken a hand in the disputed papers? The disputed papers are not at all consistent with Jay's rates, and there is no reason to question his omission from the dispute. [3]

When discrimination becomes extremely successful, the analyst faces a new problem. Are the odds that are found supported by either common or uncommon sense? If our analysis produces odds of millions to one in favor of Madison writing a certain paper, should we accept that? Or if not, what should we believe?

Probably we can believe or at least accept the idea that such odds are being produced by the specific model being used together with its assumptions. At the same time nearly all of us have believed that a certain fact was absolutely true and yet found out it was false. Millions to one is not quite "absolutely true" but near enough for a practical discussion. The point is that we have all found something we are "sure" about proved false often enough that we are uncomfortable with odds of millions to one in real life, though perhaps we are not as pessimistic as Damon Runyon's character who says nothing in life has odds more favorable than 1 to 3.

Our difficulty stems from the hazards of rare outrageous events—events that do not fit the assumptions built into the theoretical analysis being made. The general idea is that when odds are modest, say 5 to 1, we do not and need not worry much about the possible effect on the odds of rare outrageous events. But when we get huge odds—millions to one—then we need to worry.

The kinds of things one might worry about in *The Federalist* work are whether some substantial arithmetic blunder has been made, whether Madison or some newspaper editor edited one of Hamilton's papers so much that it came to seem like Madison's, or whether some forgotten unknown third party wrote the paper enough like Madison to create a mistake.

It turns out that, when there is a small chance of an outrageous event that could reverse or upset the answer, we cannot support odds much higher than the odds against the outrageous event. To make this idea more precise would require a little more mathematical formulation, but it is near enough correct to help one's thinking about long odds. When you are told that "nothing can go wrong" with odds of billions or trillions to one, you can assume that some mathematical effort has developed these odds and you are free, indeed wise, to speculate about the cumulated probability of outrageous events that might vitiate the theory leading to the odds offered. Just as an instance, could an earthquake occur that would spoil the calculations? In the case of a mechanism with backup safety devices, how likely is an event that would kill all the backups at once. They may all require electrical power, and lightning could destroy all sources. These issues are ones citizens can usefully bear in mind when thinking about safety.

Wallace and I did a lot of work on the project during summers in the early 1960s on Cape Cod at West Falmouth. In 1962–63, I worked on the final draft of the book during a sabbatical at the Center for Advanced Study in the Behavioral Sciences at Stanford, where David Levin, a scholar in history and literature, often advised me about the writing. Of course, early drafts of chapters were written separately by Wallace or by me, and then we each worked on revisions over and over.

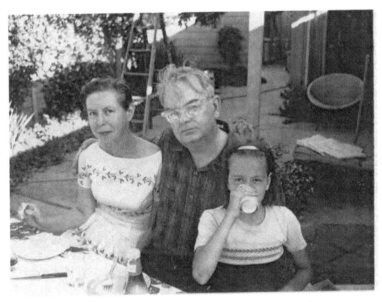

Fig. 4.3. Virginia, Fred, and Gale Mosteller in Palo Alto, 1963

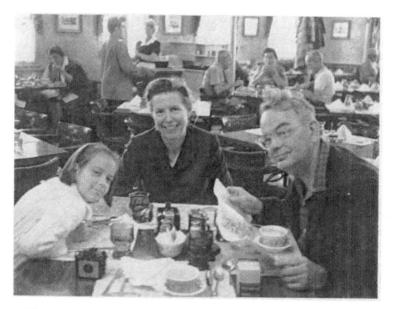

Fig. 4.4. Gale, Virginia, and Fred Mosteller at Disneyland, 1963

Ultimately the Presidents' Committee of the Joint Statistical Societies asked us to present this study at the annual statistical meetings held in September 1962 in Minneapolis, Minnesota, where we were honored with discussion by Jerzy Neyman, Douglass Adair, and Francis J. Anscombe. Being a frequentist, Neyman regretted that we had put most of our effort into the Bayesian approach. Nevertheless, he said, "They know how to do it [the frequency approach]" and pointed to the places where we had carried out that approach. We had been rather casual about that part of the work.

Addison-Wesley published the study as a book in 1964, and it was republished in a new edition by Springer-Verlag with supplementary material in 1984. The preface lists about 100 people who participated directly in the work, and from time to time I see some of them in distant places: graduate students, undergraduates, children and wives of colleagues, department secretaries, and many temporary employees.

In this study we found out a lot about Bayesian inference as well as about discrimination problems in general and authorship problems in particular. Perhaps the findings on Bayesian inference would be of importance to the reader because this method is so attractive. In most arguments against Bayesian inference, opponents raise complaints about the arbitrariness of the choice of prior distributions—how you tell what you believe in advance. But one can usually get around this by trying several and reporting the different results—a method called sensitivity testing. What we found that people had not often discussed in Bayesian work is that the shape of the data distribution mattered a lot. In technical terms this would be called the choice of the likelihood. The simple urn model versus the more nearly correct negative binomial squared the odds—thus if the negative binomial gave odds of 100 to 1 for Madison, the simple urn model gave 10,000 to 1! Choosing a model that does not fit the data may therefore give a highly misleading result; here it would exaggerate our belief in our findings. Such modeling issues have rarely been explored because investigators do not usually have enough data to investigate the data distribution.

We also found that every little question in the Bayesian approach required us, especially Wallace, to develop special mathematical theory instead of doing something rather routine in the frequency approach. The philosopher Alfred North Whitehead said that original thinking, like cavalry charges, should be saved for great occasions. Thus what we were finding was that, however attractive Bayesian methods were, they seemed not to be ready for routine use by practitioners, most of whom do not care to invent new methods and defend them, but prefer to use well-established ones. Jimmie Savage felt and many others feel that every practical problem should be attacked as a brand new research question. This is certainly appropriate for a research scholar, I like it myself, and especially valuable for the development of the field of statistics. At the same time, many routine problems must be treated over and over again. Establishing a standard attack on these can be most useful.

We complained about the computational effort of the Bayesian approach, but today that is not nearly so burdensome. In our second edition, we reviewed authorship studies made in the years 1969 to 1984. Word counts, especially filler words, seem much used in English, but the analysis usually follows the frequency approach.

More generally, I think that Bayesian inference has developed a substantial number of adherents (not yet in studies of style), though it seems fair to say that even now the theorists still outnumber the practitioners. I still see few large data analyses using a Bayesian approach. I still find the Bayesian approach very attractive and would use it when practical. The technical difficulties of imposing prior distributions are often forbidding. I have also been disappointed that more use of data to help decide on prior distributions has not emerged.

Other Discrimination Problems

Once we had finished this job, Adair wanted us to begin on a still harder problem—sorting a lot of unsigned writing in a magazine according to its authors. We might have tried if we had his help and enthusiasm, but he died before we could launch the study.

One of my students, Ivor Francis, became very interested in drawing inferences in discrimination problems and wrote a dissertation on this topic.

My discussion has emphasized methods of discrimination in deciding a dispute about authorship, but these methods have been used in a variety of fields, as I will now illustrate. Let me set the stage by indicating some simple problems that invite some methods of discrimination.

You can easily tell a dandelion from a rose, though you might find it hard to explain the distinction to a Martian who speaks your language. It would be still more difficult to explain how to distinguish between pinks and carnations, or between violets and Johnny-jump-ups. Statisticians try to develop objective ways to distinguish between such classes of plants or of people. Our reasons for developing these methods vary. Sometimes only a few experts can make the distinctions, and others want to. Sometimes the best way of making the distinction is too expensive or too damaging to the items for practical use and we need a substitute. Sometimes no one knows how to do the sorting, and we introduce formal but exploratory statistical methods in hopes of finding a reliable method.

To be successful, one needs effective variables to help with sorting. For example, striping should distinguish tigers from lions or zebras from horses. But in many situations one variable or attribute is inadequate, though several properly combined variables may give enough power to discriminate.

In a study of the emergence of the first humans (homo sapiens) on earth, W.W. Howells describes a fossil—a broken end of an upper arm—found by Bryan Patterson in northern Kenya. It was easily recognized as hominoid—primates that include apes but not monkeys (and thus a relative of homo sapiens closer than a monkey). Although the fossil could confidently be said not to be from a gorilla, an orangutan, or a gibbon, it might have been from a chimpanzee or from a human. No single measurement on the bone identified it as being from a human or from a chimpanzee. Nevertheless, by combining measurements from seven different features of the bone and comparing these with corresponding combinations for chimpanzees and for humans, the paleontologists Patterson and Howells concluded that the fossil came from a human. It was estimated that the fossil was two and one-half million years old, leading to the conclusion that humans had been around the earth for three-quarters of a million years longer than previously believed. Later it became clear to Patterson by other means that the fossil formation was over 4 million years old.

The famous British statistician and geneticist Sir Ronald A. Fisher developed a method called the discriminant function, which has been widely used in many kinds of situations requiring subtle distinctions. Patterson and Howells used it to determine that the bone was from a human. In his original scientific paper explaining the method, Fisher illustrated its use to sort three varieties of iris.

Sometimes the answers to discrimination problems lead to unexpected consequences. For a certain academic department, I was once asked to figure out what kinds of graduate students were most likely to have difficulty in completing their advanced degrees. After reviewing many properties in students' origins and preparation, I was able to report to the faculty on a class of students (about 20 percent) that had high likelihood of running into considerable difficulty during their graduate work. Sometimes long years were required for completion, and sometimes the long drill failed altogether. It was not an open-and-shut matter; some students in this class turned out to do the work with ease and turned in brilliant theses. When the identity of the class was revealed, the faculty was most upset because these students were among those they were most eager to admit, and so they certainly did not want to rule these applicants out even if they were giving trouble. I suppose it is obvious that the amount of time spent by faculty committees discussing the performance of successful students is dwarfed by the time spent on ones who are having trouble. In part this is because we believe that students we admit are capable of doing the work, and the loss of a student with good potential represents a huge loss to the system. Of course, they may contribute more elsewhere, but we are selfish about our losses.

On the positive side, now that this group was identified, and we were agreed that they should be encouraged to come, we figured out a way to help them go over the hurdles more smoothly, not by lowering the hurdles, but by making sure that they took steps early to prepare for them. Part of the faculty's problem had been that we were consistently overestimating the strength of the preparation of this group of students for meeting certain requirements of the degree, and then we often allowed them to put these requirements off until later, believing they would have no trouble. The new plan required some additional financing early on to make sure the preparation was adequate or obtained, and it reduced considerably the numbers who got into trouble.

Sometimes problems of discrimination lead to discussions about the merits of art versus science. In the medical arena sometimes proponents of clinical or of statistical methods stir up great arguments. People raise such questions as "Which is better, the clinical or the statistical method?" They think of the brilliant learned physician drawing conclusions from subtle hints given by the patient's signs and symptoms and contrast these with methods like actuarial counting or measurements built into some decision-making mechanism. Such chatter sometimes involves problems of discrimination because it is a natural approach to medical diagnosis. Indeed Paul E. Meehl wrote a thoughtful book on this topic. At least until the field of "expert systems" is more completely developed, the status might be summarized as follows: By and large we do not build a method of discrimination in medicine until the physician has described what he uses to make a diagnosis—pulse, temperature, aches and pains, or more generally signs and symptoms. Once we know what these items are and how the physician uses them, we can often create a discriminant function (or other algorithm) for making diagnoses. When that is done, a computer may turn out to perform better than the physician for two main reasons. First the computer can systematically remember to ask for and use all the data; and second, once we know the variables to enter, we may be able to put the data together in a more effective way than the unaided human mind can hope to do, essentially using better weighting. So, after being told how to behave, the computer or statistical method can be more systematic than the most careful person. I cannot see much to argue about in this machine-method-person triangle; all components have their merits.

Editors' Postscript

The Mosteller-Wallace project on the Federalist Papers *was a landmark enterprise for several reasons. First, it was one of the first large-scale Bayesian applications and one that might not have been possible without the arrival of the first modern computers on campus in the late 1950s and early 1960s. Second, it introduced modern statisticians to Laplace's method for approximating posterior distributions, a Bayesian technique that became quite popular over two decades later. For example, works such as Kass, Tierney, and Kadane (1989), and Tierney, Kass, and Kadane (1989) were paramount in popularizing Laplace's method for approximating posterior distributions. Third, the Mosteller-Wallace work was a forerunner to and exemplified the highly successful techniques of text data-mining that emerged in the 1990s using word count methods, such as those referred to as "naïve Bayes" or "bag of words." And surprisingly, the Mosteller-Wallace approach using the negative binomial distribution has produced superior results to these newer data-mining approaches, for example, in determining who wrote Ronald Reagan's radio addresses (Airoldi et al., 2006).*

Because of the work of Mosteller and Wallace, a widespread strategy for authorship attribution problems now involves using high-frequency function words. The "new field" of stylometry has built heavily on their ideas and applied them to a large range of literary genres and time periods, using an expanded repertoire of statistical tools for determining authorship. For example, the special 2003 issue of Chance *devoted to the topic contains papers (Holmes, 2003; Holmes and Kardos, 2003; Rudman, 2003) that are especially pertinent. Mosteller and Wallace's book was reprinted in paperback in 2008 by Stanford's Center for the Study of Language and Information in the David Hume Series of Philosophy and Cognitive Science Reissues.*

A recent web search produced a number of authors with manuscripts disputing the Mosteller and Wallace conclusions about the Federalist Papers, *and so the substantive issue remains alive today. None of these authors utilize methodology as technically sophisticated as Mosteller and Wallace did in the early 1960s!*

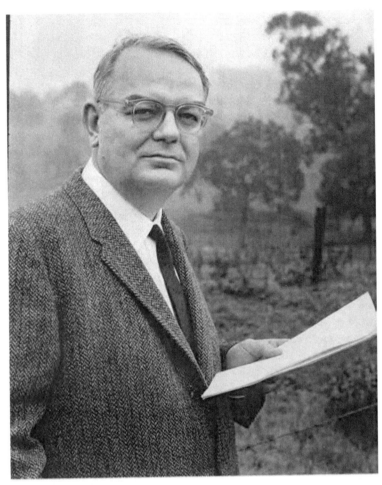

Fig. 4.5. Fred in a 1963 picture taken but not used for *Time Magazine*, which featured an article on the *Federalist Papers* Study.

Notes

1. Mosteller and Wallace (1989), pp. 116–117.
2. From Paper 14 (Madison), p. 85.
3. For a more extensive discussion of this problem, including historical details, discussion of actual techniques, and a variety of alternative analyses, see Mosteller and Wallace (1984).

References

Airoldi, E. M., Anderson, A. G., Fienberg, S. E., and Skinner, K. K. (2006). Who wrote Ronald Reagan's radio addresses? *Bayesian Analysis*, 1(2):289–320.

Cantril, H. and Research Associates in the Office of Public Opinion (1944). *Gauging Public Opinion*. Princeton, NJ: Princeton University Press.

Fisher, R. A. (1936). The use of multiple measurements in taxonomic problems. *Annals of Eugenics*, 7, Pt. 2:179–188. [Paper 32 in *Contributions to Mathematical Statistics by R. A. Fisher* (1950). New York: Wiley.]

Francis, I. S. (1966). *Inference in the Classification Problem*. Ph.D. thesis, Harvard University.

Hamilton, A., Jay, J., and Madison, J. (1787–1788). *The Federalist Papers: A commentary on the Constitution of the United States, being a collection of essays written in support of the Constitution agreed upon September 17, 1787, by the Federal Convention*. Sesquicentennial edition (1937). Washington, D.C.: National Home Library Foundation.

Holmes, D. I. (2003). Stylometry and the Civil War: The case of the Pickett letters. *Chance*, 16(2):18–25.

Holmes, D. I. and Kardos, J. (2003). Who was the author? An introduction to stylometry. *Chance*, 16(2):5–8.

Howells, W. W. (1972). The importance of being human. In J. M. Tanur, F. Mosteller, W. H. Kruskal, R. F. Link, R. S. Pieters, and G. R. Rising,

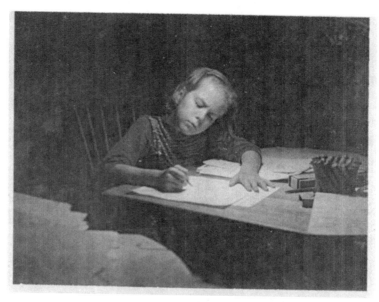

Fig. 4.6. Fred's daughter, Gale, correcting *Federalist* papers, Cape Cod, July 1962.

editors, *Statistics: A Guide to the Unknown*. San Francisco: Holden-Day. 68–76. (Also appears in the 2nd edition [1979] and the 3rd edition [1989].)

Jeffreys, H. (1939, 1948, 1961). *Theory of Probability*. 1st, 2nd, and 3rd edition. London: Oxford at the Clarendon Press.

Kass, R. E., Tierney, L., and Kadane, J. B. (1989). Approximate methods for assessing influence and sensitivity in Bayesian analysis. *Biometrika*, 76:663–675.

Meehl, P. E. (1954). *Clinical Versus Statistical Prediction: A Theoretical Analysis and a Review of the Evidence*. Minneapolis, MN: University of Minnesota Press.

Miller, G. A. (1956). The magical number seven, plus or minus two: Some limits on our capacity for processing information. *The Psychological Review*, 63:81–97.

Mosteller, F. and Wallace, D. L. (1962). Notes on an authorship problem. In *Proceedings of a Harvard Symposium on Digital Computers and Their Applications*. Cambridge, MA: Harvard University Press. 163–197.

Mosteller, F. and Wallace, D. L. (1963). Inference in an authorship problem: A comparative study of discrimination methods applied to the authorship of the disputed Federalist Papers. *Journal of the American Statistical Association*, 58:275–309.

Mosteller, F. and Wallace, D. L. (1964). *Inference and Disputed Authorship: The Federalist*. Reading, MA: Addison-Wesley Publishing Company. (Reprinted 2008. Stanford: Center for the Study of Language and Information.)

Mosteller, F. and Wallace, D. L. (1972). Deciding authorship. In J. M. Tanur, F. Mosteller, W. H. Kruskal, R. F. Link, R. S. Pieters, and G. R. Rising, editors, *Statistics: A Guide to the Unknown*. San Francisco: Holden-Day. 115–125. (Also appears in the 2nd edition [1979] and the 3rd edition [1989].)

Mosteller, F. and Wallace, D. L. (1984). *Applied Bayesian and Classical Inference: The Case of The Federalist Papers*. New York: Springer-Verlag.

Rudman, J. (2003). Cherry picking in nontraditional authorship attribution studies. *Chance*, 16(2):26–32.

Runyon, D. (1950). A nice price. Chapter in Vol. II, *Money from Home* in *The Damon Runyon Omnibus, Three Volumes in One*. Philadelphia: J. B. Lippincott.

Tierney, L., Kass, R. E., and Kadane, J. B. (1989). Fully exponential Laplace approximations to posterior expectations and variances. *Journal of the American Statistical Association*, 84:710–716.

Williams, C. B. (1939). A note on the statistical analysis of sentence-length as a criterion of literary style. *Biometrika*, 31:356–361.

Williams, C. B. (1956). Studies in the history of probability and statistics: IV. A note on an early statistical study of literary style. *Biometrika*, 43:248–256.

Yule, G. U. (1939). On sentence-length as a statistical characteristic of style in prose: with application to two cases of disputed authorship. *Biometrika*, 30(3/4):363–390.

5

The Safety of Anesthetics: The National Halothane Study

A healthy young woman accidentally slashed her wrists on a broken windowpane and was rushed to the hospital. Surgery was performed using the anesthetic halothane with results that led everyone to believe that the outcome of the treatment was satisfactory, but a few days later the patient died. The cause was traced to massive hepatic necrosis—so many of her liver cells died that life could not be sustained. Such outcomes are very rare, especially in healthy young people.

We members of the general public can take great comfort from the medical profession's attitude toward mysterious deaths in benign circumstances. Physicians hate them. One night I sat beside a famous surgeon and heard an anthropologist brilliantly describe the power of a witch doctor's spell to cause the lingering painful death of a tribesman who had offended another. My surgeon friend interrupted this moving story to ask grumpily, "Who performed the autopsy?" He did not gracefully accept the storyteller's reassurance that no autopsy was necessary, because nothing but the spell had been cast. Among students of modern magic who were present, faint doubts also swirled.

The concern of medical professionals for the tragedy of the young woman and for a handful of other patients with similar outcomes led to my participation in the National Halothane Study. This study illustrates one way that statisticians and physicians cooperate to assess a public health issue. Often, as here, such problems are complex, paradoxically involving serious biases caused by honest physician behavior. Usually the work does not move in simple logical order, but starts in one direction and then turns to another. By following this study, we observe the National Academy of Sciences-National Research Council carrying out its obligation assigned by Abraham Lincoln to help solve national scientific problems. In following this investigation, we see some dangerous pitfalls in the formulation of the scientific problem, pitfalls that, as a nation, we are frequently trapped in, such as being much more concerned with one death from an identifiable cause than with hundreds from unidentifiable ones.

F. Mosteller, *The Pleasures of Statistics: The Autobiography of Frederick Mosteller*,
DOI 10.1007/978-0-387-77956-0_5,
© Springer Science + Business Media, LLC 2010

We see how examining thoroughly about 50,000 hospital records selected with statistical care brought more useful information about the safety of anesthetics in surgery than records of many millions of operations had previously done. We see how statistical adjustments can sometimes remove or reduce biases and sometimes cannot.

In difficult problems like this one, new statistical methods may have to be developed, as they were here, and then these methods become available for applications to scientific and technological problems going far beyond the ones they were developed to solve. Thus science benefits more generally.

Inevitably, along with resolution or partial resolution of the original problem, substantial studies raise new questions, as we shall see. The questions the halothane study raised agitate us still, partly because we have not pursued them with vigor, and partly because they too are complex.

When, as here, much more than the minimum analysis was done, the findings may continue to be valuable for much longer periods in spite of intervening advances in technology.

Some Background

The young woman mentioned above had received the anesthetic halothane during her surgery. Even though it became a successful anesthetic, physicians were still concerned because its composition includes several halogen atoms. Some deadly fluids and gases contain halogens; for example, carbon tetrachloride, when used in cleaning with inadequate ventilation, can snuff out a life suddenly. Although chloroform, which has halogens, has been used as an anesthetic, it has dangers. Altering from poisons to wonder drugs, with slight changes in their composition, chemicals behave like chameleons. The chemical structure of halothane led experts to fear that it might attack the liver. Thus the condition of the young woman's liver fit in with these fears. Her death and a few others triggered the National Halothane Study, a study of the safety of anesthetics carried out on behalf of the National Academy of Sciences-National Research Council.

Before halothane came into use, its manufacturers and various biomedical research workers studied it so extensively that abstracts of the articles filled a massive book summarizing perhaps 1000 scientific papers. Curiously, I recall that only two were controlled trials in humans, neither very relevant to the question of safety. In animal studies, the liver injury observed with chloroform and carbon tetrachloride was not observed with halothane.

Why was halothane attractive as an anesthetic? For two reasons, one negative and one positive. First, it did not burn or explode. Two other anesthetics widely used at that time, ether and cyclopropane, did. Although such explosions were rare indeed, sparks could set them off. Ether sends out vapor streamers in the air which act almost like fuses, and when the rare spark hits, the flame goes right back to the patient's chest. In a cyclopropane explosion the operating team as well as the patient is in danger. These tragedies were fortunately rare, but their possibility induced anxiety in the staunchest souls.

Second, a positive reason: with halothane, the patient can be quickly brought to consciousness and can be asked to move limbs or respond to questions or other stimuli, and if necessary, returned then to deeper anesthesia, although this is not often needed. With ether, hours may pass before the patient recovers consciousness, whereas the quick clearing of halothane is a major asset. As a third benefit, some also report that halothane produces less nausea and vomiting than, say, ether.

Because of its potency some difficulties in controlling depth of anesthesia arose in the earliest operations using halothane, but these were eliminated by the design of better equipment which gave the anesthetist extremely close control over the amount being delivered to the patient.

As a result of the benefits of safety and quick clearing, by 1962 in the United States within four years of its introduction, fifty percent of all surgical operations requiring anesthesia used halothane.

The medical literature recorded several isolated cases of death with massive liver necrosis when halothane had been used. Questions were inevitably raised about its safety, and the Committee on Anesthesia of the Division of Medical Sciences of the National Academy of Sciences-National Research Council began monitoring halothane outcomes through a small study group.

Although we tend to think of the National Academy as a prestigious body that monitors scientific affairs, it actually is an honorific organization with about 1,500 members who have no real responsibility. Instead, the National Research Council (NRC) does the real work of the Academy, mainly through committees (and some other special groups) that are ordinarily chaired by Academy members and that call on experts, members or not, and Council staff as well to help resolve scientific issues. (Later the National Academy complex expanded to include the National Academy of Engineering and the Institute of Medicine.) The NRC does not ordinarily do what scientists regard as original research; instead, it usually tries to assess the current state of information by drawing on already published research and the wisdom of its committee members, staff, and advisors. The National Halothane Study was an exception because data were gathered and analyzed from record rooms of a set of hospitals distributed throughout the country.

Why did the Committee not recommend stopping the use of halothane? Answer: Numerator-only data. The classic numerator-only joke told in minstrel shows was:

"Why do the white horses eat more than the black horses?"

"Don't know. Why?"

"Because we have ten times as many white horses as black horses."

Obviously, minstrel show or medicine, we need to look carefully at rates of occurrence. If we forget to do this, we will be dazzled by meaningless incomparable counts. For example, if all the operations are carried out with halothane, it tells us little that some patients die of massive liver necrosis.

What we have described thus far are some unfortunate but rare deaths. In 1964, in the United States about 12,000,000 operations were being performed per year. Among these patients, perhaps 240,000 died, some for unusual reasons. Before indicting a procedure, we should compare its performance with those of competitive procedures used in similar circumstances. With numerator-only data, we have only the cases with bad outcomes, and thus no rate to compare with rates for other procedures. Here the numerator is the number of hepatic necrosis cases found that used halothane. We need the number of treatments all told, and we need the corresponding information for other anesthetics to begin a proper comparison. To be carried away by an argument based on numerator-only data constitutes a classic blunder that biostatisticians and epidemiologists abhor.

A second feature of the halothane situation that also leads to difficulty in interpretation is selective reporting. When observers think that an unusual bad outcome might occur in a medical treatment, they are more likely to observe and report the event than in circumstances where a side effect routinely occurs. A prominent feature of halothane use was the expectation, because of its chemical composition, of possible liver trouble, without such an expectation for most of the other anesthetics. One might therefore expect selective reporting of halothane-associated deaths with massive liver necrosis and little reporting of such events with anesthetics not under suspicion. And so both selective reporting and the existence of numerator-only data contributed to the prominent difficulty of interpreting these events.

The National Halothane Study

In the summer of 1962 John Bunker, one of the brilliant anesthesiologists who trained with Harry Beecher, stopped by the summer house that Virginia and I had at West Falmouth and invited me to join a study of the safety of anesthetics if one were set up. He made it sound both fascinating and important—they always do, and much of the fun of statistical work comes from participating in such a variety of studies. My experience has been that, no matter how boring a topic seems in advance, once I am embroiled, it becomes engrossing. Pick any ridiculous topic, such as plumbing among the Romans, and it will turn out to have all sorts of engaging ideas. For example, maybe the imperial families went mad because they used lead pipes for conveying drinking water.

At any rate, I looked forward to working with Bunker again—we had consulted on some research on pulmonary questions when he was at Massachusetts General Hospital—and he and others were assembling a strong team. Before long, the study did start, and funds were quickly found through the skill of Sam Seeley, an officer in NRC's Division of Medical Sciences. Arranging the contract took a long time, but finding the funding did not.

Originally Bunker and William Forrest, another anesthesiologist then at Stanford Medical School, had hoped to develop a randomized controlled trial, which would have been in some ways a surer kind of study than the one actually carried out. It faced several problems: the numbers of patients required to detect small, important differences would need to be about a million, and these would require several years to collect and large funds to gather.

During a pilot study at one institution a halothane death occurred, and this too discouraged an experiment. This, of course, is ironic; when half the patients are getting a treatment, why would it be inappropriate to check its safety and efficacy? One reason might be that the treatment has already been proved to be safer and more efficacious than its competitors, though that was not the reason given. The reason was the opposite—fear that the treatment was not safe, exactly why a trial would be justified.

At the same time, a study with perhaps a million patients could fall of its own weight, and the question of the safety from a public health point of view could probably be settled from a retrospective study, and that was what was done.

At one time we were informed that we would be able to tell by chemical means whether a massive liver necrosis was caused by halothane or by something else. By the time we got to the first meeting of the Subcommittee on the National Halothane Study,[1] this belief had evaporated. It is an example of a common phenomenon: many things people think they can do turn out to be impossible when careful assessments are made.

The Subcommittee on the Halothane Study held its first meeting in Washington, D.C., in the board room of the National Academy of Sciences, which has the great oil painting of Lincoln and his cabinet at the creation of the Academy. Lincoln, who had wanted scientific and technical help in winning the Civil War, looks out at the room as if he is expecting a lot from those who are meeting.

The room itself was packed, and speaker after speaker treated a variety of topics. Two things stood out, one by its presence, the other by its absence. We were certainly getting strong information about halothane and about the liver and about other anesthetics, but we were not doing anything direct about starting the study. Since then I have learned that this is a rather standard pattern for the first meeting of an Academy committee. Someone thinks of all the experts who have something to say about the problem (even if they are twice removed from it). Soon the agenda becomes crowded with speakers giving background material, and time for the committee's work is squeezed out. Having notables present lends a sense of urgency and stature to the occasion, even though the content of their discussion might be easily summarized by a short position paper prepared by the staff. Probably it also creates a constituency for the study. Through the years, I have blown hot and cold on this, sometimes feeling that the additional background material is needed and sometimes feeling that we are wasting time. I am sure that all told too much time is spent hearing from too many people with borderline contributions at the expense of time for a committee's own work. The valuable idea that committees should hold public hearings should not be confused with overstuffing the agenda of a working meeting.

The great event of that day, at least for its heat, was a series of exchanges between the toxicologist Ellis Cohen and a chemist from Imperial Chemical Industries, Ltd., who came from the home office to tell us about halothane. Cohen had done some research that seemed to show that, under certain circumstances when halothane was kept in a copper kettle and subjected to unusually high temperatures, some tiny part of the gas could change into a slightly different substance that had astonishing toxicity. Because the high temperatures described did not seem likely to occur, those findings did not appear to be of major concern for our study.

By the end of the day, it seemed clear that the primary question was whether halothane posed a public health problem. It would be the Subcommittee's job to find out. Toward 3:00 p.m., I was surprised to find that the people who had been so wise and eloquent silently slipped away with comments like "Lots of luck!", leaving only Kipling's "Thin red line of 'eroes" behind to begin to design the study. I had not realized how few we were.

How can one find out whether a medical procedure poses a public health problem? Sometimes by just sitting and thinking about it, but usually by gathering data that are not immediately available. Our study needed to get special information about the occurrence of deaths with massive liver necrosis and also, if possible, about morbidity related to the liver.

Someone suggested that liver biopsy be performed on patients having anesthetics. Liver biopsy, at least at that time, had rather frequent ill consequences of its own such as pain, infection, and death, and therefore could not be justified unless something of considerable value to the patient could be learned. Thus the biopsy would have been unethical, and so we abandoned that approach, though the suggestion resurfaced many times.

Furthermore, we knew that we needed a large data base because the rate of deaths from massive liver necrosis obviously was small or the whole medical profession already would have been up in arms. The reliability of estimates of rates of events that rarely occur is determined not so much by the sample size as by the total number of occurrences in the sample. This fact underlies all sorts of difficulties in acquiring reliability and safety information. It takes a long time (a lot of experience) under ordinary circumstances to establish the rate of occurrence of a rare event. People try various ways to speed the gathering of information. We test light bulbs by burning them continuously. We test animals at severe levels of exposure, and we try to get more information faster, but we speed up by enforcing conditions that differ from those of the real world. Events that rarely occur give us a hard time in measuring their rate, and that is part of the reality of risk assessment generally, not just medical risks.

Because the postoperative death rate in all surgery together is about 2%, and because most of these deaths occur because of the severity or advanced state of the patient's disease, we can scarcely hope to find large differences in death rates due to anesthesia itself. For example, Henry Beecher and Donald Todd in the 1950s estimated that the death rate associated with anesthesia itself might be in the neighborhood of 1 in 1500 operations, though we have evidence that this is an overestimate in 1990. By keeping track of all deaths, we know that some operations performed under general anesthesia have practically no deaths from any cause, and so anesthesia deaths must be fewer yet. Thus for total anesthesia deaths, we are dealing with a proportion much less than 0.001—less than 1 in 1000. If some anesthetic were causing more deaths than usual, we would need an enormous sample to detect the difference. We decided that a difference of 0.1% or a proportion 0.001 in the population was what we ought to try to detect. Such detection would require an extremely large sample.

We also needed variety in the institutions so as to be able to make inferences to the nation. We needed many hospitals to join the study. We had to be sure that their supporting workers were well trained in how to choose and abstract the records of the cases. We planned to take a sample from all their cases of surgery performed with anesthesia. Although 54 hospitals volunteered, some dropped out when they found their personnel or records were not suited to the task, and we ended with data from 34. They were of various sizes and kinds, teaching hospitals being one important kind, and most hospitals in the study had hundreds of beds.

Just as selective reporting can lead to biased results, so can giving selective attention to some part instead of the whole of the data. Operations analysts and economists both keep reminding us of this hazard. The problem comes up in various ways, and we often are in danger of making a bad policy mistake because of the part-whole problem. The general idea is this: treatment A is in wide use, and those who get treatment A die from a rare side effect at twice the rate of those who get treatment B for the same disease. One's instinct supposes that we should abandon treatment A in favor of treatment B. But wait! I forgot to tell you that the overall death rate from the disease with treatment A is only half as big as that with treatment B. Consequently, even though we may know that more people are going to die from the side effect with treatment A, we had better stick to A. Of course, efforts should and will be made to identify people in danger from the side effect, but this may not be possible either soon or ever.

For example, a drug warning was sent out that administering halothane to patients with liver or biliary tract disease was not recommended. At the same time, patients undergoing cholecystectomy under halothane during the period of the study suffered fewer liver deaths than those receiving other anesthetics. Similarly, according to other studies, patients with cirrhosis, a liver ailment, fared at least as well with halothane.

Although we may be able to prove that deaths associated with the rare side effect genuinely are caused by treatment A, the cause of the much larger numbers of overall deaths associated with treatment B may not be identifiable; indeed, they may never be; it may just be that more patients are saved by treatment A. People give a great deal more attention to situations where we know why a death occurred than those where we don't. If we forget that the total process must be evaluated, not just the results associated with special side effects, bad choices occur. Economists call doing well on a part of a problem while doing less well than we could on the whole problem "suboptimizing." In the medical arena, unless the quality of a death is vastly different from one disease rather than another (as it may be for cancer compared with heart attack), it is the fact of life or death that matters to the patient, rather than the reason for a death.

An example of a national situation requiring an appraisal of total versus part optimizing arose in the choice of Sabin instead of Salk polio vaccine in the United States. Sabin apparently produces a very few cases of paralytic polio in people exposed to persons recently vaccinated, whereas Salk apparently does not. Why then use Sabin? In the United States, current medical judgment says that with our rather laissez faire attitude toward vaccination we cannot expect to vaccinate all the children, and we cannot maintain the booster shots needed with Salk, and so we put up with the additional cases of polio that could be prevented. Sweden feels it can enforce the vaccination program and uses Salk. Israel has the exciting idea of using both in everyone and stamping out the disease.

Why all this discussion of side effects and known and unknown causes? In the National Halothane Study, even if it were to turn out that deaths from massive liver necrosis had a higher rate with halothane than with, say, cyclopropane, we might still find that the overall safety or performance with halothane was better, and therefore it would not be enough for the study to look at rates of massive liver necrosis associated with each anesthetic. We need to look at overall death rates. Because comparing death rates for rare events requires large numbers of cases, the Study had to be substantial in size. That total death rate was the primary issue had to be explained again and again, because for many the compelling issue was the liver rather than the total death rate. Although we needed the facts on the liver, even if they were forbidding, they might not determine policy.

A numerical example illustrates this point. Let us suppose that halothane were to cause a dozen deaths a year, and that it also cut the anesthetic death rate that Beecher and Todd estimated as 1 in 1500 operations by one-tenth. Then for 12,000,000 operations the reduction in anesthetic deaths alone would be 800. Those 800 lives saved would far outweigh the 12 lives lost to liver damage. Thus it is very important to treat the whole problem and not just a part that seems very easy to understand.

Other variables are far more influential than the anesthetic, for example, age, the operation, and the condition of the patient. Naturally other complications will occur to the reader; for example, perhaps different anesthetics might be used for different operations. If the operations had different death rates, then we would need to take the "patient mix" into account. To do so, we needed to keep track of important variables that might relate to the general health of the patient, such as age, or type of operation, or how long the operation took. In addition, we had an extra measure variously called the "physical status" score or anesthetic risk, which measures the health of the patient. A patient scoring a 1 is in fine shape except for the disease or damage leading to the operation. A patient scoring a 4 is fortunate to have gotten to the operating table alive. This sort of score along with others can be used to remove or reduce bias in the comparisons between groups of patients by adjusting for patient mix by statistical methods.

To gather the data, William Forrest, M.D., and others designed forms to be filled in from patients' records at the hospitals. We sampled 25 patients per hospital per month for the years 1959–1962. This gave us denominator information about numbers of patients falling into various categories. Our numerator data were especially good, because we could get a census. Deaths in a hospital are carefully recorded, and since happily there are relatively few of them, we were able to use the total death records for our numerators while basing the denominators on an extensive sample. For the same total number of patients for whom data were recorded, we had much more information than usual. Usually, we would have had to be content with the deaths the sample turned up, and this would have given us only about 1 in 50 deaths compared to our actual situation. Because we were able to include more of the rare events of concern, this unusual sampling scheme enormously improved our accuracy compared to that of the usual sampling study. Because we could not afford to review all 850,000 records, sampling of the population of patients was a necessity.

In 34 hospitals over a four-year period, about 850,000 operations were carried out, with about 17,000 deaths. Our sampling of total cases led to 34,000 surgical cases for our denominator data, coupled with the 17,000 deaths, or about 50,000 records in all. This 50,000 gave us nearly as much information as the whole 850,000 would have yielded.

Getting the information from the hospitals and onto the computer was next. William Forrest was in charge of this, and he soon had hospital staffs trained to gather the data, though he had to do a great deal of visiting and advising. He did a magnificent job with his staff maintaining a 24-hour turnaround, checking data as fast as received so as to ask for missing data or to catch and correct erroneous inputs.

Obviously the analysis of these data was going to be complex and extensive, and the staff needed a full-time statistician-computer person of stature. Although we had first-class people on the Subcommittee and also had other fine experts as consultants in this field, we did not yet have a full statistician-computer staff for the Subcommittee.

One of our members seemed especially ripe for the post. I had first met him at the University of Chicago, where he worked his way through graduate school doing medical statistics, and we became closely acquainted at the Center for Advanced Study in the Behavioral Sciences in Stanford. I admired greatly his computing and statistical skills, and I enjoyed his wry humor. At the Center, we began writing a joint paper, "Recognizing the maximum of a sequence"—the first of many as our careers came together. This young man was the Center's statistician, computer-wizard, and applied mathematician, John P. Gilbert. I always thought that his education at St. John's, based on the Great Books, gave him a special original way of thinking.

Lincoln Moses, the senior Stanford statistician on the Subcommittee, and John Bunker knew and liked Gilbert well. The problem was that the Center had him working for them full-time. We finally got Gilbert's permission to talk to the Center's head, Ralph Tyler. Ralph has always been a person of great vision, and so we had only to lay our problem before him. He saw our need and appreciated Gilbert's key role in the proposed study. Though he couldn't let us have all of Gilbert's time, at Bunker's request, he did give us the lion's share.

Gilbert's previous medical work ultimately made him invaluable in an additional unforeseen way. He worked closely with the pathologists in helping them design their reviews of slides to verify the diagnosis of massive liver necrosis in those who died. This study would require a chapter of its own, and so does not appear here.

At Harvard, a young woman was working toward a dissertation with me in the general area of contingency tables. Contingency tables are the tables of counts that describe relations among many variables. As an example, suppose that you have two attributes such as hair color and eye color. Then the contingency table tells for each combination, such as brunette-blue, how many in a population have both characteristics. When more than two attributes are involved, the analysis gets complicated, and such complicated situations were what we were studying. Such variables and attributes as sex, age, kind of operation, length of operation, patient's condition, all needed to be taken into account in addition to the anesthetic used and the life or death outcome.

The woman had a great deal of practical experience in the biological area, first in the fishing industry, and then in medicine and health. She quit working with the fisheries people because they did not like women on the research vessels and discriminated against them. Her medical talents and her dissertation topic made the halothane study a natural practical laboratory for her work. When bigger contingency tables came along, we were going to have them. And so, Yvonne Bishop moved to Stanford to join John Bunker and the others on the halothane project. With Lincoln Moses, Byron (Bill) Brown, and John Gilbert, this meant that several statisticians were paying attention to the analysis from close at hand. The statistical staff also included Jerry Halpern and Lawrence Tesler, who handled the data that Forrest was bringing in.

Yvonne Bishop has a remarkable ability to get things done. She pays herself off in quality of output and amount completed. Yvonne's calculations were completed and guiding our research very quickly. Beyond that, being generous and energetic, as soon as she finished her own work, she turned to helping the others get theirs done, and so she coauthored several chapters of the final work.

In the course of helping with the National Halothane Study, she produced material that completed her doctoral dissertation.

Because we sampled the cases and also had a census of deaths, a few anomalous outcomes were possible when we broke the data into many cells, as we did for analysis. It was possible for us to observe a death in a cell, where we had observed no cases. This would not be surprising because we sampled relatively few cases. If a cell had only 10 cases in the whole population, we might readily not have chosen any. Still, when computing estimates of percentages of deaths, something special has to be done about cells where deaths but no cases have been observed. Of course, many adjustments can serve; the problem is to figure out among them which may be preferable. By this time my son William had become proficient at computing, and he and I worked out together the benefits to be gained from various formulas for adjustment that would systematically be used.

As a result of Bishop's analyses and those of others, we could see the need for a book that would summarize the many methods of analyzing complicated contingency tables. A few years later, together with Stephen Fienberg and Paul Holland, she developed a book entitled *Discrete Multivariate Analysis,* which offers a comprehensive applied and theoretical guide to this area, one spinoff from the halothane study. I helped organize the work at the beginning and made some contributions to it, as did Richard Light. The practical problems we faced in the halothane study just insisted that the methods we were using be systematized for easier use in other problems.

In organizing our work toward analysis on the halothane study, we had a number of consultants. I should mention before going on that one of the benefits one gets in serving on an Academy committee is no pay. Except for people genuinely on the staff, experts serve the Academy free of charge. I sometimes argue that this is not as beneficial to the public as it sounds, but let me not derail this discussion. It offered a special benefit here. From the start one could see that the required methods of analysis were going to be arcane from the point of view of non-statisticians. In problems where the outcome has to be explained to the public or to non-experts, this leads to trouble. Everyone gets rather uneasy when data are tucked into black boxes and adjustments are used that are not convenient to describe or easy to understand. Often rightly, people worry that the data analyst will somehow make the data come out to suit himself or herself. Although in some kinds of problems that may be an appropriate concern—for example in the study of the effectiveness of capital punishment or in adversary proceedings—our situation here was different. We could make a satisfactory contribution to society no matter what way the analyses pointed. In this sort of problem, my concern arises from the possibility of gross error.

I fear that the computer system may conceal a bug that no one knows about and that is so deeply and subtly placed that we have no way to check for it. To guard against such problems, one can try to have data analyses done in more than one way—quite separate ways—so that one can look for comparability. To show that such gross programming errors are not a paper risk, let me give an example. The late Elizabeth Scott, a distinguished professor at the University of California at Berkeley, was concerned that some data that she was analyzing on the effects of sunlight in producing skin cancer were not properly adjusted for altitude above sea level. The laboratory assured her repeatedly that their computer program automatically handled it. After months of delay, she got the program and studied it. It had a nice subroutine for correcting for altitude, but the computer command to use it had never been given, and so the appropriate adjustments were not being made, just as she had feared. Most of us have more everyday problems with gross errors in computing but usually can't reach the source. For example, no matter how many letters you write explaining a mistaken bill, the computer never seems to get the message.

The halothane data offered a nice field trial for a variety of methods of analysis whose outcomes could then be compared. My statistician friends saw the value of this exercise, and so by contributing their services they were able to carry this out. In addition to the statisticians already mentioned, we had the support of John W. Tukey and W. Morven Gentleman, then a recent graduate of Princeton's statistics program. One year Tukey was driving across the country attending various statistical meetings. The statistics panel wanted his advice, and so we set up panel meetings at the professional statistical conferences, and the various subgroups had profitable meetings with him at several places including New Orleans and Phoenix.

Tukey, from Princeton University and Bell Telephone Laboratories, is one of the two statisticians awarded the National Medal of Science, the other being the late Jerzy Neyman of the University of California at Berkeley.[2] Tukey's versatility in joining theory and practice for statistics in many fields has brought him into demand by all kinds of organizations. In the halothane work he brought forward several fresh ideas, some of which have still not been fully exploited on other problems. He and Gentleman produced several chapters for the National Halothane Study as well as oceans of advice on chapters others prepared.

Let us turn now to the findings from the survey of hospital experience. At the start of the study, halothane had been given to about 10 million people in the U.S. Many of these patients had been in the 34 hospitals that joined the study. Their staffs kept good records and keenly wanted to answer the very questions we have asked. They cooperated with the Committee by sampling their records of surgical operations performed during the years 1959–1962. In addition to recording whether or not the patient died within six weeks of surgery, they gave information on the anesthetic that had been used as well as facts about the surgical procedure and the patient's sex, age, and physical status prior to the operation. Among the 850,000 operations in the study, there were about 17,000 deaths, or a death rate of 2%. The death rates, shown in Table 5.1, were calculated for each of four major anesthetics and for a fifth group consisting of all other anesthetics. Note that these are death rates from all causes, including the patients' diseases, and are not deaths especially resulting from the anesthetic.

Table 5.1. Death Rates Associated with Various Anesthetics

Halothane	Pentothal*	Cyclopropane	Ether	All others
1.7%	1.7%	3.4%	1.9%	3.0%

* Nitrous oxide plus barbiturate.

Table 5.1 suggests that halothane was as safe as any other anesthetic in wide use, but such a suggestion simply cannot be trusted. Medical people knew that certain anesthetics, cyclopropane for example, were used more often in severe and risky operations than some other anesthetics (such as pentothal, which was much less often used in difficult cases). So, as suggested earlier, some or all of the differences among these death rates might have been due to a tendency to use one anesthetic in difficult operations and another in easier ones.

Different operations carry very different risks of death. Indeed, in this study death rates on some operations were found to be as low as 0.25% and on others nearly 14%. The change in death rates across the categories of patients' physical status was even more dramatic, ranging from 0.25% in the most favorable physical status category to over 30% in the least favorable. Age mattered a great deal: the most favorable 10-year age group (10 to 19) carried a death rate of less than 0.50%, while the least favorable age group (over 90) had a death rate of 26%. Another factor was sex, with women about two-thirds as likely to die as men. Because the factors of age, type of operation, physical status, and sex were so very important in determining the death rate, it was clear that even a relatively small preponderance of unfavorable patients in the group receiving a particular anesthetic could raise its death rate quite substantially. Thus, the differences in Table 5.1 *might* be due largely, and possibly even entirely, to discrepancies in the kinds of patients and types of operations associated with the various anesthetics. Certainly it was necessary somehow to adjust so as to equalize for type of operation, sex, physical status, and age before trying to determine the relative safety of the anesthetics.

If these data had been obtained from a well-designed experiment, the investigators might have arranged to collect the data so that patients receiving the various anesthetics were comparable in age, type of operation, sex, and physical status. As it was, these data were collected by reviewing old records, and so substantial differences in the kinds of patients receiving the various anesthetics were to be expected and, indeed, were found. For example, cyclopropane was given two or three times more often than halothane to patients with poor physical status and substantially more often than halothane to patients over sixty years of age. There were many such peculiarities, and they were bound to affect the death rates of Table 5.1.

The task was to purge the effects of these interfering variables from the death rates corresponding to the five anesthetics. Fortunately, it was possible to do this. I use "fortunately" because it could have been impossible; for example, if each anesthetic had been applied to a special set of operations, different from those using other anesthetics, then differences found in the death rates could perfectly well have come from differences in the operations performed, and there would be no way to disentangle operation from anesthetic and settle the question. But the data of this study showed much overlapping among the anesthetics in the categories of age, kind of operation, sex, and patient's physical status, so that statistical adjustment, or equalization, was possible. Analysis using such adjustment was undertaken in a variety of ways because the complexity of the problem made several different approaches reasonable and no one approach alone could be relied upon. Regardless of the method used, the findings closely agreed.

A summary of the results is shown in Table 5.2. Notice that halothane and pentothal after adjustment have higher death rates than their unadjusted rates in Table 5.1. Also, cyclopropane and "all others," the two with highest rates in Table 5.1, now have lower death rates. The effects of these adjustments are quite important: halothane, instead of appearing to be twice as safe as cyclopropane—the message in Table 5.1—now appears to be safer by only about one-fifth.

Table 5.2. Adjusted Death Rates Associated with Various Anesthetics (Adjusted for Age, Type of Operation, Sex, and Physical Status)

Halothane	Pentothal	Cyclopropane	Ether	All others
2.1%	2.0%	2.6%	2.0%	2.5%

Even after the adjustments, outcomes varied from hospital to hospital. Our confidence in the validity of the statistically adjusted figures in Table 5.2 was affected by how consistent the death rates were from hospital to hospital. After all, if there were many hospitals where cyclopropane was associated with a lower adjusted death rate than halothane, even though the halothane rate was lower "on the average," we might feel uncertain that halothane was really safer just because of the difference in adjusted death rates. Some fluctuation from hospital to hospital is to be expected, of course, because of chance factors; absolute consistency is not to be expected.

The question is: "Were the comparisons among the adjusted anesthetic death rates consistent enough over hospitals to warrant taking seriously the apparent differences shown in Table 5.2?" Rather complicated statistical techniques were necessary to study this question, but the conclusions were clear; halothane and pentothal both had adjusted death rates definitely lower than cyclopropane and "all other," and those lower adjusted death rates were real in the sense that they could not be explained by chance fluctuations. The differences were sufficiently consistent to be believed. On the other hand, ether, with the same adjusted death rate as halothane and pentothal, did not have a consistent pattern of comparison. Therefore, ether could not be reliably compared with the others; we could not tell from the evidence obtained whether it was somewhat safer than it appears here—or somewhat less safe. Possibly it was as safe as, or safer than, halothane; possibly it was no safer than "all other." The findings about ether were indefinite because there were fewer administrations of ether and these were concentrated in a few hospitals; hence there was less information to go on.

What can we conclude from the findings of this study? First, and most important, is the surprising result that halothane, which was suspect at the beginning of the study, emerged as a definitely safe and probably superior anesthetic agent. Second, we see that a careful statistical study of a sample from these 850,000 operations enabled the medical profession to answer questions more firmly than had previously been possible, despite the much greater "experience" of ten million administrations of halothane and other tens of millions of administrations of the other anesthetics.

In this discussion we have concentrated on the findings from the statistical study of death rates. Some of the strength of the study came from the work of the Panel of Pathologists, who carefully studied, under controlled conditions, slides of liver tissue taken by autopsy from deceased patients. They did not find evidence of halothane's being more likely than other anesthetics to be associated with massive or intermediate liver necrosis, the two degrees of necrosis examined.

When the time came for the study to be written up, Leroy Vandam, a member of the Subcommittee and editor of the journal *Anesthesiology*, joined Bunker, Forrest, and me in assembling the final manuscript. My 10-year old daughter and I took a boat to Nantucket, and Roy and I made final editorial arrangements at his summer home.

Hospital Death Rates

A brand new question emerged with the observation that the 34 hospitals had very different overall postoperative death rates! These ranged from around 0.25% to around 6.5%. This seemed to mean that the likelihood of dying within six weeks after surgery could be 25 times as great in one hospital as in another. Just as before, however, there were strong reasons to approach this startling information skeptically. Some of the hospitals in the study did not undertake difficult operations, such as open-heart surgery, while others had quite large loads in such categories. This kind of difference alone would cause differences in hospital death rates. Further, the age distribution might be different, and perhaps importantly so, from one hospital to another. Indeed, one was a children's hospital, another a veteran's hospital. Some hospitals might more frequently accept surgical patients having poor physical status. So the same interfering variables as before surely affected the differences in hospital death rates. If adjustment were made for the interfering variables, would the great differences in hospital death rates vanish? Be much reduced? Remain the same? Or, as is conceivable, actually increase?

Lincoln Moses and I looked into this by applying adjustment procedures, and the result was that the high-death-rate hospitals, after adjustment, moved down toward a 2% overall death rate, and the low-death-rate hospitals, after adjustment, moved up toward a 2% overall death rate. The adjusted hospital death rates no longer ranged from 0.25% to over 6.5%; instead, the largest of these adjusted death rates was only about three times as great as the smallest. Almost any group of 34 such rates will exhibit some variability, and the ratio of the largest to the smallest must be a number larger than 1. Even if a single hospital were measured over several different periods, the rates would fluctuate from chance alone. The fluctuation in rate would be considerable because the death rate itself is basically low, and one death more or less makes a difference in the observed rate for the period. The fact that this ratio turned out to be 3 in these data does not, in itself, indicate clearly that there were real, unexplained hospital differences.

Careful statistical study showed that there were probably some real differences from hospital to hospital in postoperative death rates, and that these differences cannot be explained wholly by the hospitals' patient populations in terms of age, sex, physical status, and surgical procedure. Statistical theory showed that the ratio of highest to lowest adjusted rate should be about 1.5 if the hospitals were identical in operative death rate after adjustment (so that the adjusted rates differ only by chance fluctuation).

The position, then, is that we began with the large ratio of about 25 for unadjusted rates, cut the ratio way down to 3 for adjusted rates, and then compared the 3 with 1.5 as a theoretical ratio. Because the adjustments can hardly have been perfect and because there undoubtedly were unadjusted factors that differed among the hospitals, we conclude that the adjusted hospital death rates are indeed close together. Thus, what, on the basis of the unadjusted hospital death rates, looked like a shocking public health problem proved, after statistical investigation, to be quite something else. The apparent problem was mainly, though probably not entirely, a dramatic manifestation of differences not in the quality of surgical care but in the difficulty of the surgical cases handled in the various hospitals.

Concern about hospital differences prompted further extensive studies of hospitals in the United States, to determine whether the differences in surgical death rate among hospitals are as large as the Halothane Study suggested. These same follow-up studies were designed to gain further information about post-surgical complication rates, and to begin exploring the reasons for hospital differences if such differences were confirmed.

In the 1980s, when cost containment caused hospitals to reduce the numbers of patients admitted and the number of days of stay, new concern for quality of care arose. In many publications, new methods of adjustment to equate hospitals for patient mix have been tried. The Health Care Financing

Administration[3] now publishes hospital-by-hospital death rates, with some adjustments for patient mix, but hospitals complain that severity of illness has not been adequately adjusted for.

Contributions of the National Halothane Study

Although the National Halothane Study was published in 1969, it has continued to be referred to in the literature partly because it provided death-rate information for special operations and special groups, data hard to find elsewhere.

What were the main contributions of statistics in the program? First was the basic concept of a death-rate study. This needed to be carried out so that the safety of anesthetics could be seen in light of total surgical experience, not just in deaths from a single rare cause. Second, the study used a special statistical technique of sampling records, designed to save money and to produce a high quality of information. Third, special statistical adjustments had to be created to appraise the results when so many important variables—age, type of operation, sex, patient's physical status, and so on—were uncontrolled. Fourth, as a result, the original premise of the study was not sustained, but a new result emerged: halothane seemed safer than cyclopropane. This finding probably helped move cyclopropane out of the operating room.

Halothane continued to be used for some years after the study was completed, though it is now largely replaced by other anesthetics.

Let us return to the question of liver damage. The total deaths from this source were few, and the lack of autopsies for nearly half of the deaths made firm conclusions impossible.

Are occasional individuals sensitive to other anesthetics? How many people develop such sensitivity? These are hard questions to answer, and they are especially difficult to study because of the rarity of the occurrence.

It may be worth reviewing the various stages, steps, and contributions of the National Halothane Study. The matter started out as a monitoring of occurrences that might become a problem. New data arrived that led to new aims for the study and new efforts. Was halothane a public health problem? One idea was to do a clinical trial that turned out for various reasons to be impossible. One reason is that it would take a long time to gather the data and by then the object of the study might be obsolete. We seemed to need to settle whether halothane was toxic to the liver, but we also needed to know how it affected the operative 30-day death rate. And this latter issue seems more central. To get information on this, we needed to gather extensive data and develop new methods of analysis. Once developed, these showed that halothane was as safe as or safer than other anesthetics. And it also showed that hospital differences would not go away, adjust them as we would. This finding led then to a new study called the Institutional Differences Study, carried out at Stanford. Thus, although we did answer the original statistical question of the public health threat of halothane, we were led to new information and questions not contemplated at the beginning of the study. Such a somewhat wandering course is common in large scientific and statistical studies.

Editors' Postscript

The methodological lessons from the Halothane Study continue, long past the medical ones. At least three issues have persisted over the years.

This study illustrated the power of observational data to address a question of causality: Did halothane cause patients to die at higher rates than other anesthetics when one adjusts for relevant factors such as disease status and demographic characteristics of the patients? As Fred would later argue in other settings, the surest way to answer this question would be to do a randomized controlled experiment. But this was not an option in 1962. The urgent need was to resolve whether halothane was responsible for surgical deaths, and in many situations randomized controlled experiments are still not possible and one must make the best use of available data.

On a more technical level the methods for adjustment that seemed so important and promising in the 1960s for dealing with confounders have largely disappeared from the biostatistical and epidemiological toolkit, replaced by logistic regression and more-elaborate models for assessing causal effects (Greenland and Robins, 1999; Robins, Rotnitzky, and Scharfstein, 1999).

But one of the real problems that the Halothane Study illustrated has continued to vex statisticians to the present day. When we spread even large numbers of observations among many categories of a large number of cross-classified variables, many particular cells still have very few observations and sometimes none at all. For example, the National Halothane Study might have very few patients of a given age, from a given hospital, having a particular kind of operation with a particular physical status, and of these, perhaps none died after anesthesia. The study of this kind of large sparse contingency table requires special techniques (e.g., Haberman, 1977) and is an active area of research (Rinaldo, 2005).

The problem of rare events, especially associated with unanticipated outcomes, arises even in randomized controlled experiments. For example, the Food and Drug Administration (FDA) approves drugs based on extensive clinical trial data, but it can't anticipate all potential side effects or drug interactions. In 2005, the public had to be warned about possible teen suicides as a result of the use of selective serotonin reuptake inhibitors (SSRIs) to treat depression, drugs that the FDA had approved. This was not a primary outcome in the clinical trials, and the follow-up data from all clinical trials contain no suicides (Kaizar, 2006).

Notes

1. The National Halothane Study

   Members of the Subcommittee

   John P. Bunker, M.D., Chairman
   Charles G. Child III, M.D.
   Charles S. Davidson, M.D.
   Edward A. Gall, M.D.
   Gerald Klatskin, M.D.
   Leonard Laster, M.D.
   Lincoln E. Moses, Ph.D.

   Frederick Mosteller, Ph.D.
   Shih-hsun Ngai, M.D.
   Leroy D. Vandam, M.D.
   Staff:
   William H. Forrest, Jr., M.D.
   Sam F. Seeley, M.D.
   John P. Gilbert, Ph.D.

   Panel of Pathologists

   Edward A. Gall, M.D., Chairman
   Archie H. Baggenstoss, M.D.
   I. Nathan Dubin, M.D.

   Paul R. Glunz, M.D.
   Hans Popper, M.D.
   Hans F. Smetana, M.D.

   Panel of Statisticians

   Yvonne M. M. Bishop, Ph.D.
   Byron W. Brown, Ph.D.
   W. Morven Gentleman, Ph.D.
   John P. Gilbert, Ph.D.
   Lincoln E. Moses, Ph.D.

   Frederick Mosteller, Ph.D.
   John W. Tukey, Ph.D.
   Staff:
   Jerry Halpern, M.S.
   Lawrence G. Tesler, A.M.

   Consultants and Associates

   Clinical Pharmacology:
   J. Weldon Bellville, M.D.

   Clinical Analysis:
   Bernard M. Babior, M.D.
   William E. Dozier, M.D.

   Pathology:
   Charles W. Blumenfeld, M.D.
   Beatrice W. Ishak, M.D.
   Kamal K. Ishak, M.D.

   Toxicology:
   Ellis N. Cohen, M.D.

   **Project Officers, Nat. Inst.
   of Gen. Med. Sciences:**
   Ruth K. Beecroft, M.D.
   Carl R. Brewer, Ph.D.
   Louis P. Hellman, M.A.

   **Staff, Div. of Med. Sciences,
   Natl. Academy of Sciences–
   Natl. Research Council:**
   Gilbert W. Beebe, Ph.D.
   R. Keith Cannan, Ph.D.
   Sam F. Seeley, M.D.

2. They have since been joined by C. R. Rao of Pennsylvania State University and by Bradley Efron of Stanford University, who received the National

Medal of Science in 2001 and 2005, respectively. Two probabilists, Joseph L. Doob and Samuel Karlin, have also received this honor.

3. In 2001, the Health Care Financing Administration was renamed the Centers for Medicare and Medicaid Services (CMS).

References

Beecher, H. K. and Todd, D. P. (1954). A study of the deaths associated with anesthesia and surgery. *Annals of Surgery*, 140:2–34.

Bishop, Y. M. M., Fienberg, S. E., Holland, P. W., with the collaboration of R. J. Light and F. Mosteller (1975). *Discrete Multivariate Analysis: Theory and Practice.* Cambridge, MA: MIT Press. (1st paper edition, MIT Press, 1977; Reprinted 2007, New York: Springer-Verlag.)

Bunker, J. P. (1972). *The Anesthesiologist and the Surgeon: Partners in the Operating Room.* Boston: Little, Brown and Company.

Bunker, J. P., Forrest, W. H. Jr., Mosteller, F., and Vandam, L. D., editors (1969). *The National Halothane Study: A Study of the Possible Association Between Halothane Anesthesia and Post-operative Hepatic Necrosis.* Report of the Subcommittee on Anesthesia, Division of Medical Sciences, National Academy of Sciences—National Research Council. National Institutes of Health, National Institute of General Medical Sciences. Washington, D.C.: U. S. Government Printing Office.

Flood, A. B., Scott, W. R., with B. W. Brown, Jr., and others (1987). *Hospital Structure and Performance.* Baltimore, MD: Johns Hopkins University Press.

Gilbert, J. P. and Mosteller, F. (1966). Recognizing the maximum of a sequence. *Journal of American Statistical Association*, 61:35–73.

Greenland, S., Robins, J. M., and Pearl, J. (1999). Confounding and collapsibility in causal inference. *Statistical Science*, 14(1):29–46.

Haberman, S. J. (1977). Log-linear models and frequency tables with small expected cell counts. *Annals of Statistics*, 5:1148–1169.

Kaizar, E. E., Greenhouse, J. B., Seltman, H. and Kelleher, K. (2006). Do antidepressants cause suicidality in children? *Clinical Trials*, 27(3):219–225.

Moses, L. E. and Mosteller, F. (1968). Institutional differences in postoperative death rates. *Journal of the American Medical Association*, 203:492–494.

Rinaldo, A. (2005). *On Maximum Likelihood Estimation for Contingency Tables.* Ph.D. thesis, Carnegie Mellon University.

Robins, J. M., Rotnitzky, A., and Scharfstein, D. O. (1999). Sensitivity analysis for selection bias and unmeasured confounding in missing data and causal inference models. In M. E. Halloran and D. A. Berry, editors, *Statistical Models in Epidemiology: The Environment and Clinical Trials.* New York: Springer-Verlag. 1–92.

Sadove, M. S. and Wallace, V. E. (1962). *Halothane.* Philadelphia: F. A. Davis Company.

6

Equality of Educational Opportunity: The Coleman Report

In the 1950s and 1960s in the United States, social research had made considerable progress in the ability to study questions relevant to policy. Most such work had been done in economics. Advances in computers, research on sample surveys, and experience in studying complex questions provided a base for understanding strong investigations. One such strong investigation was the study made by James Coleman and colleagues, the central theme of this chapter.

Although the foundational court case, *Brown v. Board of Education of Topeka*, decided in 1954 that "separate but equal" school facilities were inherently *unequal* and required the South to desegregate schools "with all deliberate speed," nothing much seemed to have changed by 1964. Congress in the Civil Rights Act of 1964 required that the U.S. Office of Education (the Department of Education was established later) undertake a survey.

> Sec. 402 The Commissioner shall conduct a survey and make a report to the President and the Congress, within two years of the enactment of this title, concerning the lack of availability of equal educational opportunities for individuals by reason of race, color, religion, or national origin in public educational institutions at all levels in the United States, its territories and possessions, and the District of Columbia.

This mandate led to the second largest social-science project up to that time, including information on about 570,000 students, 60,000 teachers, and 4,000 schools. (The largest such study was Project Talent, largely unrelated to the present discussion.) United States Commissioner of Education Francis Keppel (formerly Dean of the Graduate School of Education at Harvard University) put this project into the hands of a team headed by the sociologist James S. Coleman, then of Johns Hopkins University, and Ernest Q. Campbell, of Vanderbilt University, and personnel from the Office of Education including Carol J. Hobson, James McPartland, Alexander M. Mood, Frederic D. Weinfeld, and Robert L. York. At Educational Testing Service, Albert Beaton played a huge role in organizing the computations.

F. Mosteller, *The Pleasures of Statistics: The Autobiography of Frederick Mosteller*,
DOI 10.1007/978-0-387-77956-0_6,
© Springer Science + Business Media, LLC 2010

Alexander Mood, a Texan whom I had known at Princeton (he was a graduate student working with Wilks when I arrived), was working at this time in the Office of Education as Assistant Commissioner of Education, directing the National Center for Education Statistics. Mood had first gone from Princeton to teach statistics at Iowa State College (now University) and while there wrote a very successful textbook on mathematical statistics. After some time at the RAND Corporation, he formed a successful private statistics and computing consulting organization in California, which he sold to a larger organization. His primary tasks as Assistant Commissioner of Education were to consolidate the gathering of statistics and reduce the burden of respondents for the Office of Education and to bring the statistical side of the Office into the computer age. The educational statistics at this period were largely collections of data on numbers of classrooms, teachers, pupils, and expenditures.

In Washington, Mood had a chance to help develop studies and carry out analyses that might help the education community improve their performance, and he had a key role in developing the government side of the study of equality of educational opportunity that Coleman implemented. Seldom does government have the services of someone who is technically trained and has an eye for the big picture, as well as wanting to improve the lot of their fellow man. Both Mood and Coleman had these qualities.

Senator Robert Kennedy was eager to know what the effect of Title I money was on pupil performance, and Mood and Commissioner Keppel saw this as an opportunity to include achievement tests in the survey. Although the schools took a lot of persuading to include these, they did in the end. The sociological questions produced more trouble, and Mood tells me that the schools withdrawing from the survey cited these rather than the achievement tests as their grounds for not participating. Midway through, Harold Howe succeeded Keppel as Commissioner of the Office of Education.

Astonishingly, at least to me, the report was released on time in mid-1966, essentially on the Fourth of July. If one studies how long it takes to carry out research and development, a rough rule of thumb I have worked out (based on Department of Defense data and my own experiences) is that on the average such work takes twice as long or two years longer than planned. Therefore this performance seems to me to be a heroic achievement, because the task was very broadly defined by the team.

Even more impressive is the actual timing of the study, because in the first year after the act was passed only surveys of a legal nature took place. Thus in the end Coleman, Campbell, Mood, and their colleagues had only one year to meet the Congressional charge, and Commissioner Keppel was unwilling to ask for an extension.

Our attention to this survey and its associated report flows, first, from its importance as a social act in itself, with social science being asked to come to the aid of policy, and second, from the seminar at Harvard that it gave rise to. This seminar in turn produced considerable research and suggested a way of working on some kinds of problems that I later found useful. From a statistical point of view, we will have an opportunity to consider what sorts of things can be learned from sample surveys and what cannot.

How can you find out about the equality of educational opportunity? Can you ask people whether they have had equal opportunity? You can, but you won't get much in return. What Coleman and his colleagues did was sample the schools in the United States and assess their quality, state, and performances on a variety of dimensions. For example, they inquired about the numbers of laboratories that were available for science classes. They assessed the amount of education of the teachers in the schools. They inquired about the libraries in each school. They queried the superintendents, looked at the buildings, and then they looked at the children themselves. How did children perform on standard tests?—standard in the sense that the same tests were used for all the children at a given level.

The children came from different home environments, and this might have affected their educational performance. It was generally believed that a home environment where learning was expected and routine would encourage pupils more than an environment that lacked this sort of stimulation. Therefore the home environment was assessed as well. Beyond this the investigators considered the children that the pupil would be educated alongside, because this educational environment in the school itself might make a difference.

The Congressional act did not define equality of educational opportunity, but left it for others to settle. In the end this led to two different ideas of equality, including a major change of mind. These definitions are based respectively on *input* and *output*. Equality of input went well with the older notion of separate but equal educational systems, though it seems from the statement of the act that Congress felt there was a lack of equality. A different definition, not much employed before this time, emerged from the report: equality of output—here academic achievement—rather than equality of input. Acceptance of this second definition, as a result of the report, drastically changed the goals of American education.

Because the ruling in *Brown v. Board of Education of Topeka* had already indicated that separate schooling was unequal, naturally the report, *Equality of Educational Opportunity*, which we call EEOR for short, explored the question of segregation. The finding was emphatic that children in schools were separated by race. From grades 1 through 12, 80 percent of white pupils attended schools that were from 90 to 100 percent white. In parallel, 65 percent of blacks in the first grade attended schools 90 to 100 percent black. At grade 12, 48 percent of blacks attended schools where at least half the students were black. This situation was expected, and its documentation afforded no surprises because "deliberate speed" seemed to mean very slow speed.

Coleman, in an interview with the press before work on the study was far along, echoed the sentiment implied in the legislation that the report would document a difference in quality of the schools. Although he might be accused of trying to use extrasensory perception to get the answers without the field work, he was expressing, if I may use my own knowledge of the views of the time, what all academics "knew"—namely, that the schools for blacks would not turn out to have facilities equal to those for whites. No one I was acquainted with expected the results to be at all close. Perhaps those who were financing educational systems knew more, but the general wisdom was firm and clear. We were not expecting anything like equality of facilities.

The actual report of the survey appeared in two volumes, each the size of a Boston telephone book, the second of which contained nothing but tables of means and standard deviations and correlations. Although the education community was used to exposure to elementary statistics, it was not well prepared for new special statistical analyses of the sort delivered in some parts of the first volume. Furthermore, the general tenor of the EEOR seemed to destroy many of the beliefs in what made for good education in schools, and the education community was somewhat confused. Such a government report may not be allowed to offer recommendations, and this prop was missing for those who sought it. A review of this work was needed, and some scholars were trying to explain to the community what the books said. They were not yet trying to reanalyze the data.

The EEOR did not find exact equality, but it did find astonishing similarity in results for the facilities. A key statement from the EEOR was

> Nationally, Negro pupils have fewer of some of the facilities that seem most related to academic achievement: They have less access to physics, chemistry, and language laboratories; there are fewer books per pupil in their libraries; their textbooks are less often in sufficient supply. To the extent that physical facilities are important to learning, such items appear to be more relevant than some others, such as cafeterias, in which minority groups are at an advantage.

It turned out that nearly all secondary schools had chemistry laboratories; 94 percent of blacks and 98 percent of whites attended such a school. In the Midwest and West both groups attended schools all having chemistry laboratories. Physics labs were not so equally distributed: 80 percent for blacks and 94 percent for whites. Some surprises were that the West had a greater disparity in such labs than the South. Language laboratories offered a reversal; 95 percent of blacks and 80 percent of whites had such facilities.

Without going into more detail, the point is that on many items the groups had nearly equal facilities, and in a few items blacks had more. Let us agree that the balance falls against the blacks, but the surprise was that anything like parity existed. This was hard for people to believe; and, if true, it should have been a cause for celebration that such progress had been achieved. Perhaps it would be fair to say that the first concept (input) of equality of educational opportunity had almost been achieved. I have not read a story putting together an explanation of just how these results came about—that is, what fundings and systematic expenditures brought this move toward equality so quietly. It would be instructive.

I shall not go into related concerns that can readily be raised—perhaps a simple count of labs and facilities is not adequate, and we should assess their newness or adequacy, and perhaps even more important how they are used. As far as I know, these matters were not assessed except in such directions as numbers of books in the library and the availability of textbooks. An additional criticism is that 21 Northern metropolitan school districts did not respond—including the schools of Chicago, for example.

When we turn to *output* of the educational system, we did not find in the EEOR the kind of good news given by the findings for facilities. Instead, it turned out that blacks, Hispanics, Native Americans, and other minority groups, with the exception of Asian pupils, scored well below whites both as a national average and region by region. For example, in the metropolitan Northeast blacks scored about 1.1 standard deviations lower than whites in the same region at grades 6, 9, and 12. But at grade 6 this represents 1.6 years behind; at grade 9, 2.4 years; and at grade 12, 3.3 years. (The standard deviation on tests scored like those used in the survey is the score we need to add to that of the middle student to get to the student at about the 84th percentile. It is a measure of variability. If we have two such populations of students with means one standard deviation apart and draw one pupil randomly from each population, then the one from the population with the higher mean will have the higher score about 3 times out of 4.)

These differences in scores on verbal and mathematics tests were regarded as substantial, and so the education system was not delivering equal output. This result was not a surprise because many small studies had suggested such differences, but now the matter was documented on a regional basis and grade by grade. The findings meant that, by the second but new definition of equality of educational opportunity (equality of output), the nation had failed. The EEOR emphasized the second definition, and it should be regarded as one of its achievements that equality has ever since been defined in terms of output rather than input, as it had previously been. Nearly everyone agreed that such differences were unsatisfactory and that something needed to be done about them.

What had happened was that, although the study had not come up with the finding that everyone expected—namely, that the schools were not equipped equally and that the teachers were not comparably prepared—it had emphasized the existence of a measurable difference in performance between the ethnic groups and, more important than measuring it, had publicized it. Data like these were available earlier from other studies, but none were so extensive or solidly based. In the end, this was the strength and contribution of the Coleman Report. The community abandoned the notion of equality of educational opportunity as providing separate but equal facilities in favor of a definition requiring equal performance, and that was the landmark change in thinking. Even though we have not been able to measure up to this new criterion, we do have the goal in mind. And so whatever else the Coleman Report did or did not do, it changed the minds of many as to the goal of the education system, and about the concept of equality of opportunity. No longer were we going to be satisfied with opportunity, we wanted equality of performance.

Lively discussions of what should be regarded as equality have continued. For example, one suggestion has been that equal proportions of students should achieve some minimum standard.

The authors (Coleman et al.) of the EEOR wanted to go beyond the findings of differences to explain them and possibly to show directions where policy might profitably move. Their approach was through a statistical method called regression analysis. Let me interrupt the narrative to explain the idea.

When an outcome like academic performance depends upon several variables, we often believe that, if we could assemble measures of these variables in a manner that would predict the performance for individuals, then we might also find out how to change the input so as to improve performance. An oversimplified example from assessment of houses may help us understand the thinking. Suppose that the value of a house in a neighborhood depends upon two features—the number of rooms and the number of thousands of square feet of land. The predictive formula might be (in thousands of dollars) ten times the number of rooms plus four times the number of thousands of square feet. Thus five rooms and 11,000 square feet would give a value of $10 \times 5 + 4 \times 11 = 94$ thousand dollars. Using this rule, a builder could figure out roughly the price of homes of different sizes on lots of different areas in the particular neighborhood during a specific period of time. If this *kind* of formula were correct, even if we did not know the multipliers 10 and 4, and if we did know the prices of houses of different sizes on different-sized lots in the neighborhood, then we might be able to derive the multipliers 10 for rooms and 4 for a thousand square feet by fitting the data through regression methods. Thus if the method works, we can sometimes find appropriate multipliers empirically. Once we know the formula including the value of the multipliers, then we know how to adjust the size of the house and the size of the lot to produce different prices. In particular we see that adding a room increases the price more than would adding a thousand square feet to the lot.

In real life we would not have these exact outcomes, though we might find that we could *approximately* predict the amount that the assessor would assign as a value for the house. Now our estimates deviate from those of the assessor, and so we are making errors in the predictions, and we would like a way to appraise how well the formula predicts. One way to do this looks at the variability of the assessor's values of the houses, measuring this in terms of the square of the standard deviation, which is called the variance. Then to see how well the prediction works, we look at the variance of the difference between the predicted value and the true value. If that is small, we are doing a good job of predicting, but if it is large, we are not. If we always predict exactly correctly, we say we are "explaining" 100 percent of the variance by means of our formula. If we have not reduced the variance at all, but left the variance of the differences the same size as the original variance, we say we are explaining none of the variance, or zero percent of the variance. If the differences have a variance half as big as the assessor's variance, we say we have explained 50 percent of the variance. The use of the word "explain" usually seems strange ("What was the explanation?" the student asks), and it just happens to be a technical word that statistics has unfortunately adopted. All it means is that when we make these forecasts, the variance of the difference has a proportional value to the original variance.

This description gives us an idea of what the total formula does when it is used to predict the value. In this uncertain world, the house builder might want to know whether rooms or whether area, when used alone, was better at predicting value, and, as before, how price would change with each. His general thought is that this information puts him in a position to make better economic decisions. This is a very simplified example. There could be more variables, and perhaps they would not be put together in just the simple way advanced here. What is believable about the example is that within limits larger houses are worth more than smaller ones and that larger lots raise prices of houses also.

The corresponding idea in the EEOR is to see what amounts of variance in school performance were explained by the several variables, and perhaps even by single variables. The EEOR did not present any information on pupil-teacher ratio because such data showed a consistent lack of relation to achievement. Earlier research had often found this lack of effect, and so it was confirmed again. (This surprising result may be the most thoroughly researched issue in all education. I used to think it surprising, but I softened when I recalled that my most successful and most unsuccessful teaching experiences have occurred in very small classes. Some of these experiences occur because the students are eager to study the material, and then they are remarkable in their accomplishments. I remember one student who managed to engage his whole extended family—those not fully employed—in supplementing his research work by being research assistants. Sometimes the course is a remedial one for a reluctant student who has no real interest in the material.)

The EEOR adjusted for six student-background variables and found that the variance in educational achievement accounted for (explained) by instructional expenditures per pupil in grades 6, 9, and 12 was a small fraction *of one percent* of the variance—nine one-hundredths for blacks and twenty-nine one-hundredths for whites. Most people would have expected the variation in expenditure on instruction to lead to a substantial difference in school performance, but these numbers make us feel that we are browsing in the round-off error.

In the example of the cost of houses, we had a fairly solid belief in the causal nature of the two variables, number of rooms and size of lot, admitting of course that they are an oversimplification. In the educational field we did not have this solid basis for the causality of the variables entering into prediction equations. It is a long chain of events from spending a dollar on education to producing improved spelling and arithmetic.

EEOR had slight findings favorable to racial integration as a way of improving academic performance when the minority-group students were not a majority in the classroom, and this integration did not seem to lower the performance of the majority. It also seemed as if a student's feeling of control of his or her own destiny was of considerable importance in explaining achievement. Many students also had high aspirations, with (unrealistically) large proportions of both blacks and whites planning to have professional careers.

The interpretation made by many readers of EEOR was that schools had little or no effect on academic performance. Naturally this is a mistaken interpretation. What seemed to be true was that, given a full-fledged school system, minor variations in the facilities and expenditures and education of teachers made relatively little difference in average performance. A better interpretation, therefore, would have been that minor variations in schools make relatively little difference. On the other hand, we know that, if we compare school with no school, we find differences. For example, a two-month teachers' strike produced a loss of two months in reading level in the city of New York in 1968–69. And we know that children do not invent algebra by themselves.

Further Analysis

After publication of the EEOR, the Office of Education continued to analyze the data in-house, and in an innovative move that deserves much praise, the Office encouraged scholars to further analyze the data. At that time it was difficult to move data from one computer to another (at what time isn't it?), and the Office went to great pains to aid scholars to get the data, whether the scholars were favorable or unfavorable to the Report and its findings. The sharing of data has been a much vexed problem in science, partly because it costs a great deal to put the data into order with good documentation even when everyone wants to make the exchange.

Encouraged by the Office of Education's helpful attitude, Harvard professors Daniel P. Moynihan and Thomas F. Pettigrew thought that an independent study of the data ought to be made, both to further the analysis and to make the findings available to educators and others. The Carnegie Corporation generously funded a faculty seminar to be held at Harvard University during the academic year 1966–67, and later extended funding for the seminar's further work. Originally it was planned as a rather small and specialized group, but the Cambridge community took a strong interest (we all think we know about elementary and secondary education and how to fix it) that led to 50 to 60 faculty members and other interested persons joining panels and committees.[1] Gordon Ambach and Robert Schwartz acted successively as executive director to the group. Marshall Smith was the research director, and Betsy Harshbarger provided clerical and management support. Because questions raised in the panel were answered within one or two weeks, the seminar always seemed to be moving briskly.

Moynihan, then a professor at Harvard, later was ambassador to India and still later was elected to the United States Senate from the State of New York. His writings on the family were widely read and controversial. He had had much practical political experience. Pettigrew, a professor in the Department of Social Relations, was a former student of Gordon Allport, who, like Pettigrew, had strong interests in problems faced by minorities. Although at Harvard the idea of a university-wide seminar to study a specific topic was not unusual, the size and extent of this seminar were. It attracted people from all over the University—the Graduate School of Business Administration, Medical School, Law School, Arts and Sciences, Divinity School—and the Graduate School of Education, where part of Moynihan's appointment lay, played a key role. The seminar met regularly, about once every two weeks, and people often came from Washington to attend. Many researchers who were looking into educational questions participated. Coleman and some of his colleagues came and lectured and debated on the methods used and the meaning of the findings. Alexander Mood and others from the staff of the Office of Education sometimes attended, including Commissioner Howe.

The meetings were usually held at the Harvard Faculty Club on Quincy Street in Cambridge. Ordinarily the evening began with visiting speakers followed by a question period, then a light supper, which led into meetings by the many little groups that were specializing in particular problems. After the group meetings some people stayed late to hold discussions with members of other groups, encouraged by Amstel and Tuborg beer and soft drinks.

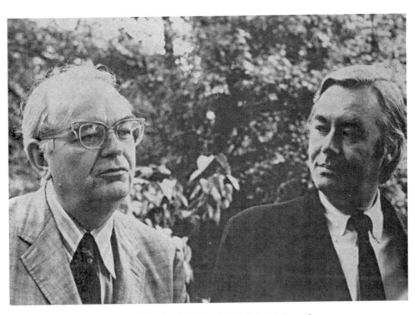

Fig. 6.1. Fred with Daniel Patrick Moynihan.

Engaged with such a mixed body of outstanding people, one begins to appreciate the great gaps of understanding between professionals. One realizes that adult education is both necessary and extremely difficult when groups of brilliant people can continue to misunderstand one another week after week. None of this is helped by the confusion created by such statistical expressions as "explained variance." Most groups had as members both graduate students and faculty members, and usually one of the students acted as staff for the group, writing minutes and sometimes providing new materials. Some faculty members who were currently working on research in education found this a good milieu for discussing other work and its relevance to educational progress. Others were hoping to use the data from the Coleman survey for new analyses as soon as the data became available. These analyses took some time and did not begin until the seminar was about half over.

Several professional groups, including lawyers, asked for and received special classes in interpretation of statistics to help them with the readings in the seminar.

Some members of the seminar wrote and published papers while the seminar proceeded. Members continued to rework the analyses, and gradually a book began to take shape, but the manuscript was not completed until the close of 1970. Pettigrew had some large projects taking up his time, Moynihan was commuting to Washington, D.C., and I was asked to help put the manuscript together and write with Moynihan the opening paper for the book entitled *On Equality of Educational Opportunity*. It consisted of papers deriving from the seminar and largely from the reanalyses of the survey data, though some material came from outside.

The book contained 14 papers in all, four of which are labeled appendices. The analysts did not like the EEOR method used to attribute school-to-school variation in achievement to the various variables such as teacher's education, facilities, and community, and therefore they used other techniques, though usually regression methods. The original method of analysis had the drawback that its answers depend upon the ordering used to ask about the effects of the variables.

To return to our house valuation example for illustration, the value per 1000 square feet of lot would differ depending on whether you appraised it first by itself alone as the only predictor of housing value or asked what it was additionally worth as a predictor after having first used the number of rooms in the house for the estimate. Part of the problem is that the sizes of the houses are correlated with the sizes of the lots, and so when you use the number of rooms alone, you have stolen some of the predictive power of the lot size, and vice versa.

What did the reanalysis of the data find, and how did it differ from the original? Let me give some highlights from the book. Part of the difference had to do with the firmness of the findings. There was considerable nonresponse to the questionnaires—not only from whole school districts, but also from individual pupils, teachers, principals, and superintendents. The nonresponse left more room for variation. Some kinds of questions, such as father's occupation and education, are often omitted, and young children may not be reliable in answering them. Because of the timing of the survey, the teachers could not be related directly to the pupils they taught except through the schools they were in. Thus our ability to relate teacher effectiveness to pupils actually taught was totally frustrated. David K. Cohen, Thomas F. Pettigrew, and Robert T. Riley, who believed that integration of schools would benefit the academic achievement of blacks, were unable to untangle the effects of social class (socioeconomic status) from that of race. Although they probably still believed in integration, they found that their analysis did little to support its educational value.

Christopher Jencks concentrated on northern urban elementary schools. He thought that many people distrusted the findings of the EEOR: (1) that blacks and whites had nearly comparable school resources within regions, and (2) that once one takes account of race and family background, academic achievement is weakly related to school policies and resources. His reanalysis found little racial bias in allocation of resources among schools he studied, and in addition found little social class (socioeconomic status) bias in allocation of resources. And he reported that, after taking student background into account, the relation of school facilities and programs and even of teacher characteristics to academic achievement was slight, just as EEOR had said. (Recall that characteristics of the individual teacher did not have much chance to show their value because they were averaged over all pupils in a school.) Moreover, he disagreed with EEOR on the issue of whether blacks or whites were more influenced by school policies and resources; he found blacks less influenced where EEOR found whites less influenced.

Jencks found a strong relation to social composition of classmates even after taking account of a pupil's own race and family background. But he did not know what to conclude from this finding. Was it the schoolmates of the lower-class pupils who also attend the middle-class school who help them, or the family that sent them there? We see here the error in the common saying "You can prove anything with statistics." Instead, it is very difficult to prove anything by any means, and proving something with statistics requires much preparation and analysis. I will return to this issue later.

Eric A. Hanushek and John F. Kain attacked the EEOR for trying to do more than it could possibly achieve. Instead of emphasizing only inputs or inputs and outputs, by trying to find what elements would improve education if changed, the EEOR overreached itself and so failed of its purpose, they said. But Coleman argued back that, if one does not know what inputs are important to performance, one cannot know what opportunities are equal. We see again that equality is being defined in part on the basis of the data rather than from some overarching principle.

David J. Armor analyzed the data by school rather than by individual pupils. As did the EEOR, he found on many input measures that schools with almost all black students seemed no worse off than schools with almost all white students, though there were important regional variations. Southern schools were more disadvantaged than schools elsewhere; and Armor pointed out that, because blacks were so numerous in the South, they as a group were therefore more disadvantaged than whites. During the period studied, many blacks migrated north, where they had to compete with the products of the better northern schools, better in the sense of facilities and the strength of their teaching personnel.

Black schools sometimes had teachers who were far ahead of teachers in white schools on the basis of their years of educational training but were behind them on the basis of teachers' verbal achievement. This finding argues for integration: if blacks are trained by teachers with low verbal skills, they will be handicapped. Armor also attended more to the initial disparity between black and white children in first grade. He found that in some samples the initial difference was 1.5 standard deviations and that this gap widened to 2 standard deviations by the sixth grade. Thus the schooling did not narrow the gap, as some people believed the public schools were designed to accomplish. (One argument for public schools has been their equalizing effect. Whether that idea works is really an empirical question. Most of us would not approve of a training system that worked by holding some people back and pressing others forward. Although it could be that groups starting with a disadvantage would reduce the gap through training, that was not what Armor and others found.) He found that family inputs were more powerful predictors of achievement than school inputs for both blacks and whites.

Marshall Smith reappraised several of the more controversial findings of the EEOR. He found one of those computer errors that I am always fearful about. By some chance, the EEOR had made a mistake in entering some variables in some of the calculations, with the result that family factors had their importance underestimated. When Smith corrected this, the effects of home background turned out to be 3 or 4 times as large as had been reported in EEOR. Many had feared that home background was given too much credit compared to schools or teachers. Instead, it was grabbing even more with the corrected data. Smith, like Cohen, Pettigrew, and Riley, could not find support for the position that characteristics of other members of the student body influenced verbal achievement. None of these authors denied the possibility, but they felt the data were not behind it in EEOR.

Smith also raised an important point that related to the high-school years especially. He noted that self-selection practices and school placement practices might have effects on the inferences about the relations between school resources and achievement. The EEOR did not distinguish among trade, academic, and comprehensive high schools in the analyses (nor alternatively the programs students were in). This made certain types of analysis impossible. Also EEOR did not distinguish between junior and senior high schools. As a result the question of the relation between resources and achievement at the secondary level was left very open.

The struggle to analyze the survey for hints about policy was a struggle to do more with the data than a single survey was likely to be able to do. One-shot surveys are at their best telling us what the state of a system is. For example, EEOR did a reasonable job of telling what the ethnic composition of classrooms was and how various grades and ethnic groups performed comparatively on verbal and arithmetic tests. On the policy side, if lots of schools needed textbooks, that information could have told what to do—get more texts.

To find out what would happen if specific changes were made requires something like an experiment—that is, an investigation where the investigator has control over the treatments being studied. Although regression situations may give one the illusion of finding out what would happen if we changed something, in the absence of an experiment they merely offer guesses.

Let me illustrate. We are all familiar with the idea that we can estimate height in male adults from their weight. We can explain a substantial percentage of the variance in height in this manner. The implication too is clear: the greater the weight, on average the greater the height. But not one of us believes that adding 20 pounds by eating and by minimizing exercise will add an inch to our height. This relation between height and weight is a descriptive idea, an association, and it does not imply that increasing one's weight will do a thing for height. Ideas of what happens when we change things may be different from those that show how things stand.

To be effective with regression, we have to know that changing the value of one variable does influence the value of another. Experimentation gives the primary evidence for such relations. George Box, a statistician from the University of Wisconsin writing about the design of investigations, said, "To find out what happens to a system when you interfere with it, you have to interfere with it (not just passively observe it)."

In later years, assessments were made of such important educational programs as Head Start, Planned Variation, and Follow Through. These attempts were weakly evaluated because the investigators did not, possibly could not, use experiments. The Headstart evaluations tried to match up control groups with those in the program, but they were not very successful. Part of the problem was that many children in the control groups would not have been eligible for the program itself. The various studies in the Planned Variation program were more like demonstration projects, and from them Marshall Smith found that one got little information about their contributions to achievement.

Nevertheless, major difficulties face the experimenter who is trying for information that will be helpful to policy. In brief, one wishes to institute a treatment in one school and not in another, and the schools should initially be comparable. Trying to arrange this in the same school system may create grave problems for the school superintendent. He or she will be perceived as favoring one school over another. The likely outcome is that the superintendent will find funds (other than from the experiment) to institute some program into the control school and thus upset the experiment. As this example shows, the path of the experimenter may be very rocky.

While the members of the seminar were putting finishing touches on their papers, and Cleo Youtz and I were completing the editing of the manuscript with the help of the authors, the school system of the South underwent massive change. In the spring of 1970 the dual school system was largely in place; in the fall of 1970 it was almost all gone. In October the Secretary of Health, Education, and Welfare reported that 97 percent of the 2700 school districts in the 11 Southern states had desegregated. Expressed in percentages of 3.1 million children rather than districts, 27 percent had desegregated before 1970, 63 percent desegregated in the fall of 1970, and 10 percent were not desegregated but living in the 76 districts not in compliance. A new era was beginning.

Although the completed scholarship from the seminar was slow in coming, I was impressed that, when masses of scholars focused on a common question of considerable social concern, the process was educational to the participants, and much work was completed. It seemed to me to offer a way of working that was pleasant and productive and brought together people who might not otherwise join forces. The experience encouraged me to try to develop similar efforts in later years.

The EEOR group was not the only one to use wrong variables. When the time came to print the results of the seminar, the publisher picked up the copy of the manuscript that Moynihan had sent him from the White House rather than the carefully edited one Cleo Youtz and I sent from Harvard. The typesetters were halfway through the book before we discovered the error. They started over.

Further Concerns about Education

As a consequence, probably, of this seminar experience I was asked to serve on the National Advisory Council on Equality of Educational Opportunity and learned a great deal about the further activities of the government in educational affairs. Through this Council, I learned more about American Indian affairs and about the Hispanic groups.

In order to preserve their cultural heritage, and to give children speaking only Spanish a good start in schools, and not leave them behind in all subjects, the Hispanic groups wanted to maintain bilingual programs. In theory, the bilingual program was to continue for a while and then move the pupil into English as the primary language, but many schools maintained the bilingual, usually Spanish, program for a long time. Both in the Council and among outside black groups, the attitude toward the bilingual program seemed to be that it prevented the pupil from focusing on the primary language, English, and therefore made it difficult for the pupil as he or she became older to enter the economic mainstream. It is easy to see merits in both positions. Even without trying to maintain a cultural heritage, many immigrant groups need to begin schooling in a language they can understand, and so bilingual programs have had to be offered in many languages for beginning school children.

Although the EEOR dealt with colleges and junior colleges as well as with elementary and secondary schools, our Harvard group had not looked at the results of that work. During the work with the Council, I did have an opportunity to observe a college science program for minority youth. These students were taking a regular science program, mainly in biology, but with a solid set of mathematics and other science courses. To help them financially, they also had paid jobs in the laboratory, but not just washing test tubes and beakers. Instead, part of the program required the faculty to organize sequences of experiments these students could carry out and write up individually under faculty supervision. I heard several of them give rehearsal speeches for a scientific conference where they were going to present original papers. I had also the opportunity to interview several of them individually. A common notion many of them expressed in different ways was the surprise and tremendous gratification they felt that they were able to master this scientific material and keep up with the mathematics and other courses. "I had no idea I could do things like this" was almost a common quotation. I was moved and excited by this program, and I hope it worked out as well as it appeared to be doing.

Heartwarming though these experiences are, society may still ask how to assess the success or contribution of the program. When some groups are contributing no new members to an occupational area and then a new program produces a substantial number from those groups who enter and continue in that field, that is one form of success. It is not so easy, though, to respond to a skeptic who says, "these people you chose for your program would have done well without the program's intervention." To investigate that would require something close to a randomized experiment.

In the years since desegregation, the nation has continued to worry about the state of the school system. Many reports have shown us that the general level of education is low and that our pupils' performances compare poorly with those of pupils from other developed countries. Because our concern is partly related to the economic state of the country in an international situation where many countries are performing better than we are, and where the competition is expected to become more severe as the European Economic Community accomplishes its goals, we have every reason to be troubled.

We put very little into research and development in the area of education, especially considering its importance to the whole national future. Some estimate that one-tenth of one percent of the budget for education from kindergarten through 12th grade goes into research, an amount that any industry would find minuscule. And this goes on in a dynamic environment where the knowledge base affecting us all changes at an enormous rate.

We have not paid attention to the life cycle of the student. One part of the cycle, early adolescence (10–14), seems to have a gap in academic psychology, jumping from little children directly to teen-agers. In elementary and secondary schools, students go through a 12-year cycle, and so that has to be considered when we are trying to improve a system. It takes a generation to make a complete change.

I do not observe, though, any attack that seriously deals with all of the interrelated components of the schools, including curriculum, teacher competence, learning materials, working conditions (of teachers and pupils), standards of achievement, location of authority, organization of space and time, behavioral problems, updating of and maintenance of buildings, curriculum materials, libraries, computers, and continuing education and recruitment of teachers. Because of interrelationships, attempted solutions to one problem may thwart those of another. For example, if we raise standards for children in science education, we will need more and better trained science teachers. If we simultaneously raise the standards of competence required of science teachers, we reduce their pool, so that attempts to raise standards of teacher preparation and pupil performance simultaneously will need at least some third input to offer success.

Returning to the general point, we have general attacks on the problems of space technology, on warfare, on poliomyelitis, on cancer, and now, after some stumbling, on AIDS. May it not be time for us to put a major effort into education?

Part of our problem with improving education can be traced to the level of responsibility for education. Up to now, education of children has been a state or local responsibility rather than a federal one, and this task seems likely to remain so placed. Not only do people feel that education of their children is a local matter, but also, converting elementary education to a federal responsibility would make a very large change in funding; and, as far as one can see, no part of the U.S. government wants to take on such a financial burden. Some congressional representatives might be willing to increase substantially the federal share of the costs of some programs, but which ones is an open question. The federal funding for schools has generally declined because of changing tax structures, and the state contribution has increased.

When William Bennett was Secretary of Education, he emphasized the need to evaluate and improve the performance of college and university education. This is a reasonable activity, and something useful may be coming of it, at least at a few institutions, but it does not much address elementary and secondary education. Hand-wringing, such as we have steadily been doing, after the first few years, does not accomplish much. We know, apparently, that when we decide on a big and concrete goal like putting a man on the moon, we need to have a major long-run program, one that may take much longer than the persons in governmental offices will all see during their tenure or even their lifetimes. When this is so obvious for a technological program like space exploration, why can we not see it for education? Some reasons are obvious. The payoff may be very slow. We hope some miracle like computer education will solve the problem, just as in medicine antibiotics came along and cured many ills. Instead, we have had computers now for a long time, and though we are using them, they are not solving the problem of pupil education. Perhaps part of the reason lies in the contrast between space exploration and education. Our knowledge of physics and technology was sufficiently great that we could be pretty sure that, given time and resources, a man would get to the moon. We do not know enough about the educational process to make the comparable claim, and so many things are wrong that we scarcely know where to start. The decentralization puts a great many individuals and institutions in the path from the president to the child in the classroom, and many of these have a very effective veto on school initiatives. Authority and resources are widely dispersed, and therefore the processes of decision making and follow-up of implementations and their consequences leave much to be desired. Vetoes are easy, launchings are painful.

The nation has to face up to the idea that it does not understand with its present social, economic, and family structure how to improve education. It does not have a solid list of what it wants to accomplish, even to meet economic goals. I do not mean that some groups do not have ideas, but I do mean that we are not tackling our whole problem. We know several symptoms of our problem. We know that some classrooms are total chaos. We know that many people cannot read. We know that test scores in standard subjects are low. We know that fewer mathematically trained people have recently been available for teaching in the schools. We know many things about the system that seem unsatisfactory. But we do not have a list of things we are trying to accomplish, with a notion that they will contribute to the goals the society wants to set in the light of its coming difficulties in international competition.

Even if this list were available, we do not know what steps we should take—what changes to make—in order to bring about and maintain a better product. It is possible that the whole society must change and that this will happen, if at all, only after crippling economic consequences. At any rate, we should recognize that we do not have an overall organization, and that we do not know what works on a national scale. This is not to ignore places where good education is being delivered, but these systems appear to be somewhat special and isolated. So many things are the trouble with our system that nothing short of a broad, long-range system of investigations and implementations has a chance to solve our problem. Educators, parents, and industrialists all have ideas for programs that might be valuable in improving education. Taking a small set of these and implementing them in a variety of places, so that their performance can be compared and so that the possible special effects of place and pupil can also be assessed, could in a few years give us evidence of the comparative effectiveness of various programs. Where research must be done to find out what variables are important, there are not promises of success. We have had some success in the past, however, with trying to do better by examining whole systems. We could begin with that optimism.

Inevitably the reader's response to such complaints will be to ask for the writer's program. When I served on the board of directors and later as president of the American Association for the Advancement of Science (AAAS),

I pressed for additional efforts to engage elementary and secondary school pupils in mathematics and science. AAAS already had a substantial program related to museums and special lectures as well as informative guides to literature useful for teachers and students. After several years AAAS launched its Project 2061 (date of next return of Halley's comet). Naturally I have no program to sell, but I do care about the problem, and so I have discussed it with James Rutherford, who directs Project 2061, a project intended to improve mathematics and science education from kindergarten through secondary school. My comments on national education both above and below have been improved by Jim's criticisms and suggestions.

It would be unfortunate if I gave the impression that nothing is being tried or investigated in the educational area. Many ideas are being tried, and some will work. For example, I have heard of a program in university mathematics for students who came poorly prepared. The idea is, instead of asking for remedial mathematics, to call for high achievement by these students because their standard test scores are high. The students see this as a matter of practical importance because continuing in mathematics maintains their career options. Let us suppose for a moment that this program has been a success as has been reported. The difficulty is that without funding other institutions are not going to pick it up and use it. And even in the institution where it currently flourishes, we can expect it to be abandoned after a modest period. The nation does not have a method of maintaining strength when it gets it.

If a good program is developed under sponsorship of the government or of a private foundation, after a few years the funding source will either move the funds to another institution so as not to favor one over another, or it will go out of the particular business and move to another. This mobility arises from an announced goal of supporting innovations and from limited funds. Thus again we have no good way to maintain strength when we find it. The popular expression in both government and foundation language is "institutionalization." The idea is that the new program will ultimately be absorbed and paid for by the local institution. Unless the program actually replaces at the same or lower cost activities already being carried out by the institution, it is most unlikely that the program can be maintained.

Businesses set aside funds for capital development, but schools do not. Such organizations as the World Bank, the Fund for Small Businesses, the Trust Funds, or funds for a savings and loan bailout have no parallel in education.

Although many good ideas and programs are being tried out in the nation, we do not have a system in place for taking some advantage of the total effort. Even if most of the programs were successes, we have not a method or a system or an organization that has responsibility for moving these good ideas into the educational system. We do not have a way to develop national reform in education. With all the methods of communication and publication we have available, we have no way to make new ideas available to schools or to encourage them to update and improve their curricula on a regular basis.

In the field of teacher education and recruitment we have no action to produce minority role models for students who are behind in their educational attainments. My understanding is that the school teacher population is becoming if anything more white, just when the population is becoming more mixed.

Among the possible resources in the nation for improving schooling is the large collection of agencies in the federal government whose work depends heavily on the products of the school systems. Just to mention a few, the National Institutes of Health, the Department of Energy, the Department of Labor, the National Aeronautics and Space Administration, to say nothing of the Department of Agriculture and the Department of Defense. Although these organizations need the product of a good educational system, at the moment they are taking very little part in the formulation of the product or in aiding its improvement. The Department of Defense does a great deal of training by itself after it enlists its forces. The Department of Defense uses a considerable amount of technology in its training. As far as I know, the school systems do not have access to such equipment and materials. No organization has responsibility for helping to bring the national system into the twenty-first century.

Throughout the nation or its regions we do not have a system of schools organized to try out cooperatively new materials and technologies and to train teachers in their use, with the further responsibility to make available to the rest of the nation the fruits of their work. Although our medical system is decentralized, hospitals do pull together for multi-institutional trials of important medical technologies where gains may be small in size and therefore hard to detect, but very valuable when well documented, disseminated, and widely implemented.

The changing social structure, smaller families, less supervision, and more television are all part of the collection of issues needing to be faced. Probably we need many changes that are compatible with one another. The system we have now does not take advantage of the technologies that are available for direct teaching of the students nor for recruitment and preparation of teachers. Teachers themselves have suffered as part of the social structure. Half a century ago the teacher was a respected member of the community; today the teacher is rarely recognized in our highly urban environment.

The American Association for the Advancement of Science has a long-run program of curriculum development that involves many helpers from many strata of education—schools, colleges, universities, businesses, and government. Their program is developing slowly. Its first phase has taken several years, and now it moves into a second phase to see whether the science, mathematics, and technology in the proposed program is teachable and whether some methods are preferable. Although this work will be informative, the nation has no way to pick up this program if it should be successful and help implement it. The point, though, is not that the AAAS program would not be picked up and promoted, it is that we are not set nationally to take advantage of any organization's good ideas, and we need to be.

Editors' Postscript

The faculty seminar model that emerged from this project underwent repeated refinement as Fred carried it forward to the School of Public Heath in the 1970s and 1980s, and it led to many other edited volumes (e.g., Bunker, Barnes, and Mosteller, 1977).

During the 1990s, despite his putative emeritus status, Fred continued his work on research synthesis and remained an advocate for evidence-based decision making for policy making. He remained an advocate of randomized experiments in various settings (e.g., Moses and Mosteller, 1997, and Mosteller and Boruch, 2002), following the prescription in his chapter with Gilbert in the Mosteller-Moynihan volume. He was particularly enthusiastic about the Tennessee class size experiment, which actually randomized children into small vs. larger classes in the early grades and traced the effects of that differential treatment through their years in public school, finding that the beneficial effects of being in a small class persisted for many years, even after students were integrated into normal-sized classes (Mosteller 1995, 1999). "His imprimatur reportedly helped spur President Bill Clinton's request for 100,000 new teachers to reduce classroom sizes" (Bernstein, 2006).

After 2000, the controversy over the need for experimentation to support changes in educational practice became part of a political debate that reverberated in the social science and education communities. Both sides of the debate cited Fred's work.

Note

1. Partial List of Attendees at the Harvard University Seminar on Equality of Educational Opportunity

Gordon M. Ambach	John D. Herzog	Howard Raiffa
David J. Armor	Eugene Hixson	Robert T. Riley
Albert Beaton	Harold Howe	Kristine M. Rosenthal
James M. Beshers	Herold C. Hunt	Robert A. Rosenthal
William G. Buss	Christopher S. Jencks	Paul F. Ross
Clark Byse	John F. Kain	Richard Rowe
Robert Campbell	Sydney J. Key	Albert M. Sacks
Jeanne Chall	Frederick R. Kling	Nancy H. St. John
Abram J. Chayes	Richard Leone	Robert B. Schwartz
Antonia Chayes	J. Leeson	David S. Seeley
William G. Cochran	Gerald S. Lesser	Florence Shelton
James S. Coleman	Seymour M. Lipset	Charles E. Silberman
Vincent F. Conroy	Gordon MacInness	Nancy Sizer
Andre Daniere	Roland McKean	Theodore R. Sizer
Henry S. Dyer	James McPartland	Gene M. Smith
Jason Epstein	Frank I. Michelman	Marshall S. Smith
Mario Fantini	John U. Monro	Robert J. Solomon
Judith Fellows	Alexander M. Mood	Frank Stefanich
John P. Gilbert	Donald R. Moore	Susan S. Stodolsky
Fred L. Glimp	Anton S. Morton	Nathan B. Talbot
Cliff Goldman	Frederic A. Mosher	Marc S. Tucker
Edmund W. Gordon	Frederick Mosteller	John W. Tukey
Neal Gross	Daniel P. Moynihan	Ralph W. Tyler
Charles C. Halbower	Charles R. Nesson	Frederic D. Weinfeld
Eric A. Hanushek	Thomas F. Pettigrew	Sheldon H. White
Elizabeth Harshbarger	H. Douglas Price	Dean K. Whitla

References

Bernstein, A. (2006). Mathematical theorist: Frederick Mosteller. *Washington Post*. July 25, 2006, B06.

Box, G. E. P. (1966). Use and abuse of regression. *Technometrics*, 8(4):625–629.

Bunker, J. P., Barnes, B. A., and Mosteller, F., editors (1977). *Costs, Risks, and Benefits of Surgery*. New York: Oxford University Press.

Civil Rights Act of 1964, P.L. No. 88-352. 78 Stat. 241 (July 2, 1964).

Coleman, J. S., Campbell, E. Q., Hobson, C. J., McPartland, J., Mood, A. M., Weinfeld, F. D., and York, R. L. (1966). *Equality of Educational Opportunity*. 2 volumes. Washington, D.C.: Office of Education, U. S. Department of Health, Education, and Welfare, U. S. Government Printing Office. OE-38001; Superintendant of Documents Catalog No. FS 5.238:-38001.

Moses, L. E. and Mosteller, F. (1997). Experimentation: Just do it! Chap. 12 in B. D. Spencer, editor, *Statistics and Public Policy* (Festschrift in Honor of I. Richard Savage). New York: Oxford University Press. 212–232.

Mosteller, F. (1995). The Tennessee study of class size in the early school grades. *The Future of Children*, 5:113–127.

Mosteller, F. (1999). How does class size relate to achievement in schools? Chap. 6 in S. E. Mayer and P. E. Peterson, editors, *Earning and Learning*. Washington, D.C.: Brookings Institute Press and Russell Sage Foundation. 117–129.

Mosteller, F. and Boruch, R. F., editors (2002). *Evidence Matters: Randomized Trials in Education Research*. Washington, D.C.: Brookings Institute Press.

Mosteller, F. and Moynihan, D. P., editors (1972). *On Equality of Educational Opportunity: Papers Deriving from the Harvard University Faculty Seminar on the Coleman Report*. New York: Random House.

Part II

Early Life and Education

7

Childhood

Although I was born in Clarksburg, West Virginia, my family did not stay there long. We lived briefly in Parkersburg, West Virginia, and then in the general area of Pittsburgh, Pennsylvania, primarily Wilkinsburg, until I was 12.

My father, William Roy Mosteller, became a master glass blower at age 17. He traveled all over the country, making fine wages for the early 1900s. His family came from Williamsport, Pennsylvania, where Mostellers are more numerous than Smiths. He had less than a high school education in formal school—it was vague whether he finished fourth or eighth grade. Later he took correspondence courses. During World War I, he left the glass trade and made artillery shells. After the war he went into the trucking business and later branched out into road building, mainly in western Pennsylvania, but later he built in the eastern part of the state as well. My mother, Helen Kelley Mosteller, was born in Ladoga, Indiana, and raised in Indianapolis. She was the oldest of three children, and she may have had a part in raising the two younger children. Her father died early, and her mother remarried. My given names, Charles Frederick, are in honor of my step-grandfather, whose last name was Hartung.

My mother admired education and learning and cared a great deal about pronunciation, grammar, and spelling. She was proud that she had had some German language courses in high school even though the language became unpopular with World War I. I do not think she finished high school—perhaps the 11th grade. She was a loving, strict, protective mother. She did not allow me to go out and play in the streets with the other children, partly because she did not think they were well behaved, and partly because she did not like me to get dirty.

My father was rarely home during the day except on Sunday, when he always slept until noon. My father read a good deal. He read the *Saturday Evening Post* stories, and he liked to read cowboy stories in pulp magazines. He and my mother read newspapers religiously. Radios were just coming into

F. Mosteller, *The Pleasures of Statistics: The Autobiography of Frederick Mosteller*,
DOI 10.1007/978-0-387-77956-0_7,
© Springer Science + Business Media, LLC 2010

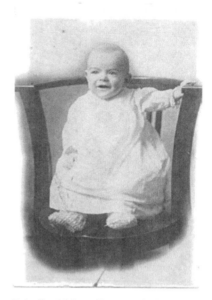

Fig. 7.1. Fred Mosteller as a baby, circa 1917.

fashion. Early on, we had a crystal set with earphones and listened to station KDKA in Pittsburgh.

My mother had worked for various businesses in Pittsburgh as an accounting clerk, but as I got older she stayed home and took care of the house and the bookkeeping for my father's company. We had relatively few friends, and until I went to school, I had none. I had plenty of toys, and I had a good time with them, and my mother was often in a wonderful mood and would play cowboys and Indians with me in the apartment. She could shriek with the best of them. The main things I remember at this time were living in a third floor flat and walking on the streets of Wilkinsburg with my mother to the bakery, bank, library, grocery and dry-goods stores.

My father was excellent around machines, but not much on carpentry or handyman sorts of work. My mother was just the opposite. She was skillful and bold on all household crafts such as painting, varnishing, and wallpaper hanging, though slender, the kind of person who could build a house with a pair of scissors, a screwdriver, a saw, and a hammer.

My father was an extremely intelligent man, but his education did not allow him to discuss matters. He liked to "argufy," essentially taking a position and defending it for no very good reason. He did not find discussions where everyone was trying to reach a solution to an intellectual problem an especially attractive exercise. If he had a problem, he expected to solve it himself.

I was always in awe of him, though he rarely struck me, whereas my mother took a well-deserved stick to me very regularly. Of course, I was with her more. Occasionally she wanted him to punish me when he came home, but I can see

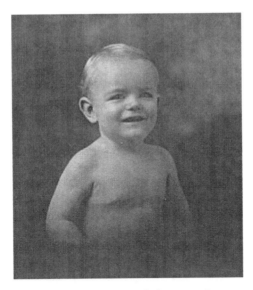

Fig. 7.2. Fred in a baby portrait.

now that his heart was not "in the work," as Andrew Carnegie might have said. Besides, a gruff word from him was a severe chastisement to me. He did not, though, pay much attention to me, except one Christmas when he bought me an electric train and set it up firmly by driving nails through the carpets ("We won't tell Mama"), and we played with it by the hour. Sometimes he was home a lot in the winter because road building was impractical in icy weather.

On my first day at school our teacher taught us to spell "picture." I was delighted and so was my mother. I entered McNair Elementary School at the age of six, and two things happened. First, I turned out to be left-handed, and my sweet old-lady teacher did not think that was satisfactory for writing. She would sneak up behind me with a ruler when I was writing left-handed and whack my writing hand a good one. I don't think it hurt so much, but it startled me and scared me out of my wits. Actually, I think it did hurt, though not as much as when my mother took a stick to my legs. The teacher did it regularly. I told my mother, who went to the school and discussed it with the principal. The principal told her that "We do not believe in changing children's handedness here," and she was sure this was not being done. On the other hand, the old lady who was teaching me did not seem to know about this policy, because while denying doing it, she continued to whack me every day until I learned not to write with my left hand. I personally think this set me back a great deal, and my school work was not satisfactory until the fifth grade. But statisticians and educators know that cause and effect are hard to prove, especially in individual cases.

The second big event was that about midway in the semester I became ill from many different diseases, one right after the other and all very severe. Chicken pox, pneumonia, pleurisy, and so on. I was home from school for months. These illnesses may have hit me so hard because I had been isolated from childhood diseases. It seemed best to start the first grade over because I had missed so much of the first half. The same elderly teacher, who was otherwise a sweetheart, continued to whack my hand from behind with a ruler whenever I used a pencil, pen, or crayon with the left hand.

My recollection of school from the first grade through the fourth is a bad blur. The teachers seemed not to like me, and I seemed to be afraid of them, and I was not very good at my work. My work was never neat, my numbers were in irregular columns, and except perhaps for memorizing poetry, I do not think I understood very well what I was doing. Flashcards did not help me. I just guessed wildly when they were shown. I think I did not understand what was required, and I certainly was not prepared, although my mother tried hard to get me in shape and I tried too, or thought I did. I may not have understood the difference between working out arithmetic answers and just knowing them. Today I appreciate the value of both abilities.

About the time I was finishing the first grade, I still loved to have my mother read stories to me. One evening she was terribly busy preparing a complicated dinner for my father and me, and she was in no mood to be bothered by my pestering. She announced that I could read perfectly well by now, and that I just was not trying. She turned off the stove and spent about ten minutes showing me how to sound out words (as we had been doing word by word at school) and said, "now get going." So I began, out loud, and she helped for a few weeks after that, and from then on I got so I could read speedily. This got me into trouble at school because in reading class we were forbidden to read ahead in the book. But who could bear to wait once the reading started? I would, of course, read way, way ahead. And I was bored with the agony of other children reading out loud, and I no longer liked to be read to.

Furthermore, my mother always got books for me from the library, taking me along. And so I read a great deal from this time on, even though I was not performing well at school. And I enjoyed reading. In these years, no one ever gave me anything technical to read, or anything other than stories.

When I was young, sometimes I spent part of the summer with either my father's mother in Washington, D.C., or my mother's mother in Indianapolis, Indiana. My father's mother spoiled me, but my mother's mother did not. She treated me very sensibly. My main recollections of these summers are seeing my cousins on both sides of the family and seeing something of Washington, going to Glen Echo Amusement Park in Washington, and to Kennywood Amusement Park in Pittsburgh. I saw little of my father during this period.

When I was very small, the tradition was that the President of the United States shook hands with visitors on the White House lawn on fair summer Sunday afternoons. When one of my grandmother's roomers took me, the

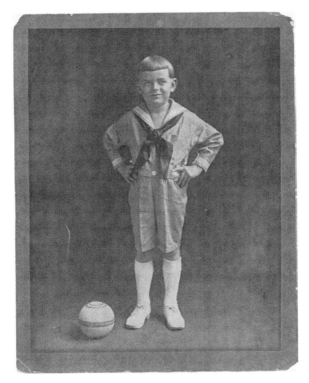

Fig. 7.3. Fred in his early childhood.

secret service men kept making me take my hands out of my pockets. In this way, I met Calvin Coolidge, and he told me that I would never forget that day, and I haven't.

Although I wasn't doing well in school, it was not for want of help from my mother. She made things like the multiplication table and spelling good fun. Each evening she washed and I wiped the dishes after dinner, and during this period we would make a game out of spelling, and in this comfortable atmosphere, I learned to spell very well. Why wasn't I getting good grades in spelling? For one thing, we had to write in ink with steel pens, and I see now that we should have practiced that at home, but we didn't. I was always blotching up the paper. Furthermore, my handwriting was so bad that teachers often did not accept responses as correct. Even though I could see how the teacher could make these mistakes, I did not realize that a teacher with 30 or 40 papers to read for each of several classes could not give a lot of time for special consideration.

My father spoke of men who wore glasses as sissies. And so when I realized that I couldn't see very well from the back of the room where the taller pupils were often placed, I said nothing about it. At the annual checkups for vision in the school, I would sit on the bench awaiting my turn and memorize the

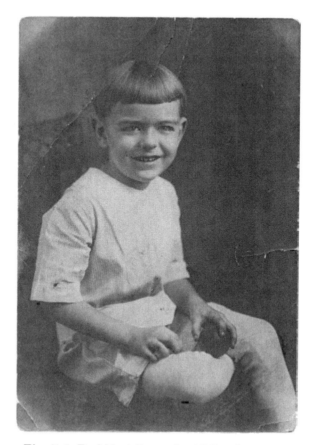

Fig. 7.4. Fred Mosteller, early childhood portrait.

letters. This worked until I was 10, when we were asked to wait outside and the door to the examination room was closed, so that one could not even hear the letters being spoken. Consequently I couldn't read any lines, and I was given a note to take home to my parents, but I was ashamed to carry it and never delivered it. Soon my mother received a note in the mail from the school notifying her that I needed glasses "as you will already have been informed."

Everyone was upset that I had not brought the note home, but I soon had glasses fitted. When I went to get them, the optometrist had a hard time getting them on my head, and I had a hard time seeing through them. I kept telling him that they were unsatisfactory and that I couldn't see through them, and that they hurt, but he was sure that I would get used to them in no time. I tried and stumbled into a tree on leaving the building. It was my first experience with lenses of any kind. It's always hard for children to get adults who are professionals to listen to them. Often adults have the same problem with professionals. When I got home (only by removing the glasses), I felt miserable. My mother was very understanding (she had worn glasses from the age of 7) and went to bat at once. She realized that my eyes could not have needed this substantial a correction if I could nearly see. I had received the wrong glasses.

We soon got it straightened out, and thereafter I was surprised at what a difference it made. I was impressed that it was easy to see the board from the rear of the schoolroom without squinting. Other boys chanted "four-eyes, four-eyes" for a day or so, and then my shame was over. My father said nothing about it, then or ever.

Although this vision problem is confounded with my early childhood performance at school, I do not think it had much to do with it. Though I had trouble seeing the board, I could squint my eyes enough to make out what was going on.

Before long, during summers I usually worked on my father's road construction jobs, carrying water for the men during the earliest years. I got to know the men on the road job, especially the men who ran the equipment or who were foremen of the various gangs and who worked year around and every year. I never saw a great deal of my father because he had much to do on the road job. He must have been an excellent manager, and he loved his work. He liked to go out to the job on a holiday or a rainy day or in the evening and talk about what he planned to do next. He kept no notes; everything was in his head.

In the fifth grade we had a new teacher from Texas, a Miss England, and I especially remember her teaching me arithmetic, perhaps short and long division. Among all the teachers I had ever seen, Miss England was the youngest and most beautiful, and best of all she did not seem to dislike me. Indeed, she went to a lot of trouble to take us weaker ones off into little groups and show us the mysteries of division, and how to check it, and why it worked. I fell madly in love with her. And I was also eating up arithmetic. Unfortunately for me, Miss England married before the year was out and went back to Texas. She was, however, the turning point in my school life.

Shortly after this I changed schools again and had a new start with a pleasant older teacher. As I moved from class to class and teacher to teacher in this new school, I at last felt entirely different. I suddenly was on top of the material, other pupils did not know it any better than I did, and although some of the teachers were mean (a word we pupils used among ourselves), I understood what they were doing and did not care much what their attitude was.

It was a strange turn of events for me, both with respect to intellectual things and with respect to the teachers. Suddenly they were just people to whom I owed certain work, but they were now real people, and I saw them as human beings with aggravations and likes and dislikes and problems of their own. Until then, except for Miss England and the sweet old lady with the ruler, they had all been monsters.

On the darker side, my parents' marriage broke up shortly after this. I stayed with my mother. Naturally, I had realized that we had a great deal of tension at home, but without much experience with other families, I supposed life was like that. The actual breakup was a shock to me. At that time, children of divorced families weren't very popular with intact families.

After the divorce my mother opened a hemstitching shop. By chance, one day, she looked through a tube a calendar came in, first through one eye and then the other, and found that one of the eyes was not delivering much of a signal. The oculist told her that she would have to give up the hemstitching business, and that she could work for him as a secretary, where there was not much close work to do. And so she gave up hemstitching and went in for secretarial work. As I recall, she did not have any shorthand, but she did know how to type.

While my mother was having her eyes treated by the doctor and working as his secretary, she had Saturdays off. On this day we ran a small food business. After my father left, to make ends meet she had split our apartment in two. A couple came and lived in the main part of it, while we lived in the two rooms remaining, but we did not have a stove, only hot plates. Nevertheless, we ate most of our meals there, and in the mornings I would make my own breakfast after she had gone. She would set up the oatmeal, and I would cook it.

On Saturday, we would get out the hot plates and bowls and make mayonnaise, Boston brown bread, cakes, muffins, cookies, cole slaw, and potato salad for people who had ordered them from my mother. I don't know what grapevine brought her these orders, but she did go to church a lot, and perhaps people there knew her. At any rate, I became good at mixing mayonnaise and baking cakes and muffins. She always took them out of the pans herself and did the final touches on the frosting.

In the afternoon, when all the cooking was completed, I would walk all over town delivering the goodies. I soon grew sorry to see a woman come to the door to take the food, because it almost certainly meant there would not be a tip for delivering. Men usually gave something, mostly a nickel, sometimes a dime.

My mother generally worked in areas related to food. She took a correspondence course in hotel management and as a result of that got a sequence of posts.

When my mother's sight apparently returned, she got a post as director of a high-school cafeteria. This work paid remarkably well as I recall, but the hours were long. She had to get up before five in the morning and take a long streetcar ride to the school and get the staff organized for the day. In the evenings, we did the bookkeeping together. It took long hours by hand, and frankly I was a great help. She had to make up the menus for the week, order the food, hire the cashiers (pupils at the school), and so on. The school frequently put on banquets for civic and other groups. So in addition to the regular lunches, often extra meals were prepared, and my mother would have to stay late for these.

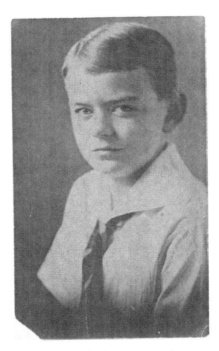

Fig. 7.5. Fred as a young boy.

She wore a sort of white nurse's outfit, except for the cap, with a starched collar that stood up in the back. Her red hair and hazel eyes always made her look attractive. She was quick in her movements and once in a while would slip and fall and get badly bruised—not just at this time, but all her life.

As the year went on, this effort was clearly wearing her out, and she decided she could not handle it. And so at the end of the year, she resigned and we went to Williamsport to live with the Dangles, who were related to my father. She and they got along well, and they were most generous people.

In Williamsport, my mother worked for the YMCA at the desk for boys. They had two pool tables and two table-tennis tables, a basketball court, and a swimming pool. And so for boys my age it was a center of activity. I had plenty of time and opportunity to play table tennis because I usually stayed until my mother was ready to leave and walked home with her.

I also attended a typing class for a few weeks, and this did me some good several decades later.

We lived with my uncle Hiram Dangle and his wife and children Louise and Earl. Hiram was a brilliant man who taught school near Williamsport. He lent me an algebra book and showed me how to get started, though we had some trouble over the issue of what x was, as have many others before and since.

8

Secondary School

As a result of my early illnesses and the move to Williamsport, I had lost a full academic year of schooling compared to my age-mates. My mother then took a position in Delaware, Ohio. I realized at once that what they were studying was material I had already covered. Arrangements were made to give me special state examinations to see whether I could skip the eighth grade. I did well in all but perhaps English. And so I started the ninth grade several weeks late.

Nothing was any trouble except Latin. Starting several weeks behind, I had a great deal of memorizing to do, and Latin was all I ever worked on in study halls. The competition in the school was stronger than I had met elsewhere, because a great many of the children were related to people from Ohio Wesleyan University. Some were related to the staff, and others were children of missionaries who had returned for a sabbatical year. In this atmosphere so favorable to academia, lots of pupils thought that learning was something to like, that they were good at it, and that it would pay off. Many had special talents.

In Delaware, Ohio, I joined the debating team as a high-school freshman. The state of Ohio had a very active debating program in both secondary schools and colleges. I spent a great deal of time working on this. The topic that year was chain stores. Although I can't recall the wording of the proposition, essentially it said that chain stores were a bad institution. I read hundreds of pages about chain stores. Our coach decided to put freshmen on the team for the first time in a building program that would give him and the school an outstanding team by the time they were seniors. Poor fellow—nearly every freshman he put on left town the next year. I was not as good at debating as I had expected to be, and I needed criticism. The coach was wise. He got the more experienced members of the team to consider our work and give us criticism.

My first debate was "away" from home, and my side lost. I had had to take the affirmative side of a proposition where I really preferred the negative. I now realize that the older members of the debating team all took the negative

F. Mosteller, *The Pleasures of Statistics: The Autobiography of Frederick Mosteller,* 123
DOI 10.1007/978-0-387-77956-0_8,
© Springer Science + Business Media, LLC 2010

side for the same reason. They sometimes won. Our young affirmative team never did. I learned a lot that year. I spent long hours in the Ohio Wesleyan University library working hard on debating. I learned about losing, but I did not find out why we were losing. In retrospect, I think we didn't have either good arguments or good rhetoric, and that the issue itself was biased by the grinding poverty of the times. I got a letter for my sweater at the end of the year, a lovely orange gothic "D" which looked beautiful on black.

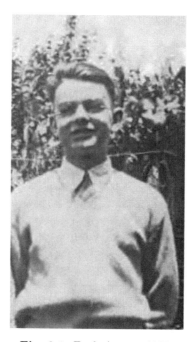

Fig. 8.1. Fred, August 1930.

The year was important to me in another way. The job at Delaware did not pay my mother enough to support us, and she had to take another in Watertown, New York. She decided that, rather than change schools twice, it was best to leave me at Delaware to complete the year, and she went on. This was a very maturing year for me. Although I again had very few friends, lots of people were friendly. I ate and lived with an invalid woman. She was an intelligent, well-educated, much traveled person with broad literary interests, and we discussed many things. She was very considerate of my youth and never made fun of my ideas. I read a little of Sigmund Freud, though I didn't understand it very well, and I tried to talk with her about this, but it was not successful. I was not ready, even though she was.

I enjoyed all my courses except Latin. Latin did begin to make me understand what the English class was attempting to teach—the structure of

English, through a method called diagramming. Though, in spite of this, I found no attraction with the technical side of English. I was surprised and impressed with the idea that one could take a course that led to reading novels. I liked that and tore through them at a great pace, not only the assigned novels, but others by the same authors. This was the first time I had gotten out of the Tom Swift, Edgar Rice Burroughs, Rover Boys, Horatio Alger, Albert Payson Terhune rut. But still no one suggested to me that I read anything in particular except in regular assignments. Or if they did, I did not take notice. I read some books about magic, and they were hard to understand because they were about anthropology, and I could not understand what it had to do with magic. I wanted to be magician, not a witch doctor. I felt that there was something wrong with the cataloging system at the library. The librarian tried to explain, but I misunderstood.

And I tried to read about religion. My aunt belonged to a Swedenborgian church, and I looked at some of Swedenborg's writings. I could not understand a word of it. I decided it was too old for me. I could have used some intellectual guidance. It impresses me that libraries today have vast amounts of material prepared for young people in all fields. Things are much better at least in the materials available for young people.

When the time came to go to the annual state competitions in different disciplines, I had a great disappointment. I had hoped to represent the school in mathematics in my grade. By working ahead, I had completed the entire textbook for the year in preparation for the possibility of being chosen. I had solved every problem in the book and memorized the proofs. But my English teacher picked me to go in English! Nothing I could do could change this. I went to Columbus, Ohio, with the rest and tried, but we did not win in that category, nor in mathematics either. We were given no idea of where we had placed.

I came out of the year well prepared in English, science, and mathematics, fuzzy on Latin—indeed, about in the state I always found myself in languages: I was not quite sure of the prepositions or adverbs, vague about the tenses, but rather quick translating from the foreign language to English, though not the reverse.

I was reading widely and had many classmate acquaintances, but no close friends. I did get to know one boy who played chess, and we played a few times. Still, I cannot recall being homesick during the year.

When the year was over, my mother and I returned to Pittsburgh, where she had decided to open a rooming house and tea-room. My father's mother had always been successful with rooming houses, and my mother felt that she could be too. In the middle of a depression, it was not so easy. We lived within walking distance of the main Carnegie Library, Fine Arts Museum, and Natural History Museum, where I spent a good deal of time. Many of us Schenley High students worked there every evening. At school all went well, except of course the second year of Latin: as usual, I was good at translating Caesar from Latin to English. At Schenley, I benefited from a remarkably talented collection of teachers. Those at Delaware, Ohio, had been very good, but Schenley seemed to me then and seems to me now to have provided the most outstanding collection of teachers I have ever had relative to their mission. Of course, since then some single teachers have stood out, but as a group, the Schenley teachers exuded competence. They were reasonably demanding of the stronger students and considerate of the weaker ones.

Our geometry teacher was a woman, gruff, perhaps a little mean, and superb. An exam every day—learn the theorem, learn to prove it. Most people do not realize what a great thing it is to have mathematics at one's finger tips, and on the tip of one's tongue. It is all very well to be able to figure it all out, but when you want to build on knowledge quickly, it is well to have it deeply in one's mind. This woman sold me this idea in a most impressive manner—strict, fair, and forward moving.

Our Latin teacher was the first scholarly teacher I had ever had. He always had a lot more to say about the lesson than could be found in any books we had available. And I remember a Latin motto he had in a plaster of Paris mold: "Disce ut semper victurus, vive ut cras moriturus." (Learn as if you would live forever; live as if you would die tomorrow.) I liked it, and used it years later in the final TV program of a probability and statistics course on Continental Classroom. It produced a great many letters, not only from those interested in the mathematics, but also from some Latin teachers, to my great delight. I could not believe that one of them would be viewing, but one should never sell school teachers short. They are a dedicated band.

English was all right. I enjoyed reading the Shakespeare plays, but like most other students, I disliked studying the footnotes. I gradually realized that the source of the difficulty was that I was engaged in reading a foreign language under the guise of its being my mother tongue. I felt then and feel now that, if I am going to have some fun reading a play, I ought to read it and get the idea of the play. If, on the other hand, we are to go into literary criticism, that is another game, and one that we ought to have some motivation for. We seemed to me to be doing the latter all the time under the pretense of learning to appreciate literature. Nothing slows down appreciation like a lot of footnotes. Footnotes are fine when you have fallen in love with a set of material and want to know more and more. The falling in love part was what was being omitted.

I had an absolutely marvelous homeroom teacher, named Rose Stewart. She was a tall, gawky, thin woman with nerves of steel and a wonderful smile. She insisted on having nothing but boys in her homeroom. They ran from sophomores through seniors, about 40 or 50 of us. The administration sent her the rowdy ones being kicked out of other rooms. She enjoyed boys, and tough as they tried to make it for her, she was always able to cope through a joyous quiet sense of humor, a complete understanding and sympathy for the underhandedness of young males, and personal brilliance and confidence in the rightness of what she was doing and of her ability to outmaneuver any boy. She was making young men out of young boys, and she would, over a three-year period, create respect and affection for her among even the most unruly. They were always coming back to see her.

She was a history teacher who believed in making history personal. Every day was an important historical day to her and so to us. Our homeroom had a most complicated mixture of ethnic groups and of immigrant children as well as children of wealthy many-generations-in-America families. She would tie a boy's name to his ethnic background, and when the birthdate or other celebration date of a famous person from the same ethnic group occurred, that boy had to go to the front of the class and tell what this person had done. Sometimes it was something for America, but sometimes not. We all razzed the person who had to go forward, but he always had a good story to tell because Miss Stewart made sure of it. And so we heard about Cavour from someone of Italian descent, about Pilsudski from a Pole, George Washington Carver from a black, and so on.

At this time the reading of the Bible was still allowed in public school, and though I'm not much for formal religion, I must say that the failure to continue this seems to me to have eroded an important aspect of our culture. At any rate, because our class was made up of about a third each of Catholics, Jews, and Protestants, Miss Stewart ordinarily read to us each day from the Old Testament. Then at key times of the year, such as Christmas and Easter, she would announce that she was going to read a passage from the New Testament, explaining that those who did not regard it as an appropriate part of a religious belief could well appreciate it as a legend of another culture and that it would do them no harm. We never had any objections from parents or students as far as I know, and I never heard any murmuring about it in the homeroom. She did not always read the Bible. Sometimes she would find something of special historical significance, such as a passage about the moment that the guns became silent at the Armistice in World War I, or the flight of the passenger pigeons and their ultimate extinction.

We heard rumors that, during summers, Miss Stewart and her sister acted as American missionaries in Tennessee (or maybe Kentucky) where feuding was still extant, and that they held church services there on alternate Sundays for two feuding families. They personally escorted the family members to church so that the other family would not shoot them on the way. She was a great woman.

Some mathematics and science teachers stand out. Mr. Veverka taught algebra, trigonometry, and a little calculus, so much that when I went to college, I had had the whole first year before, though Carnegie Tech would not admit it. I enjoyed his teaching. Indeed, all the mathematics and all the teachers impressed me. Veverka had an enthusiasm for what he did that I had not observed before. And he had a lot of enthusiasm for what the students did as well and sarcasm for those who did not try.

Paul Dysart was marvelous in physics. He was very mature, very deep, and solemn though he had a good sense of humor—a little like Miss Stewart's, in that he knew boys would be boys, and he knew in advance what they were about to do. He believed anyone could learn anything given enough time and given some incentive, and so he arranged his classes so that the student could go in a rather self-paced manner, getting whatever grade he or she wanted to achieve by taking exams over and over if the first exams did not go well. It was great for both his mathematics and physics students.

His laboratory and classroom were a gathering place after school for all the boys (girls did not stick around in the afternoon) who were in the science and mathematics mode. We loved this quiet, dry man. He reminded me a little of my Uncle Hiram, he was so all-knowing. And he showed us marvels of light and waves and levers and electricity. What a great show! In the physics course, for the first time in my life I kept good notes. I took them home and transcribed them into lettering—none of my illegible handwriting. I worked all the problems and enjoyed them thoroughly.

The last two years in high school I took German. Somehow it was like Latin. I never could buckle down hard enough to spend the time memorizing the important features of the language in the way I had appreciated the need for total recall in the geometry class. And so again I was good at translating from German to English but not the other way. It all helped me a lot later, though, and turned out to be a useful choice.

Where did all the time go? Aside from waiting tables, chess, for one thing. Schenley had a chess club when I arrived consisting of eight members, and I became a ninth. We played together once every two weeks. On a Jewish or Catholic holiday not enough were in school to make a good meeting. I wanted to play more chess. I thought that I was learning how to play and wanted to do more of it. Suddenly out of the mathematics classes sprouted a whole group of young fellows who wanted to play chess. Soon we were all playing every afternoon in Dysart's physics laboratory. We decided that we would make something of the chess club by acquiring more chess sets and increasing the activity. We had two sets of avocational clubs at school, and they met on alternate weeks. We asked and the school allowed the chess club to meet every week. We began promoting chess and soon had 50 people attending the chess club, and we also opened up into two sections. We were giving instruction to new people all the time, and some girls were beginning to join. Furthermore, we began scheduling matches against other schools and clubs. Soon we were playing against several other high schools and the local college teams, as well as the district and industrial men's clubs. After a year or two, we were very strong, because we had a lot of tournament experience, and we went into matches in our knee pants expecting to win. I realize now that older men who would insult us by cautioning before the match that we had to play "touch-move" were underrating us so severely that they did not do nearly as well against us as they should have. We had an unfair advantage.

The school paper advertised the chess club with regular stories about its matches and about the size of the membership, and by the time we graduated there were three hundred in the chess club, including about one hundred girls.

I had then, and have now, great admiration for the school administration in this connection. In 1933 we were deep in depression in Pittsburgh and everywhere else in America, and we went to the administration to ask for about 100 chess sets. I recall that Walter Reid, another chess friend, had shopped very hard to find an inexpensive but adequate set, but even so, where could the school find the money? I have no idea, but they did. All the mathematics teachers went to bat for us.

Working Summers

When I returned to Pittsburgh, my father got in touch with us again, and during the summers I began again to work on the road construction jobs, first as a ditch digger, then as a semi-skilled laborer such as mason's or carpenter's assistant, and then later as foreman on various gangs, rough grading, clean-up, stone-laying, and so on. And as time-keeper on some jobs.

Although my mother had instilled the idea of going to college in me from the earliest age, my father was not pleased with the idea. Because I knew a great deal about building roads, he felt that in a few years I could be a superintendent in my own right. He saw no reason for going to college. I would profit more financially in the road construction business. He had been successful with little schooling, and so could I be.

Although he had a good point, one difficulty was that I disliked working on the road jobs. I prayed for rain. One summer it did not rain from the first day of summer until after I had left to return to school. We worked overtime. I had charge of 50 trucks. At the beginning it was dry, but it gradually became dusty, and then after a while the dust in the road itself became so fine that it behaved like water—it flowed, and we had to buy special coal scoops to remove it because we were not allowed to lay stone over it. It just slipped off regular shovels.

The only thing I really liked about the road jobs was playing poker. I enjoyed this very much, and I hoped for rain so we could rest up and play. Most summers it rained a lot, and we played a good deal in the evenings or under some shelter when it rained.

People often discuss key events in their lives, and I suppose knowing Miss England, Rose Stewart, Paul Dysart, and Mr. Veverka was among these for me. With respect to my father, one event stands out as most influential. It taught me something I've never forgotten, and it has influenced my working behavior. One summer as carpenter's assistant, I was helping to build headwalls—some people call them culverts. The runoff of water from the road into the ditches on the sides is likely to erode the berm (the earth shoulders beside the paving) and ultimately undermine the road itself unless drainage has been properly constructed. To handle this, at various spots, large pipes are put under the road crossways so that water from the high side can flow under the road to the low side where it is removed, perhaps down the side of a hill. At the spot where the water collects to enter the pipe (I am talking about pipes at least a foot in diameter), a concrete structure is built to guide and control the water so that it doesn't undercut the roadbed or the pipe. These structures have various shapes and sizes, one at that time being a simple good-sized vertical wall surrounding the pipe opening and shoring up the earth around. Others were more complicated, like the "box culvert," which in addition to having a vertical wall has a large box-shaped bottom perhaps four feet by six feet by four feet high. Water flows down into this box and then into the pipe. It prevents the water from overshooting the drain and continuing on the same side of the road.

To make these headwalls or culverts, one had to construct wooden forms, oil them, insert structural steel, and then tighten them up to just the right width with wire, and then finally pour in concrete. Once the concrete hardened, the forms were carefully removed and cleaned up for use wherever possible on another headwall, because the wood was worth a lot and the carpentering took a lot of time.

It was a reasonably satisfactory job for a boy or young man, whichever I was. One had to put up with the usual apprenticeship nonsense that every such occupation offered, but I had been through that with each job each summer, and so I was rather untroubled by the usual jokes on the neophyte, the hunt for the skyhooks, the left-handed crowbar, and so on.

The head carpenter, Jesse, liked me and I liked him. We roomed together and became fast friends. He used to try to stump me with problems such as how long the side of a right triangle would be if its two legs were 1 foot and 12 feet long. It bothered him that I could do calculations like this in my head. I gradually realized that he did not so much want to show me up with these difficult problems as to proudly show me his solution, which used his carpenter's square. His method was very good and practical when you were out on a rainy, damp road jobs and had to figure things out accurately.

He taught me a practical use for a mathematical theorem. When the form for a box culvert was put in place, we had to be sure it was "square" (rectangular). We built the outer shell outside the hole and then wrestled it in. He told me to check that it was "square," meaning a perfect rectangle. I borrowed his beloved carpenter's square and tried its 90° angle on the corners. He just laughed at me and got our rulers out and measured the two diagonals, and then we adjusted the box (which would be a parallelogram not quite rectangular) until the diagonals were equal. We had built opposite sides equal, and so with opposite sides equal and diagonals equal, we then had a perfect rectangle.

The largest culvert we ever built had a pipe about 7 feet in inside diameter. None of our other culverts had pipes more than 3 feet in diameter. The large pipe was especially curious, because there never was any water in the ditch that led up to the pipe. And so it seemed rather a waste, but as a way of making a small bridge inexpensively over a ravine, one could readily understand it.

We worked on it for some weeks, because it was an enormous task for our small gang. Finally, the whole structure was in place ready to pour concrete on the day before the Fourth of July weekend. No one had had a day off for weeks, all had been working weekends, and the men were planning a trip to Pittsburgh. My father came around to talk to Jesse late in the day and said, "Don't you think you ought to pour tomorrow? The plant would stay open for you, even though they would charge double-time." (This referred to the ready-mix concrete company.) Jesse felt that the men had not had a day off for a long time, and they all had outings with their families planned. My father clearly felt this was a mistake, but he didn't insist. He personally was a great fan of the Fourth, of Memorial Day, and of Labor Day and loved to go to a baseball game, usually to see the Pittsburgh Pirates as a sort of picnic on these days. I think these outings were the happiest times I had with him, except perhaps when we were playing poker.

Sunday and Monday were holidays, and on Monday night it rained torrentially. It had not rained much all summer except for dampish sorts of days. When we went to see our headwall, we understood why the large pipe was being installed. Trees with trunks two feet in diameter had come down the ravine and slammed into the forms, destroying them. And since the forms blocked the entrance to the pipe, we had created a dam, and the silt that comes with such a runoff piled up deeply on the forms, covering much of the trees. Not only had everything we had done been wrecked, but we were much worse off than when we started, because the silt and mud was six or seven feet deep in the neighborhood of the form, and it extended back up the ravine. Before we could remove the old form, we would have to dig out. Furthermore, at that time we had no equipment to help dig—the power shovel would not reach. It was back to ditch digging for all concerned. But whereas the digging of the footer for the headwall was a fairly modest job in the first place, just a couple of feet deep, now we had long hard digging. The least sentimental man there must have been sick about it, because we had all been so proud when we left on Saturday night.

My father had a somewhat one-sided discussion with Jesse. One could tell even from a distance that he was not pleased. And he rarely suffered in silence. On the road jobs he often used very bad language, though practically never in front of women. Although I had had nothing to do with this decision, he took me for a ride, unusual during working hours, and explained his dissatisfaction at length. Although I tried to say things such as that Jesse couldn't help the rain, my father said Jesse didn't have to stop the rain, he just had to finish his job instead of going off to play. "By God, finish the job!"

Later he left me off at the ruined culvert, and I returned to digging out. We had to get trucks and the roller to help pull out the trees. Although I was full of resentment against my father, I was aware enough to make some rough calculations of what this waste effort was costing. I knew roughly what a truck cost per day and what the men and Jesse cost. And I had a vague idea about the lumber—which had been broken and twisted. And it was taking us longer, because of the clean-up, than to build the original form. It was costing thousands of dollars. I lived with my mother, who got no alimony, and we never had a thousand dollars. I worked all summer, and even with the poker, by the time I paid room and board I never had a thousand dollars. To be involved in losing thousands of dollars was genuinely appalling. I was deeply impressed, by nature's destruction of our intricate piece of work, by my father's rage and invective, but mostly by the magnitude of the loss, and all because we hadn't finished what we could have finished the next day. All those "stitch in time" and "lack of a horseshoe nail" stories came true in our ravine.

Ever since, when a project comes near to completion, I have an irresistible urge to move heaven, earth, and colleagues to complete it. I am comfortable with a project that has a three-year plan, but if it is within two months of completion, absolutely every effort should be bent to completing it. By chance, through the years, occasional bad events such as illnesses and crises have reinforced this attitude. Of course, part of this behavior is pure superstition, part the marks left by this event, and I surely know that part is that "finishing" always requires many times as much work as one expects. Thus something to be done in two months won't be done in eight unless everyone speeds up. "Finish the job that's nearly done" is high on my list of "do's."

Entering College

In the fall of my senior year in high school, applications for college were due. My hope was to go to Carnegie Tech. I knew nothing about it, but my father thought highly of the school. He knew nothing about it either. My mother had no views. No one counseled us. I had no valid reason for wanting to go there, but my heart was set on it. Naturally, I applied to other schools as well. Early on, Carnegie notified me that I had a scholarship for the first year. I was delighted and told them that I would come.

A special state representative scholarship competition was based on an all-day set of examinations. It offered one scholarship for each state representative. I received the one from my district. This gave me something toward college tuition each year. All told, these scholarships did not pay all the tuition charges for the four years, but they helped a lot, and the first year was entirely covered.

As an aftermath of the state representative's scholarship, many letters from colleges in Pennsylvania offered a partial or full scholarship to their institution. Very flattering.

9

Carnegie Institute of Technology

College for me was different from the experience for many other students because I was a "townie." I lived at home, though most students lived in dormitories. As a consequence, I did not develop many new friends in college, though some from my high school days were also in my class. Pittsburgh was very different then from the clean city of today, and the education of an engineer at Carnegie Institute of Technology—now Carnegie Mellon University—was different too. Some of this may be worth recalling for reality rather than nostalgia.

In my freshman year the course in engineering drawing and descriptive geometry met nine hours a week and had plenty of outside work as well. We learned about hardness of pencils, how to use sandpaper to make leads into points or wedges, and gained skill with T-square, ruler, engineer's triangles, steel drawing tools, and some students, but not I, became skilled with India ink. No one ever called me neat in my work, not even my mother or my wife, and these instructors prized neatness.

At that time Pittsburgh was grimy—large chunks of soot worked their ways through windowsills and after floating down on a drawing, needed then to be blown carefully away. These large chunks were merely symptomatic of small chunks you didn't notice which gradually blackened your sheet. One classmate was a professional at drawing, and he washed his T-square and triangles before every class, his hands every half-hour, and kept a cloth over all parts of his drawing that he was not penciling or inking. I learned to wash my hands often, but the rest was too much. Grades were based on a total of 100 for an assignment. I usually got high marks for problems solved, but 30 off for "arrowheads" or for "lettering" or for "sloppy drawing" or just "technique," whatever that was.

We had shops. Andrew Carnegie thought that we should have practical work as well as labs and classes, and over the first two years I believe that I had four shops: masonry and carpentry, both of which I was good at because of my experience on the road-building jobs, and sheet metal and welding, which were new to me.

F. Mosteller, *The Pleasures of Statistics: The Autobiography of Frederick Mosteller*, DOI 10.1007/978-0-387-77956-0_9,
© Springer Science + Business Media, LLC 2010

In welding, we had a graduated series of projects for both electric and acetylene torches. The electric went like a charm. Acetylene welding went well through the first four projects. The fifth was a T-joint, a pipe welded onto another pipe perpendicularly. To test a project, the instructor took a heavy hammer and broke it while the student stood proudly by, proud unless it broke at the weld—the weld had to be stronger than the metal, or the project failed. This seems a little unreasonable even now, but that was the rule, no doubt a good one. When a project failed, you did it again and again. After a few weeks redoing project five, the instructor invited me to his office for a personal conference. I had a good attendance record and had failed project five about six times despite good effort. "I think," said he, "that we will give you a C in this course, provided one thing, you do not take Advanced Welding." It was a deal. For my mother, though, the course had a major success. We had a pencil sharpener with a broken cast-iron handle. She wondered if I could fix it as long as I was taking welding. After I burnt quite a bit of the metal away, some knowledgeable student informed me that instead of welding I should be brazing, a skill not taught in the course, or at least not to those still on project five. And so I tried brazing, and suddenly a great glob of metal fell into the pieces and joined them. An hour or so at the grinding wheel and we had a useful handle. I was amazed and my mother was sure that my instructors must be delighted with my work.

Parts of the English course I enjoyed because our instructor was a man with a somewhat sardonic sense of humor. His special field of study was Jonathan Swift. We wrote a 1000-word theme each week. I handed in a carefully counted 1000 words each week and usually got back a grade of B or B+ and occasionally an A−. At first the papers had no comment whatsoever, but some time in the first semester, the notation "Write longer sentences" began to appear. I tried, but each week the same notation appeared. It got to me. Finally I decided to write a theme with few sentences. With some effort, I wrote a three-sentence 1000-word theme. It came back with no comment and an A, the only outright A that I got the whole semester except for the final grade. Thereafter, I lapsed back into what I suppose was my short-sentence writing style, and he quit asking for longer sentences.

The second semester of the English course was devoted to reading a book a week. Though for the most part I enjoyed this reading, I had two shocks. Usually I left the reading to the night before the weekly quiz and whipped through it easily. The first occasion that there was trouble was when we read *Tom Jones*. First, it turned out to be a more slowly reading book than I expected, and second, it had crazy, puzzling introductions to the chapters that seemed to have little to do with the story. Naturally, I skipped them as any sensible reader would have done. Strangely, our instructor wanted to know about our interpretation of these parts and had no interest in the rest of the story. Although taken by surprise, I could see in retrospect that perhaps that was what the assignment was all about; when you got to college, people weren't going to pay off much for your reading amusing stories.

The second shock came when I was given a rather thin book to read that I knew wouldn't take long, John Stuart Mill's *On Liberty*. I was late getting in from a chess match and had to begin reading the assignment that same evening, perhaps 10:30 P.M. or 11 P.M. I began, and found that the wording was difficult and headway slow. After a while I had read only a few pages, and I could see that the possibility of finishing and understanding anything about this work was not available in the time I had. Even peeking at the back pages didn't help. I decided to go to sleep and forget it. This troubled me very much because both my mother and my father were very strong on the idea of finishing everything. And while I must at some other time have failed to complete assignments, this is the first time I ever recall deliberately deciding not to complete one. Next day there was a quiz on the book, and I just wrote that I hadn't read it, and that I was sorry.

Years later this failure came back to haunt me. I was on the board of an organization deciding about awarding grants. One came up about "liberty," and I listened to the discussion with some unease. Everyone there seemed to know a lot about this field, and Mill's book *On Liberty* was absolutely central to their discussion. When the discussion ended with only one silent mouse, we were asked one by one, an unusual procedure, what we thought, and the mouse was the last one asked. He said that he was sorry but that because he had not read the book he had no opinion. Embarrassing. The others didn't let it go at that but ground it in with a good deal of chaffing.

The mouse went home determined to read this book. To be embarrassed twice in one lifetime by the same little book was too much. People said this was a great book, clear and easy reading. How then was it that I found it slow going the first time? An illness kept me in bed for several weeks, and so I took the book home and went to work. Mill's teacher told him to write long sentences, and he never forgot. It was so bad that I would fall asleep after nearly every paragraph. Furthermore, I soon found that I couldn't recall a thing about what I had read. How could I be the only one who ever found this book hard to read?

I started over, and after reading each paragraph I would write a sentence or two saying just what the paragraph said, but in my own language. It still put me to sleep a lot, but over a period of days I finally got through the book and produced a manuscript of what it was all about, including a critique of the logic of the effort. There is a little circularity in the argument right off the bat. Copies went to the friends who had chided me. Unknown to me, one of them sent a copy to the scholar who was going to study "liberty," and the latter one day mentioned to me that he had found the document extremely helpful because it had saved him an enormous amount of time. Gratifying. At last this assignment had been carried out. My mother would still be disappointed that it hadn't been done properly in the first place.

As for extracurricular activities, Carnegie had a School of Drama. Tickets were free and I began to go. My mother usually couldn't go because her work often took her out of town, and so I often went alone. This was much stronger fare than most movies and often more moving. *Liliom* was the most touching that I recall. A friend gave me tickets to an opera, which bored me, and to *The Green Pastures*, which I thought was great.

In my sophomore year, I had calculus, mechanics, French, quantitative analysis, and physical measurements. The French was like Latin and German. I didn't enjoy it though I was sure I needed to study it, and that ultimately turned out to be correct though not until graduate school.

The physical measurements course had the most engaging set of laboratory exercises I had ever participated in. Not only did we measure all sorts of unusual things—heat, electricity, mass, light—but we were honestly trying to measure how accurate our work was. Physics was for me, and I became a physics major. This was what Dysart must have been pointing us toward in high school. No course ever engaged me more by its variety and ingenuity and by using the principles we learned in other courses in the most amazing ways. Every meeting offered happy puzzles. For example, I was astonished to find that a small light source 30 feet away was essentially at infinity as far as our mathematics was concerned.

★ ★ ★

A little statistics and probability entered the physical-measurements course, and somewhere along the way we were asked to compute the probability of casting a total of 9 and of casting a total of 10 using *three* ordinary dice rather than two. Because each die has six sides, one must account for $216 \, (= 6 \times 6 \times 6)$ possible outcomes, and although most students found the answers, the problem troubled me. When the class discussed this problem, I said to Dr. Pugh, who was excellent at keeping us motivated and moving an extra step, "Most of us got the answer mainly by counting on our fingers. But, if you had asked about 6 dice or 15 dice, we'd still be counting. Is there a better way to do it for larger problems?" Pugh's greatness as a teacher came through. He said immediately, "I don't know how, but I think I know a man who might, Dr. Olds. Why don't you ask him about it?"

Among the mathematics professors at Carnegie, Dr. E. G. Olds was one of the few doing original research at that time. He was also teaching me calculus, and he had a huge voice, was very good humored, and had astonishingly big teeth. He reminded me of other loud voices in my life, and I did not follow Dr. Pugh's advice, though I saw Dr. Olds nearly every day.

One day soon after, I was working in the silent library when Dr. Olds came in and shouted in his usual conversational tone of voice, "I hear you want to know about the dice problem. You must come see me some time about it." Me, whispering, "Yes, one of these days."

He then said, "Well, you're not doing anything important right now. Come along," and led me off to his lair.

After a little, I got over my embarrassment and began thinking, and he began showing me slowly and carefully how to do the three-dice problem. The amazing feature, as I look back on it, was that I had all the technical manipulative equipment required to handle the mathematics of this problem. Some of it was algebraic trickery that I had enjoyed learning in secondary school but had been sure would never have a practical use (perhaps because I hadn't seen any).

The method was that of generating functions, and it magically, and I do mean magically, counted how many ways there were to get each total with the dice. Although I had loved mathematics all along, this was the first time I ever felt that I'd been working with a peashooter when I could have had a cannon, and furthermore, that the tricks I had learned could produce such a marvel. I thanked him sincerely and got ready to hurry off to class, but before I reached the door, he said, "Just a moment, young man. Come back."

He quickly pulled a book off the shelf, turned to the end of the first chapter and marked off ten problems. "If you liked the probability problem and the generating function, you'll like this. Bring the problems back in two weeks." Authority meant a lot then, and so I did. Each week he'd check off problems in another chapter, book after book.

I complained to my mother that I was taking an extra course and not getting credit for it, and why did I have to do it? "I don't know, dear, but I'm sure he wouldn't ask you to do it if it weren't good for you."

Soon I was a mathematics rather than a physics major. If week after week, year after year, and book after book, you study a chapter and solve ten problems in a subject, it's hard not to have some feeling for it and investment in it. Furthermore, I could see how it could help my poker playing. When I mentioned this to Olds, he seemed uneasy but did not reprove. He was a serious churchman. Despite this, one summer I wrote him from the road job about a poker problem I had found instructive and how I had gotten an approximate answer. He responded with a long letter bringing up a point I had missed, though it luckily didn't matter a lot, and showing a way to do the problem exactly. I believe his own doctoral dissertation was on probabilities in bridge. And he was a bridge player.

In part of his research, he was engaged in finding the exact distribution of the rank correlation coefficient for samples of size 7 and 8. This led to enormous piles of paper on each of which a substantial array of numbers were written—oh, for today's high-speed computer! The hitch was that he could tell from looking at his answer that there were some mistakes in the counts, more than one.

Some governmental funds were available for students to earn by helping professors do research, and so he unleashed me on this pile to check the answers. I did this by merely redoing his calculations, a method that for various reasons is not likely to be a good check. It is too easy to be asleep at the switch at the key moment, especially when nearly every line is correct. As safety inspectors know, alarm systems that are not much used are rarely in good working order.

Another difficulty was that it was boring, endlessly tedious. After a while, I began noticing something of a pattern—something familiar page after page.

What was I noting? It couldn't be very complicated or I would not be noticing it. I quit doing the actual work and began playing around with the numbers, and sure enough, the totals always provided a special pattern. If they didn't, then something was wrong. Now I had a theorem, could I prove it? As often happens when you know the answer, the proof comes rather easily.

When I showed Dr. Olds the result, he was clearly pleased. He also was able to turn the task of checking over to a clerk because now all that had to be done was a series of additions to get a definite check. And the new check was much faster and more reliable than the repeated calculation. I suppose this was my first research experience in mathematics. It did use some of the mathematics I had learned in my special readings assigned by Dr. Olds, and I probably could not have done it with the equipment I picked up in my regular course work. Most regular work emphasized calculus or geometry; the discrete mathematics I learned with the outside readings was what was required.

★ ★ ★

In my sophomore year, my mother and I lived again in Wilkinsburg, and I rode streetcars to Carnegie Tech. I observed an attractive young woman who got on at my stop at the school and who often was on my streetcar going into school in the morning. She did not, however, respond to being greeted. No doubt she was deaf and could not read lips.

In those days an institution called a tea dance occurred regularly on Friday afternoons, and when I attended one of these and invited this same young woman, Virginia Gilroy, to dance, she accepted, and we had a good time. Her hearing had improved. She was taking the four-year course in Secretarial Studies at Margaret Morrison School for Women—the Radcliffe of Carnegie Tech.

Soon we became close friends, and this continued for years. We went to many dances and plays together and even took a one-semester course in psychology together.

★ ★ ★

I studied both scientific German and scientific French. In the German course, Philip Morrison, who later edited the book-review column for *Scientific American*, and I were two of only three students outside the field of metallurgy. The third studied biology. We read small books from the series known as *Sammlung Göschen*. These books ran about 120 pocket-sized pages each. Since the Department of Metallurgy had about 30 students in the course, we read two volumes on the metallurgy of iron, then four on metallography, and after that one on biology, one on astrophysics, and I read one on projective geometry. Years later, having read the projective geometry was a great help. It also was a help in an undergraduate course in projective geometry, and vice versa, knowing the English words helped the translation.

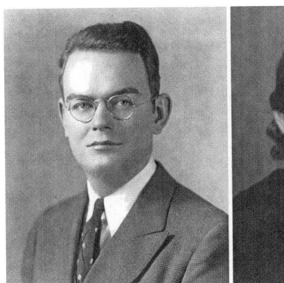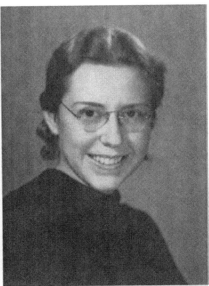

Fig. 9.1. Fred Mosteller and Virginia Gilroy in their college years.

The German professor made us read the legends of the tables and the footnotes and translate the endless abbreviations. With the right kind of dictionary, I began to find that one could in a few days become enough acquainted with the vocabulary of a subject to read along at a satisfactory pace for scientific work, especially mathematical work where a page in an hour or two may be appropriate. In other words, without being extremely facile, one's speed was not much less than it would have been in English. The main trouble would be the difficulties of subject matter, rather than those of language.

And so later when I studied from Courant and Hilbert's *Methoden der mathematischen Physik*, I was not bothered that the text was in a foreign language. This surprised me. I still was a one-way translator. But the mathematics required attention, not the German.

As I look back on languages: Latin, German, French, and a smattering of Russian, I am annoyed both with myself and our educational system. All over the world people learn to speak two or more languages fluently and many to read them with genuine appreciation. Yet I have put in small amounts of time for several years without having even the goal of fluency. Yet I know that under forced draft people learn languages well in only a few months. Is it all my fault or should our public education get a complete body-and-fender job in language training? Our nation needs languages for diplomacy and international trade; yet it has practically none. When I consider the success of language education in other countries, it makes me think that this must be a problem readily fixed.

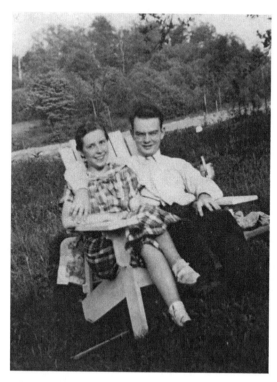

Fig. 9.2. Fred and Virginia at the home of her parents in Butler, Pennsylvania in 1937.

$\star\,\star\,\star$

When I first went to Carnegie Tech, which is located in the Schenley Park district where I lived at this time, our chess team from Schenley High School moved almost bodily to Carnegie. We found a chess vacuum and filled it at once. Walter Reid was our leader, active in trying to get sponsorship from the school and in arranging meets and correspondence games.

He arranged simultaneous matches for us so that we played perhaps 20 people at once. There is nothing difficult about this unless they are as good as you are, and then you tie or lose. By and large, though, people who are fairly good do not come out to play unknowns, and so we were in little danger and won nearly all the games.

In college, we helped organize and maintain a city-wide league of chess clubs with regular matches. We won several matches just because we all always showed up and the other club forfeited points because someone didn't come. In our junior year, Walter organized a trip for the team to New York City during the Christmas season. He had discovered a collegiate chess tournament for us to play in. He got Carnegie to put up a small sum of money for us to go. The ride to New York was terrible because at all times two of the five of

us had to ride in an open rumble seat, and it was snowing all the way. By the
time we got there I had a bad cold.

We played in at least one match nearly every day except Christmas itself.
In addition to the regular matches, Walter had organized some special matches
for us with West Point—we went up there and played on the grounds—and
with Columbia University at the Marshall Chess Club. I think we won one and
tied one; both matches were close, and I do recall that I won one game and tied
one. The match at the Marshall Chess Club was more memorable because we
got to meet Frank Marshall. Marshall was one of the great American masters
and had played Capablanca for the world championship and lost. He wore
a big silk bow tie, very flourishing and *fin de siècle*, and long hair, most
uncommon at the time. His attire and toilet were what I imagined a Parisian
artist would fancy, though I had never seen one, except in paintings of an
atelier.

Because of the Christmas season, some of the Columbia players and one
of ours had engagements that would require them to leave the game at a
given time, and Marshall agreed to adjudicate the games that had to be so
ended. One game came to this. Our player was a piece down, though he was in
an extremely strong position. Marshall asked each what he wanted from the
game, the Columbia man said a win, and our player said a draw. Thereupon,
Marshall took over our player's pieces and said "What were your next few
moves?" and they quickly played out a sequence at the end of which Marshall
had a winning game. He then put the pieces back and said "Let's try that
again," with the same result. After repeated trials he said to the Columbia
player, "You don't even have a plan, and you're lucky I don't give the other
player a win. I declare it a tie." And that was the end of that, and no one
even murmured.

In these early matches, we had been warming up for the college tournament, which was played at the Manhattan Chess Club, a much more austere
place like a business office than Marshall's, which was like a very plush men's
club. The teams entered, in addition to Carnegie as I recall, were New York
University, City College of New York, Yeshiva, Cornell, Columbia, either Harvard or Yale, and perhaps a couple of others. We soon found that some of
the players on the New York teams were old-timers with very tenuous ties
to the schools they represented. All told, I believe, I got less than half the
possible points, and our team placed below the middle—maybe fifth or sixth
out of about eight. The top teams had much better trained players than we.
Whether we could have been trained to the corresponding levels I do not
know, but clearly they knew much more about the game. Reid persuaded
Samuel Reshevsky, another great American master, to play him for a dollar,
but Reshevsky wouldn't play a second time because Walter played so slowly.
Reshevsky couldn't afford it.

For me the most fun was watching famous players playing "skittles." Essentially, it is ten-second chess. After a move, the referee waits a little, then
says, "one, two, three," with a pause between the numbers, and then "forfeit,"

if the player has not already moved. Spectators stood around and bet with one another on the outcomes of the games. The matches I enjoyed most were between Isaac Kashdan and Israel Albert Horowitz (a great chess editor), and one of their games left me with a lasting impression. They were playing for a dollar a game, and spectators were betting much more (big money in 1936). The game went very fast until there were relatively few pieces on the board, but Kashdan had an extra knight, and I thought a sure win, and apparently so did he. He said, "Why don't you resign?" Horowitz said "Oh, it's a draw, White vs. Cohen, London, 1912," or some such reference. "Oh," said Kashdan, "that's right," and swept the pieces off the board.

This conclusion had a profound impact on me. Not only were these men miles ahead of me already in the study of chess, but, in addition, it was a scholarly occupation offering no future except for a few stars. It already was taking a great deal of my time, and so I decided then and there to go home, play out the year in the league in fairness to the other members of our team. I resolved to do nothing more, and play no special matches. I would then quit playing chess, and I would use the time in more profitable pursuits. We won the league championship again, but I never played what I would call a serious game of chess after that season. At the time, I believed I decided all this almost immediately as a result of the Kashdan-Horowitz game, but it seems more likely that the time-consuming nature of chess had been getting to me for a long time. I needed more time to be with Virginia.

Once in a while I have the urge to play over a few games published in the paper or in a book. One summer, Lincoln Moses gave me a book of end-game problems that were just superb training, so much so that as I worked through them, I gradually became very good at solving the mate-in-two chess problems in the newspapers. Finally, after I had solved about 300 of the 1000 problems, I managed to mislay the book and fortunately have not come across it again. What a time eater! "Just this one more problem," and another half hour is used up.

And so chess was out of my life, and that left room for many other things.

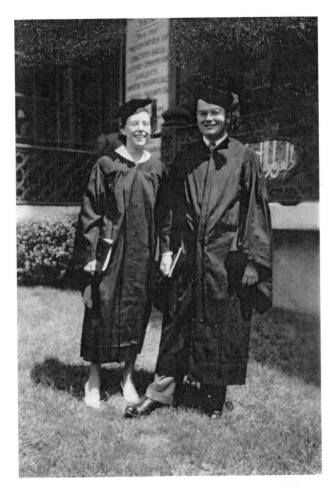

Fig. 9.3. Virginia and Fred at graduation in 1939.

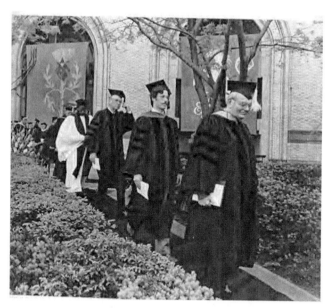

Fig. 9.4. Fred (followed by Jay Kadane) at the commencement ceremony at Carnegie Mellon in which he received an honorary degree in 1974.

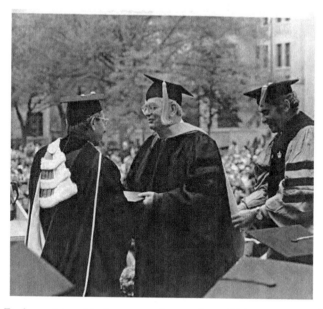

Fig. 9.5. Fred receiving his honorary degree from Richard Cyert, President of Carnegie Mellon University.

10

Graduate Schools: Carnegie and Princeton

All through my undergraduate years, Carnegie had not had a winning football team although it had some first-class players. Two of these players—Kawchak (a guard) and Miskeviks (a center)—were in my class, majoring in mathematics. They were not only first-class players, but they were also doing satisfactory work in the mathematics department. In one year or another each was mentioned on an All-American team. After we graduated, Carnegie decided to have a further fling at big-time football and had recruited many bright small players to the team. In the year I was in graduate school at Carnegie, they won practically all their games. They went to the Sugar Bowl. I was one of the tutors in mathematics for the members of the team. What impressed me was that these athletes needed very little help. They were strong students and mainly just needed time with their books to do well. And so it was enjoyable to tutor them.

For me the key mathematical work in 1938–39 during my graduate year at Carnegie was learning about real variables, an advanced course in analysis very different in tone and idea from the problem-solving courses in calculus, advanced calculus, and mechanics that I had been used to.

I was the only person in the course, and Professor Moskowitz gave his personal time to this tutoring. Because it was a reading course, there were no lectures, and the discussion developed entirely from whatever difficulties I had in writing out solutions to the problems or in reading and understanding the material. Likely a regular class would have been better for me, but I got into the spirit of it after a while, though I could see that it was not the sort of mathematics that I got a lot of fun out of, except for paradoxical matters having to do with sets and infinities. Moskowitz was a very gentle man and very competent. He always wrote very large and legibly. I would remember that years later when I needed to try to correct errors in my derivations.

I had a further enormous human benefit from my experience with Moskowitz. Hitler was gathering himself to seize Europe and to annihilate the Jews, and Moskowitz explained in a passionless but impressive manner some of the horrors that were going on at that time.

F. Mosteller, *The Pleasures of Statistics: The Autobiography of Frederick Mosteller*, DOI 10.1007/978-0-387-77956-0_10,
© Springer Science + Business Media, LLC 2010

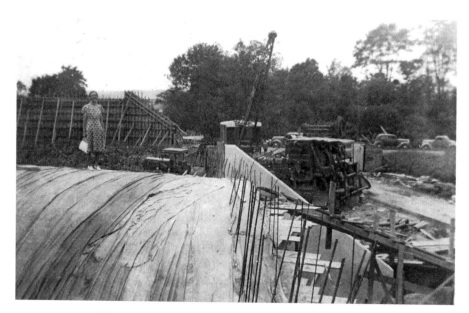

Fig. 10.1. Virginia at a road job in the late 1930s.

★ ★ ★

Near Christmas of 1938, Dr. Olds told me that the meetings of the Institute of Mathematical Statistics were going to be held at the Book-Cadillac Hotel in Detroit and that he thought I should attend. I said that I didn't know whether we could afford it, and he, in his bluff way, said that I couldn't afford not to go. And so my mother and I worked it out. The meeting was very exciting for me. The first person I heard speak was William G. Cochran, who had just come to Iowa State College from Rothamsted Experimental Station in England. I was delighted to realize that I could understand the speaker's presentation very well in spite of my rather meager training in statistics. Little did I realize how rare were speakers with Cochran's clarity.

In the course of a few days I met many statisticians including S. S. Wilks of Princeton, Harold Hotelling of Columbia, Daniel DeLury from Toronto, Allen T. Craig from the University of Iowa, Cecil Craig from the University of Michigan, and many others. Olds's hope was that I would be given a fellowship at Princeton and go there to work with Wilks, but of course money was scarce and so we discussed other possibilities like Michigan and Columbia as well. Wilks was very much in demand at the meeting because he was editor of the journal *Annals of Mathematical Statistics* and one of the principal organizers of the then very small Institute of Mathematical Statistics. When we were sitting beside each other at lunch, Wilks asked me what I was working on. I explained about my master's thesis, which was on kinds of rank correlation coefficients.

Later I very fortunately got an award for Princeton that took care of room, board, and tuition, and in return I had certain duties such as teaching or assisting Wilks edit the *Annals*.

When my mother figured out that I was going to Princeton, she also could see that we were not likely again to be together as we had been for the previous 10 or 11 years. She organized a trip on a ship for us—neither of us had ever been on a ship before. The ship embarked from Philadelphia and went to Boston and then returned to Philadelphia. We went to Philadelphia from Pittsburgh by bus. The trip on the ship was more exciting than we expected. The food was unbelievably extensive in both variety and quantity. After we got used to the roll of the ship, we enjoyed walking about and playing the various games they had available. One day the waves were fairly high and few people came to meals. The great excitement was that the European war was declared while we were at sea. From time to time submarines from different countries would surface suddenly and take a good look at us and then submerge, giving the passengers some thrills and scares. In Boston, we had lunch at the Hotel Vendome. In the end, we went safely back to Philadelphia. My mother went home to Pittsburgh, and I to nearby Princeton.

★ ★ ★

My first two years at Princeton I stayed at the dormitories of the Graduate School. At the graduate dormitories in 1939 and for the next few years, dinner was held in a great hall, and all attending wore black gowns, usually shabby and secondhand. Seating was open, though some groups tended, of course, to sit together. My roommate, Robert Nulsen, was an economist and sometimes we sat with his economics friends—among them Lionel Mackenzie later at the University of Rochester. Nulsen was from California, and I learned how differently people from Los Angeles felt about the weather than we did. We got along very well together and have kept up our acquaintance through the years. He was more interested in practical economics and decided to go into business, where he has been very successful. I sometimes sat with the mathematicians and physicists including Tukey, Richard Feynman, Bryant Tuckerman, and Charles Dolph.

In the spring of my first year at Princeton, Wilks inquired what I planned to do in the coming summer. I said that I would probably work on the road jobs as usual; otherwise I wouldn't have funds to return to graduate school. Departing from his usual roundabout treatment of anything he was not pleased with, Wilks grumbled that this did not seem to be an effective way to become a professional statistician. He said he would be back to me in a few days. He returned with the opportunity of a summer job running IBM punch cards through a counting sorter for Professor Hadley Cantril, social psychologist and head of the Office of Opinion Research.

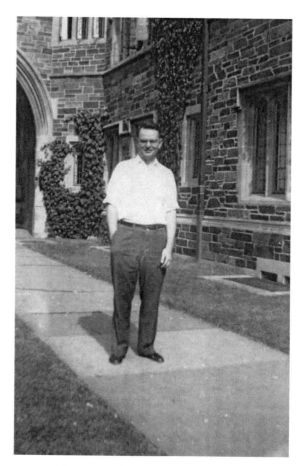

Fig. 10.2. Fred at Princeton, 1940.

Hadley was the first social scientist that I came to know, and he profoundly influenced my life. First, he was important intellectually because he aroused my interest in the affairs of people and encouraged me to develop quantitative approaches to social science problems; second, he started me carrying out research on quantitative matters with substance of more than technological interest; third, he introduced me to teamwork as a way of getting research done; and fourth, he introduced me to many social scientists, one of whom (Samuel Stouffer) ultimately moved me into that professional area.

The summer of 1940, though, was one of running the punch cards through a sorter so that Hadley could analyze the data. One of his students was writing a thesis on the kind of people who respond to polling questions with "don't know" and "no opinion." This seemed a strange question at first, though eight years later I was moved by it in the 1948 elections. Hadley would give me sets of questions and variables that he wanted run as pairs, and I would produce

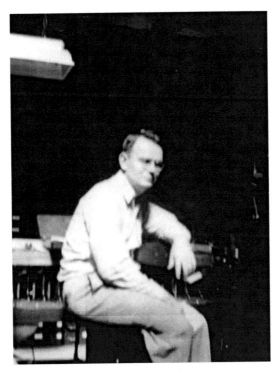

Fig. 10.3. Fred working for Hadley Cantril with the counting sorter during the summer of 1940.

the required contingency tables, relating opinions and preferences to age, sex, education, and socioeconomic status.

In addition to the results from the sorter, he sometimes also wanted a little statistical work—wanting to know what sort of variability the results were subject to. Or he wanted to know whether the relationship that he had found was substantial, or whether it could have come about readily by chance even if there were no relationship. Usually these problems were routine, but I found it exciting that applications of textbook formulas were of genuine concern to a professional psychologist and not merely mathematical exercises that I had done as algebra or probability problems. Now and again, the problems were just enough off the mainstream to make it fun for me to work them out, but not so hard as to be discouraging.

During the summer Virginia came to Princeton for a visit, and just at that time the people running the other IBM sorter were going to take a trip. So Hadley said perhaps Virginia would like to come and run the other sorter while she was visiting. This suited us very well, and we had additional fun while being productive, though we worked in an oven-like attic. Hadley was a behavioral scientist as well as a scholar. He was one of those wonderful people everyone liked from the moment they met him—tall, good-looking, always passing out praise and encouragement, always in good humor, and very patient even when he was in a hurry.

Soon he was organizing teams to write a book about public opinion— *Gauging Public Opinion*—and we wrote many papers based on the data he had collected or obtained from the Gallup organization.

After the summer, he asked me to continue helping with the statistical work, and I did. When World War II started for the United States, he lent me sometimes to Samuel Stouffer at the War Department. That is how I became acquainted with Sam, and probably the primary reason that I went to Harvard in the Department of Social Relations.

By what means it occurred I do not know, but Hadley once a month produced the result of a question asked on a national poll for Franklin Roosevelt. I think the White House set the question, but I am not sure. A lot of thought went into the analysis. On the basis of this one question, the results were set out on one page, often with a graph, just a histogram. Whatever text Hadley prepared had relatively few words, margins were wide, and the page had a great deal of white space. It would have been hard, and would even now be hard, for me to exercise such restraint and trust the reader to supply so much of the interpretation.

★ ★ ★

That summer the psychologist Launor Carter, later of Systems Development Corporation, and I shared an apartment. Through him I met many then young psychologists mentioned in this book.

The second year I roomed with a young man from Texas who was related to friends of Sam Wilks. His name was Ernest Villovasso. During the year we were together we had a happy time. He was studying statistics and making wonderful progress. He especially liked the analysis of many variables that Wilks specialized in. An unfortunate accident led to recurrences of malignancies that caused his early death.

When I went to see Wilks, I had not recalled that he was so young. Indeed, he looked younger than any of his students. In the class ahead of me were George W. Brown and Alexander Mood. My own class consisted of Wilfrid Dixon, a married graduate student, and Philip J. McCarthy. Dixon came from the University of Oregon, where his father-in-law was a mathematics professor, and McCarthy came from Cornell University. Later from conversations with Henry Scheffé, I realized that Dixon and Scheffé had had a very strong course in real analysis back at Oregon, and as my high-school sophomore geometry teacher had enforced with me, they had memorized the important definitions and theorems so that they had them on the tips of their tongues.

The mathematics program was very simple. Nothing was required. Take any courses you want, and prepare yourself in about 4 or 5 fields and pass the language examinations and you are then ready for your orals and you proceed to the dissertation. Sam Wilks taught the one graduate course in statistics.

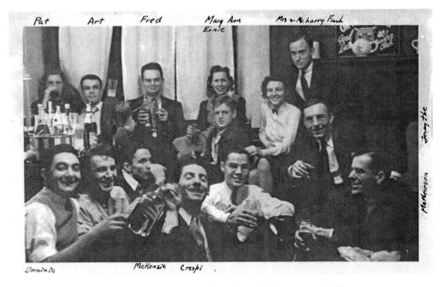

Fig. 10.4. Fred and friends at Princeton, 1940.

When it came time to attend the real variable course at Princeton, probably about 20 years more modern than the one I had had at Carnegie, the teacher told the class that we could have a regular real variable course, but wouldn't we rather have a course on Gödel's new book on the *Consistency of*

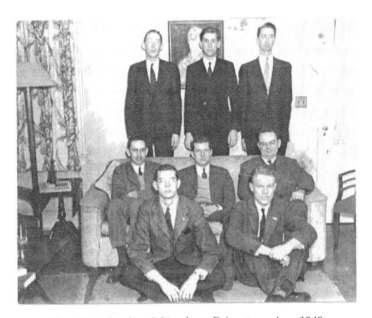

Fig. 10.5. Fred and friends at Princeton, circa 1940.

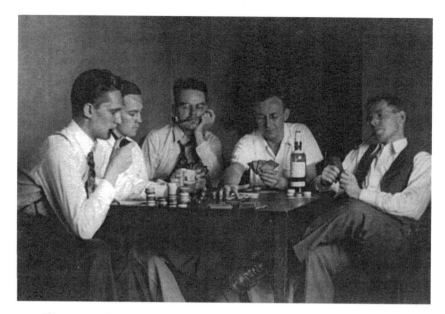

Fig. 10.6. Fred playing poker with friends at Princeton, circa 1940.

the Continuum Hypothesis? As I recall, I was the only voter for the regular course. Most of the students were so far advanced that it was sensible of them to want to get right to the exciting frontiers of the field. I needed more of the equipment most of them had come with.

For learning modern algebra, the primary books were in German by Van der Waerden. Reading this material was satisfactory.

Professor Salomon Bochner was in charge of the graduate student enrollment in courses. He reviewed with each of us what we planned to take in the second semester. I planned to take Bochner's own course in complex variables. When I presented my schedule, Bochner asked about my plan to attend his course in complex variables. He noticed that I had not yet had a course in complex variables, and I said, "Well, if I had already had a course in complex variables, why would I take yours?" Without any affect at all he said, "I don't know, but all the other 30 students have." So again I found out what not being well prepared was all about.

Nevertheless, he called on me in class whenever he was sure that I knew the answer. His was the most educational mathematics class I was ever in, and I have to explain this. He was the first professor that ever tried to tell me what the proofs were all about. He would say, "Here is the idea of the proof for all things like this," and then he would lay out the plan. This was marvelous. And yet there were feet of clay too, because whenever he actually tried to prove something in class, it didn't work out. In this kind of mathematics, you were always supposed to prove that something was going to turn out to be less than a small quantity called epsilon. For Bochner in that first year, it usually turned out to be larger, and he would tell us to go home and figure out the error.

All the professors were very kind to the graduate students. The Albert Tuckers and the Bochners invited us to their homes, and Gena and Sam Wilks had us in frequently, as did a young instructor, Tommy Tompkins, whose course in calculus of variations I took.

My statistics reading at this time was of two kinds outside of class. Because I was helping Wilks with the editing of the *Annals*, I was familiar with nearly all the papers that were being published there. One picks up a great deal even when one is just copy-editing a manuscript and marking it for the printer. I also read a great deal in the wonderful mathematics and physics library in the old Fine Hall. I mainly read *Biometrika* and the *Journal of the Royal Statistical Society*. Everything about the library, the tables and chairs, and lighting, invited one to read and study.

Wilks had given me a specific paper to look up and report on in a journal called *Terrestrial Magnetism*. Margaret Shields, the small woman who was librarian, was a new sort of person to me. I innocently asked where this journal was. This was my first occasion to speak with her. She told me exactly how many columns of shelves to pass, and I began to go where she told me when she passed me like a whirlwind (she did wear tennis shoes). By the time I got there, she was scolding more or less as follows, "I told Professor Lefschetz we would get into trouble by buying a broken set even though it was inexpensive, and now you want Volume 1 and we do not have it. This is just terrible. I'll have to inform Professor Lefschetz at once." I didn't want Professor Lefschetz, head of the department, bothered on my behalf at all, but she was not to be stopped. In a very few hours I had a note from her in my mailbox telling me when a copy of the first volume would be available for me. Over the years she did many wonderful things for the graduate students. Library problems were her pride and fun.

⋆ ⋆ ⋆

Virginia and I married in the summer of 1941, and I moved out of the graduate dormitories.

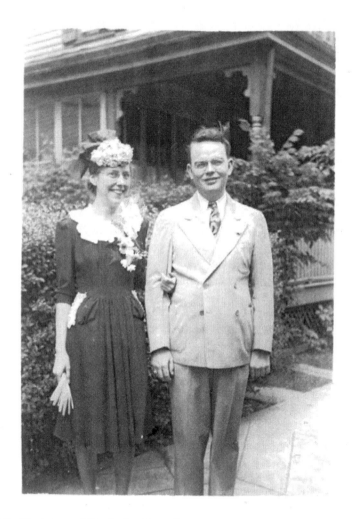

Fig. 10.7. Virginia and Fred, the Mosteller newlyweds, in 1941 on their wedding day.

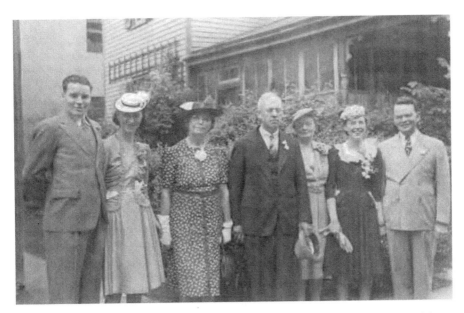

Fig. 10.8. Charles and Mary Lou Jeffrey, Virginia's brother-in-law and sister; Mary and Alfred Gilroy, Virginia's parents; and Helen Mosteller, Fred's mother; with Virginia and Fred on their wedding day, 1941 at The Manse, Princeton.

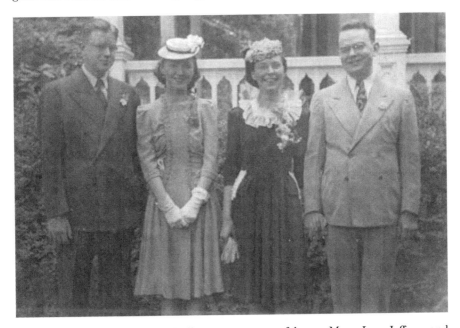

Fig. 10.9. Best man Ernest Villovasso, matron of honor Mary Lou Jeffrey, and Virginia and Fred on their wedding day in 1941 at The Manse, Princeton.

★ ★ ★

Between classes, travels, committee meetings, and long-distance phone calls, one rarely could catch Wilks doing his own work, but a glimpse at him getting out final copy for an issue of the *Annals* may provide some insight. Since the Wilks family loved to give hospitality, on a typical evening a visiting fireman would have been encouraged to stay on for yet another train (because Sam had no plans at all for the evening), and the guest was finally taken to Princeton Junction about 10 P.M. As the train pulled out, Sam would begin to express uneasiness about the need to get out the next issue of the *Annals*. He would wonder whether he shouldn't spend a few minutes on that yet tonight, and conviction would grow in him that he should, indeed. He supposed that his graduate assistant would not care to join him because the hour was so late. Surely a half hour or so would do the whole thing. Driving to the office, he would begin to list the dozens of little matters that needed attention. And finally after a furious half-night's work the packages would be mailed at the Princeton Post Office around 3 A.M. The next morning he was likely to be on the 7 A.M. train to New York City.

References

Cantril, H. and Research Associates in the Office of Public Opinion Research, Princeton University (1944). *Gauging Public Opinion*. Princeton, NJ: Princeton University Press.

Gödel, K. (1940). *The Consistency of the Continuum Hypothesis*. Princeton, NJ: Princeton University Press.

11

Magic

One day in 1941 when Fred Williams and I were organizing some public opinion data by using IBM sorters, he delighted me by doing a magic trick with a cigarette. He said that, if I wished, I could join a magic club on the campus. It met about every two weeks on Sunday evenings. The price of admission was a trick that you performed yourself. Although I had no trick, after I came the first time, someone lent me a book, and I was soon studying hard.

When I was a freshman in high school, the year I spent alone in Delaware, Ohio, I had tried to find out about magic both at the town library and at Ohio Wesleyan University's impressive one. Although both libraries had substantial holdings in the anthropological areas of magic and religion, I could not find anything that would help me learn to do things I had seen Houdini do back in Wilkinsburg, PA., or Thurston in Charleroi, PA, or Blackstone in some other little town where I worked in the summer.

The intellectual leader of our magic group was Professor Frank Taylor of the Department of Psychology at Princeton. He was a wizard at sleight of hand as well as an inventor of commercially sold tricks. Among these was the Taylor Peek Deck. The effect is that the participant chooses a random card from a deck, and the magician reads his mind and names the card. In another lengthy routine, he manipulated half dollars so that they multiplied their number and divided again to the accompaniment of a continuous flow of amusing patter, some of which mattered. For example, at a key moment he said, "At this point other magicians put a hand in a pocket, like this, but I don't do that, instead ... ."

The club was not large; it had a few undergraduates, one or two faculty members, and one or two graduate students. We also had frequent visitors who were club alumni, just passing through town. I do not know whether the club had an official existence at the University.

At first, it was all I could do to perform the preset tricks described in the book I had borrowed. I began buying inexpensive devices from magic shops and generally having the lark I had hoped for when I was younger. After

F. Mosteller, *The Pleasures of Statistics: The Autobiography of Frederick Mosteller*,
DOI 10.1007/978-0-387-77956-0_11,
© Springer Science + Business Media, LLC 2010

buying some beautiful little, shiny, red billiard balls, a delight to handle, I
tried to learn how to make them multiply and disappear.

For anyone starting on magic late in life, as I did, it probably is wise not to
plan on being a great sleight-of-hand artist but some other kind of magician.
Even after long hours of practice on billiard-ball tricks or manipulating cards
before mirrors, I was dissatisfied with my performance. These concerns flowed
not only from lack of smoothness in the execution, but also from the failure to
perform what I regarded as a genuine miracle. Although I admired, enjoyed,
and was entertained by sleight-of-hand work when done by others, for me to do
it was not personally satisfying because I would always say to myself, "It isn't
a miracle because it's sleight of hand." This attitude still seems ridiculous,
but how can one account for one's scruples and aspirations?

As time went on I worked on "true" miracles. When they speak of tricks as
having "effects," magicians refer to the way someone who saw the trick might
reasonably describe the conditions under which it was done and what the
consequences were. At the same time, the effects do not necessarily describe
the true or relevant conditions any more than an autobiography is the truth
about a life. For example, I had invented a good trick whose effect was that
the subject called a randomly chosen phone number (three digits in Princeton
then) and asked the person who answered to tell what card the subject had
chosen from a well-shuffled ordinary pack of playing cards, and the correct
answer was forthcoming. This trick couldn't be used regularly, because how
often can a random phone call bring one's wife to the phone? Still, it was good
enough for our little club because the members appreciated the preparation
others put into their illusions. One young man, after a miracle he did not
fathom, used to say, "I'm going to shoot myself."

Although I wanted to create miracles, I knew that the general public could
not distinguish one set of conditions from another. For a lay audience, the most
trivial trick well done has just as high astonishment value as a miracle done
under ironclad, Price-Waterhouse audited magical conditions. For the most
part, the viewer has no notion of what the outcome of a trick is to be, let
alone a checklist of conditions or time to pull wits together amid deliberate
distractions. Therefore a true miracle cannot be appreciated by a general
audience, and so what is the payoff for the inventor? Two come to mind.
When a perfect trick is built, it walks its way through the steps with the
overpowering inevitability of the proof of a mathematical theorem. It gives a
satisfaction of total control, a warm, finished feeling. Second, you baffle your
professional colleagues, or at least win their respect and attention.

It surprises me today that, after only a few months as a total amateur in
magic, I knew exactly what I wanted to do, whereas at the same time, though
years more mature in my professional life, I was just wandering and had no
clear purpose in mind. How was I to create a true miracle, especially when
my sleight of hand was bound to be weak? I read about a few tricks that
depended on mathematics, but I didn't care for them because the bones of
the mathematics protruded enough that for me they marred the effect even

though a layman might enjoy them. After all, in principle it's the performance that counts, not the trick, but I could not accept that for myself. I struggled to think how to create a miracle, and found it hard to get an idea.

I explained my frustration to Taylor, and he solved the problem. Taylor advised me to think of an effect I would like to create, and then to figure out a way of doing it. This advice appealed to me: think of the theorem, then try to prove it. After a week or two, I was able to think of effects I wanted to create, and then turn to the research problem of finding a way. From that time on, I had no more trouble thinking of tricks to do and inventing them, though the inventions were slow—miracles don't reveal themselves overnight. Taylor's secret is to think of a miracle you would like to perform and then just treat it as a homework problem. After a while you will likely solve it. Starting with the answer was a major breakthrough.

My first miracle was that the subject should merely think of one of the 52 cards in an ordinary playing deck, and then the magician would identify it. It took me some weeks to work out a method, and when presented at the magic club it received tremendous applause, because not only was one person's card identified, but several different persons' thoughts could be read simultaneously. That is, several people could simultaneously and independently think of a card, and all their cards would be identified. That's real mind reading!

About this time our club members met Bruce Elliott, who, with Walter Gibson, edited the magic magazine *The Phoenix*. That was a labor of love. To make a living, Elliott at this time wrote pulp stories and scripts for radio. For example, when Walter Gibson, creator of The Shadow, went on vacation, Elliott would take over and write stories about The Shadow, one magazine-length story each month and a script a week for the radio program. Elliott would add these to his other writing and editing chores. Gibson was also a magic buff. Taylor had me show Elliott my trick, and he published it, and I received some free issues of *The Phoenix* in return for what is now known as the Mosteller Spelling Trick. I would say it is the finest of my four or five published tricks. In all modesty, I can say that it is a true miracle, though I'll never perform it again. One reason is Elliott's preliminary explanation to the reader of *The Phoenix*. After puffing the effect of the spelling trick, which he called "Bravo," he says, "We are positive that our readers are going to scream with anguish when they read the amount of preparation necessary," and then later, "If you can crawl into the room under the weight [of the equipment], the trick works automatically."

The reader may feel thwarted that I do not explain how the tricks are done, but magicians never tell. They are happy to have you read the explanation in a magic book or magazine, but disapprove of telling how. What the origin of this morality may be, I am not certain. Perhaps long experience has shown that when a person has been told how a trick was done, he or she then backlashes with "Oh, well, if that's all there is to it, anybody could do that," or some similar deflationary remark. Then, one wishes one had not told. When you have to learn it for yourself, it doesn't seem so easy.

The mentalist and magician Dunninger adapted the spelling trick with an improvement which left the subject with a souvenir of the occasion and incidentally made it a little surer that the subject didn't make ruinous mistakes. Subjects often destroy miracles by forgetting or by making little errors. Dunninger's addition was a little printed card that said something like DUNNINGER WILL SPELL YOUR CARD, with spaces on it for the spelling. What a proud moment when a genuine professional uses and improves your trick! My statistician and magician friend Persi Diaconis, who keeps up to date in magic, tells me that the spelling trick is widely performed even today; with new variations being introduced, it has had a revival.

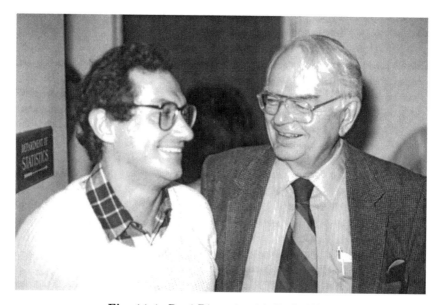

Fig. 11.1. Persi Diaconis with Fred, 1987.

On TV one night, I saw a mentalist performing my Book Test. From a library, a random book, page, and line is chosen, and the magician turns out to have pre-identified the statement found there; at least that is the effect. Needless to say, such a miracle takes a little preparation, and this one has, when I performed it, a scary moment for the magician when it can all come unstuck, and so it does not have the steady inexorable movement I prize. If it had not been for this unique and difficult move, I could not have recognized my Book Test in the TV show because there are many book tests. When the move came, I could only gasp in admiration because the mentalist had fitted that move into his whole pattern of behavior, and for him there was nothing jerky about it, whereas the move did not suit my personality. I guess I never enjoyed the performing as much as the inventing.

When I was teaching courses in quality control, my friends encouraged me to do some magic along with the statistical ideas. And I used to do that. The students seemed to like it. Later I did a little magic during my regular classes just to liven things up. I like to present students with actual demonstrations of random events such as drawing random collections of balls of different colors out of a box to illustrate statistical principles—not only to show with formulas what sort of variation we can expect with various sample sizes but also to give demonstrations that show what happens when we try to practice what we preach. When you mix magic with proof, you are expecting too much of the audience—they cannot be expected to believe that you are being honest about the demonstrations one minute and that you are fooling them the next. Therefore one has to choose between entertainment, which helps instruction a great deal, and squareness if one wants belief. And so I stopped doing magic in class.

After that, I stopped doing magic altogether. Like piano playing or any other skilled activity, it requires time to maintain skill and to keep in touch with the profession, and I had a profession already.

Although I never do magic any more, watching others do it still is great entertainment. Sometimes I know how a trick may have been done, and sometimes not. I feel sorry for people who are concerned when they can't figure the trick out, or who want to do something to mess up the magician's act, and make the trick fail. Tricks fail often enough without meanness. Perhaps such viewers would be helped by remembering that magic is entertainment rather than an insult to one's intelligence. One should realize that a magician may go to enormous trouble to create an effect. If you have a chance to help a magician, give him or her a lift.

When my daughter Gale was about six, she complained that she wanted me to do "the real magic." Today's real magic comes from science and technology. Who would believe that we can hear someone speaking from 10,000 miles away, or that they could see the actions of someone thousands of miles away, or that water would flow out of a hole when you turn a knob, or that you could go around the world in a couple of days? Or that you could float a rock on water and it would point south? Although as a child I saw Blackstone, Thurston, and Houdini perform more than once, and they pleased me, nothing they did is as impossible as what an airplane does, zipping along with no visible means of support. Still, as Persi Diaconis reminds me, people have been comparing magical entertainment with science and technology for hundreds of years, and like me they still enjoy these illusions.

When I worked in New York City in the 1940s, I came across an erudite book by Erdnase on card magic, or possibly how to cheat at cards. Jimmie Savage wanted to learn a little about magic, and so I lent him this book. Jimmie loved it for two reasons. First, the author said he wrote the book because he needed the money. Second, Erdnase treats each problem much like a mathematics text would. He has names for various devices such as false shuffling (riffling cards but leaving them in the original order), and he tells

12

Beginning Research

At Carnegie, working with E. G. Olds, I had a small taste of research, partly from my work for Olds and partly from my master's thesis written with him. Still these did not do much to prepare me for research later. At Princeton, Wilks's idea was that his students should produce a research paper early on to get them into the swing of such things and also to put Wilks himself in the position of being able to prove to the mathematics faculty, when the question of advancing to the doctoral dissertation came up, that the student could do publishable research. He proposed that I examine the distribution of runs above and below the mean.

The general idea was that one took measurements, say on successively manufactured objects; these measurements are ordered in time. The measurements divide themselves into two classes—those higher than the mean (the average of all the measurements) and those lower than the mean. For example, there might be only two runs in a set of 12 measurements, such as LLLLL-HHHHHHH with L standing for a measurement lower than the mean and H for one higher than the mean. In this notation a run is a succession of identical letters; the example has one run of Ls and one of Hs. Such a sequence would rather suggest a time trend in the data. Or we might have a different sequence, like LHLHLHLHLHLH, showing a great many runs, here 12. Such a sequence would suggest something jumpy about the manufacturing process.

This distribution problem proved rather difficult to solve, but I found it comparatively easy to solve a problem very similar to it. This second problem asked for the distribution of the number of runs above and below the median (the middle measurement in an odd-sized sample, or the average of the middle two for an even size) rather than the mean. For example, with 4 measurements 2, 3, or 4 runs are all equally likely. To see this, we can write out the six possible equally likely arrangements together with their numbers of runs:

HHLL 2	HLLH 3	LHLH 4
HLHL 4	LHHL 3	LLHH 2

F. Mosteller, *The Pleasures of Statistics: The Autobiography of Frederick Mosteller*, DOI 10.1007/978-0-387-77956-0_12,
© Springer Science + Business Media, LLC 2010

Each number of runs 2, 3, and 4 occurs twice, and so each has probability 2/6 or 1/3 of occurring.

I produced tables to go with the formulas that I worked out and gave them to Wilks so that he could see what they looked like and could decide whether he wanted something more or different from what I had done. When I asked him after a couple of weeks of silence how he liked them, he said, "What tables?" Somehow they had vanished, never to reappear, and a couple of weeks' worth of calculation on an old-style mechanical desk calculator had to be done over. That evanishment taught me an important lesson. Make a copy—in those days a carbon copy. Copying was not as easy or inexpensive as it is now. I had given him a handwritten table, not a typed one.

When the paper was ready for publication, Wilks showed it to Walter Shewhart, who in turn showed it to Paul Olmstead. Shewhart provided a footnote about his own contributions to the use of runs in quality control. Olmstead produced some tables somewhat different in plan from mine, but based on the same formulas and requested that I publish them along with mine; otherwise he said they never would be published because, at that time, publishing a paper through his organization was too laborious a process just for these tables. Encouraged by Wilks, I added these materials to the paper, giving credit to Olmstead. Today I don't know how I would feel about adding all these things without offering coauthorship to the other participants, but then I was too innocent to give the matter a thought. I just wanted the paper accepted for publication—what every author wants.

The problem about runs above and below the mean was ultimately solved, I believe, by H. T. David in his doctoral dissertation at the University of Chicago.

After my paper was accepted, it occurred to me that a nice topic for a doctoral thesis would deal with the distributions of runs up and down. For example, suppose we have measurements in a sequence as follows: 1.4, 2.5, 5.1, 10.3, 7.6, 8.4, 9.7. Among these 7 measurements, the first 4 rise, the next one falls, and then the rest rise. In runs, depending on how you count, we have a run up of 4 $(1.4, 2.5, 5.1, 10.3)$, a run down of 2 $(10.3, 7.6)$, followed by a run up of 3 $(7.6, 8.4, 9.7)$. One question is, under random arrangements of the values, how often is the longest run of at least 4? Or how many runs are there on the average, and so on? I made considerable progress on such questions for runs up and down.

I heard that W. Allen Wallis and Geoffrey Moore were giving a paper at the 1941 annual meeting of the Institute of Mathematical Statistics in New York City exactly on the topic of runs up and down. New York wasn't far from Princeton, and so I went to the session where Wallis presented a paper very beautifully. So beautifully that it was sickening. Wallis and Moore had half the results I had worked so hard to get. It was nice meeting Wallis because he was so enthusiastic about everything. Wallis and Moore were analyzing economic time series, whereas I was thinking in terms of quality-control problems. One participant complained that von Bortkiewicz had done all this work before. In a characteristic move, from his briefcase Wallis pulled the book referred to and said that he had looked for these results and had not found them there, and offered the book to the participant to peruse. The latter didn't try, claiming that you had to read between the lines.

Not long after that meeting, Jacob Wolfowitz published one of his many papers, and this one carried the rest of the results I had found together with much more. Thus, that thesis topic evaporated. It was not such an unusual tragedy. Mathematicians who work on well-known problems have this difficulty all the time. Because a problem often takes a very specific form, it is not like painting a picture, where another painting of even the same cathedral can be original (though sometimes the new proof of a theorem can be). Mathematicians often work on exactly the same question, and so it is not surprising that multiple inventions occur.

An extreme example occurred when Alexander Mood worked on his thesis. He had worked on an important problem on distribution of several variables. Naturally, an important problem in any field does not go unnoticed, and the strongest people in the field try to solve it. About the time Alex handed in his thesis, four different famous statisticians published the essential results in three different journals around the world: R. A. Fisher, A. Girshick, P. L. Hsu, and S. N. Roy. In those days, this sent the student back to the drawing board.

Fortunately, Mood had another thesis topic he was working on—the general theory of runs of several kinds of elements. The simplest of these is the distribution of the number of successes and failures that occur in a row, just as in the runs problem I described earlier. For example, suppose S stands for success and F for failure. Then a sequence like SSSFSSSSSFFFSF has in all 14 trials and 6 runs, 3 runs of Ss and 3 of Fs. The longest run, 5, consists of Ss. Mood had a general theory of how runs would behave for given numbers of trials, even when there were several kinds of elements—like balls being drawn from an urn with replacement, the balls being of various colors, say, red, blue, yellow, and so on, and each having its own chance of being drawn. For example, if the number of trials is large enough, runs of almost any length will be sure to occur. This means that, if we maintain a longstanding sequence of records as we do in baseball, it is almost certain that a record will be tied or broken sooner or later.

Later in my life I often came back to runs of various kinds in practical problems, and a graduate student, Mikiso Mizuki, wrote a thesis with me on runs occurring in more complicated processes. For example, suppose that categories a, b, c, d can occur with various probabilities; then we might have a sequence like abacccdaabcbad.... If the sequence is 1000 letters long, how many times will the sub-sequence abcd occur in successive letters, or how many times will baaad occur? Mizuki studied such run problems under much more general conditions than Mood or I did. Mizuki does not assume independence between successive outcomes but allows more complicated relations.

When I wrote this chapter in 1988, the Boston Red Sox had broken their own all-time record for the number of games won in a row at home, and they were tied with the most games won in a row at home in the American League. It is astonishing that this should be true when they had had a most mediocre first half of the season, but the idea that *they* might break a record is surprising—not that *some* team should break a record. It is the business of sports statistics to make records that can be broken. That is part of the excitement of the game.

New York in 1944–45

During the early part of the United States's involvement in World War II, I was teaching algebra and trigonometry to Navy and Marine students, helping Hadley Cantril at the Office of Opinion Research, and consulting for the Research Branch of the War Department designing sample surveys and occasionally participating in carrying them out. Through this consulting I met Samuel A. Stouffer. He was Director of Professional Staff of the Research Branch, Information and Education Division, in the War Department (later at Harvard he led the writing team that prepared three of the four volumes on the American Soldier).

At the same time I tried to work on my thesis. Wilks was not around much because he traveled a lot to Washington and elsewhere at this time, and so I had little intellectual support. The new thesis moved very slowly. Under Wilks's direction, the Statistical Research Group of Princeton included, among others, William G. Cochran, Philip J. McCarthy, and Alexander M. Mood. They worked on many sorts of problems, one being to design efficient attacks on submarines.

Also in Princeton, George W. Brown, Wilfrid J. Dixon, Paul Dwyer, Albert W. Tucker, John W. Tukey, and Charles P. Winsor, among others, worked under the direction of Merrill Flood at Fire Control Research, an organization that researched a variety of problems for the Army and Air Force. Virginia was Merrill's secretary. We lived on Bank Street, a narrow one-block-long street beside the building where she worked.

Wilks decided to set up an additional branch of the Statistical Research Group of Princeton in support of the strategic air force. (Among ourselves we called this branch SRGPJr.) This office, under the direction of John D. Williams, was stationed in New York in the same building as the Statistical Research Group of Columbia, which was a titan. Williams was an astronomer with a considerable engagement in statistics—astronomers have lots of statistical problems.

I had gotten to know Williams between 1939–41 through Brown and Mood, because they liked to play bridge. I knew little about bridge, but I enjoyed playing, and so sometimes we would have a foursome at Williams's home. Mood was a mad bridge player. He felt then that if you were playing bridge, you basically should be playing for slam or at least game. Scores ran high

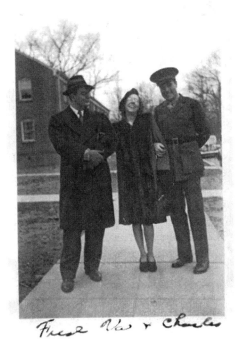

Fig. 12.1. Fred and Virginia visiting with Charles Jeffrey, Virgina's brother in law, who was in the Marines, in 1944.

both ways, for he often failed to make his contract, though it was a great deal of fun because we never played for money, only for bragging privileges.

Wilks and Williams told me that I would be moving to the new office in New York to work with Williams. This was a surprise and a twist, but Virginia and I packed up and left, and Virginia became the secretary to W. Allen Wallis, head of the Statistical Research Group of Columbia. It wasn't quite that fast; I commuted for some months by train before we moved to New York City. Housing was scarce.

The group I worked in was small and young. It consisted of Olaf Helmer, a German philosopher of science and a mathematician; Cecil Hastings, Jr., a man who loved to work with numbers and tables; Jimmie Savage, borrowed from SRG-Columbia; Stewart Cairns and Edwin N. Oberg, who usually worked at Air Force bases; and John Williams, with his wife Evie as secretary. John rented a house owned by the statistician C. J. Clopper, who with Egon Pearson had published charts of confidence limits for binomial proportions (proportions of successes).

John liked to go to airfields to gather problems for our shop directly from experienced officers there, though sometimes problems came through other channels. He brought many concrete problems with strict deadlines. This feature was a very important part of my education.

John would launch the problem by going to a chalkboard and giving us a short statement. Sometimes he used his sense of humor in the introduction—essentially saying that we were not going to believe that this is what they want to know, but they do. Then after he had described the problem, he would sit down and sip coffee for the opening part of the discussion, answering what questions we had, but not offering comments on our proposed plans. He liked to soak up the discussion, then come to some conclusions about it and deliver some pungent views at the end. Sometimes he chose among approaches, and sometimes he condemned some because he could see that we hadn't time before the delivery deadline to carry out some of the more ambitious programs.

In our discussions we would try to pull the problem apart into workable chunks. People would volunteer for parts. Then we would go away and work on volunteered or assigned parts. One idea that was new to me was having problems that had to be done by a given date. You might think that ordinary homework problems in my courses would have given me this idea, but homework problems are ordinarily fairly short with definite ends. Moreover, they have usually been designed so that the reader using the methods he or she has just learned can solve them fairly readily. Thus the idea of delivery of all or nearly all homework problems finished by a given date was not out of line. When research questions are new and the problem has to be created from scratch through mathematical modeling, it is not so easy to tell how long it will take to solve the problem, or even whether it has any solution. We learned quickly that, because all the problems had a deadline, it was important to make workable assumptions. And we learned to do what we could in the length of time allotted.

Thus, we turned out many small reports which went to the particular officer or branch that had ordered the work. We had only a few of the larger telephone-book-size reports that other organizations turned out. This happened because John was willing to work on very specific problems thrown out by the operating people even though the problem seemed not to have general mathematical, statistical, or operations research interest.

Before we came together, others had done a great deal of work on train bombing. The idea was thus: an airplane is going to release bombs one after another. What spacing is best if a target is to be hit by at least one of the bombs, allowing for both aiming error and variability in the behavior of the bombs? The trouble with this problem was that the forces in the field weren't using train bombing. Instead, bombers went over Europe in formations and dropped their bombs more or less simultaneously on a signal from a leader, using a single aiming point for all the bombers in the group.

I worked with Jimmie Savage on several problems. He was a brilliant mathematician who loved to solve every problem from scratch, ideally by himself, while giving little lectures to his colleagues. Solving out loud had the effect of both maintaining communication and also preventing others from thinking of an alternate approach. One problem Jimmie, John, and I worked on to-gether dealt with the merits of using an airplane full-time to assist in weather forecasts—a weatherplane.

The problem arose because weather in certain Pacific areas was very un-certain, and a bombing raid in bad weather was likely to produce a very large aiming error. This had been one of the findings in a regression model relating size of aiming error to many variables for describing the flight, such as the altitude from which bombs were dropped, airspeed, and strength of fighter op-position. The equation clearly showed that the amount of fighter opposition influenced the size of the error: the more opposition, the smaller the error! Unless one noticed that the equation contained nothing about the weather, this was hard to fathom. When the weather was highly overcast, why send fighters against the bombers? The bombers weren't going to hit a target of military value anyway. Thus the amount of fighter opposition was probably measuring weather rather than improving the aim of the bombardiers. (A re-gression equation with 10 predictors took a day or two to compute with a desk calculator then.)

Because it was SRGPJr's first big effort in connection with the Pacific war, and a job for an air-force organization new to us, we had worked for several days and long evenings trying to get this report into shape. Although we had drafted a solid story about the weather plane, Jimmie was dissatisfied. We had the paper written, typed, and reproduced, and Williams and I were going together to Washington to explain it in case someone wanted a briefing. Jimmie believed that we had a much better way to evaluate the merits of the plane than we had carried out. We had more or less proved that the weather plane was worthwhile, but Jimmie wanted a more decision-oriented approach that better explained what would be gained—a sort of cost-benefit analysis. This we had not provided. Von Neumann and Morgenstern's work on game theory was new at this time, and Wald's work on decision theory was just being written. Abraham Wald was a member of the Columbia Group.

This new way of putting it intrigued Williams, and so he proposed that we all take the train together to Washington, discussing the matter as we went; we'd make any changes in the report on the way, get any required new typing at dawn in Washington, and deliver the report on time. Of course, this wrecked whatever plans Jimmie and his family had for a couple of days, and Jimmie didn't like working late hours. He rose early like many scholars and others who feel that they do their best work in the morning. In contrast, I always liked to work late and often worked all night. Being an astronomer, this may have been natural for Williams as well. He too was a late worker. Anyway, we all went. (Years later, after Jimmie gave the Ronald A. Fisher Memorial Lecture to the statistical societies, Jimmie told me, "I did a John Williams to get this lecture done. I couldn't write it down though I had done the reading, and so finally I stayed up all night to finish it.")

It may sound as if we were in agreement that Jimmie had a good idea. That was not quite the situation. What was before us was that Jimmie felt the report was unsatisfactory as it stood and needed this new approach to deliver the goods convincingly. Neither John nor I felt that was true, but we couldn't convince Jimmie. We knew Jimmie was opinionated as well as brilliant, but not mulish. When you had an argument with Jimmie, he loved to help you with your side of the argument as well as delivering his own, and sometimes he found that he lost. Consequently, it was unwise to overrule him when he was so adamant. On the train, we buckled down to work, and after a while Jimmie persuaded us to use his approach. Then we had a great flurry of rewriting the report. I was not as quick at composing then as I am now, Jimmie was then a slow and painful writer, and a bouncing train didn't help. When we got to Washington in the evening, we still had a good bit to do, and it was 2 A.M. before we got to bed. Early to rise, we rushed out to a place where John had mysterious friends who would help with typing and reproduction, and we were able to take the report on time to a beautifully dressed Air Force colonel. He took it and thanked us, saying "I hope it wasn't any trouble." Nobody wanted a briefing. As with many of our reports, we did not find out the consequences of our work.

Trying to meet firm deadlines by doing late night work once led to some embarrassment. We had a problem about the effectiveness of air-to-air bombing (one airplane trying to bomb another with both in flight) that became urgent for us to complete. We went to work to find out how likely a B-29 was to be hit in a bombing attempt. Once we got the assumptions in good order, it was not hard to simulate the procedure, because we had special graph paper that helped us a great deal.

Around 2 A.M. as we were completing the runs for the last few tables, I had a thought, and I turned to John and said, "Is there any possibility that the Air Force doesn't want to bomb B-29s but was thinking about enemy planes?" John thought about this for about ten seconds and said, "Colonel X is probably going to be surprised to get a call at this time in the morning." Then he mercilessly drove the call to Florida through a lot of officers who couldn't believe the Colonel wanted to hear from us at that time. It turned out that the Air Force was not asking about the danger of B-29s but did want to consider attacking enemy planes in this way. It was not hard to redo the tables because we knew how to handle the problem.

John never understood people who talked about the need for courage to make suggestions or deal with authority. His view was that the difficult matter was to get wisdom and facts and originality. Anybody could have courage he believed, and should not get extra credit for it.

In any large organization special groups tend to be viewed as a nuisance and any excuse can serve to get rid of them. In the bombing field at that time, special missiles had been designed to improve the probability of hitting special targets. Three of these were called Azon, Razon, and Felix. Azon was a bomb whose flight could be somewhat controlled in azimuth (left and right) and so could be used against a long narrow target like a road or a railway. Razon was a more complicated version; it could be somewhat controlled in both range and azimuth (forward and backward as well as left and right) so as to hit small targets such as a bridge, even a short one. Both Azon and Razon were controlled by an operator in the plane dropping the bomb. Operators were helped by a flare in the tail of the bomb, and they moved a small "stick" to various positions to guide the path as the bomb fell. Operators were trained in simulators on the ground. Felix, named for a cat, possibly because it could "see" in the dark, was a forerunner of some of the missiles available today. It was a heat-homer, that is, it hunted for spots where the change in heat was greatest. It might be useful for attacking a ship because of the differential between the temperature of the water and that of the ship.

Our group, SRGPJr., had some responsibility for helping to design experiments on the optimal handling of such special weapons, and my first airplane ride was to Florida from New York for such work. Forty-five years and hundreds of flights later I know now that this was the worst flight I have ever had; nearly everyone on the flight was ill, and I was very uncomfortable as well as terrified. I said to Jimmie, "How can they talk of how beautiful flying is?" He looked up from the bag he was depositing his breakfast into and mumbled, "It isn't always like this."

To get back to the bombs, at the office we got a call from Washington that someone from our group had to go to testify before a top scientific panel about the value of these special weapons. It seemed that someone had found out that the average aiming error (distance from target) for some of these guided missiles was larger than that for ordinary bombs. If that were true, then surely these weapons had no special value and the whole program could profitably be wiped out. John Williams was far away in the field, and so I was sent to report what we knew. It is a standard statistical difficulty that having just one statistic about a problem may not be adequate. People often say that averages may be misleading, and for many purposes they are right. In the instance at hand, when I came to testify before the panel led by Warren Weaver, they asked me first whether it was true that the average error was bigger or at least as big for Azon, say, as for ordinary bombs. I had to tell them that we had some data to that effect. Next they wanted to know how it was possible with average aiming errors of, say, 500 feet that we could have much chance of hitting a road, say, 25 feet wide.

The answer, of course, lay in the temperamental nature of the mechanisms. The bombs were controlled by radios and mechanical fins. Although the equipment people worked hard to make sure they were in good repair, sometimes the mechanisms failed, and when they did the fins tended to lock into an extreme position. Then the bomb would go as far from the path of the plane as possible. Before dropping the bomb, the plane ordinarily lined up on the target road if possible, and so when the mechanism failed, the error would be huge—much larger than an ordinary bomb would have produced. When the mechanism was working properly, the average error was very small, on the order of 10 or 20 feet. When one averages a few errors of 5000 feet with small numbers like 10 feet and 20 feet, the result can readily be 500 on the average. For example, if 10 percent were 5000 and 90 percent were 0, the average is 500. Thus this huge aiming error could reflect 90 percent hits and 10 percent wild misses. That example would be a bit optimistic, but it carries the idea.

The committee of distinguished scientists went over this carefully and asked what data we had. I always thought that these scientists probably understood this whole story before I came, but they had been asked to investigate and so they did. The example illustrates well the problem with averages when averages are not the proper payoff.

Williams developed big treatments when we had a general problem. Sometimes John's problems were very difficult, and we twitted him that some day he would bring Fermat's last theorem to be done by Tuesday. Williams took me to see Warren Weaver (whom many people spoke of as Uncle Warren, and whom John revered), who was head of the Applied Mathematics Panel of the National Defense Research Committee. John mentioned that his staff had worried that he would bring home such a problem, and Weaver laughed and said essentially, "Well, John, if I thought it were possible to actually answer some of these questions in a reasonable length of time, I wouldn't ask a statistician at all, but since the answers are not likely to be gotten, we might as well ask a statistician to make a good guess because that's what he is trained to do." John enjoyed this.

Right after this John did bring home a terribly difficult problem, one we had known for some time that we did not know how to handle. The bombing people wanted to know how often a place would have to be bombed if a given piece of it had to be hit repeatedly, say three times, before it was destroyed. The general idea is that a pattern of bombs is laid and that this forms a region of destruction. If patterns are dropped, then because of aiming error, they would not hit the same place but there might be some overlap. The overlap region then would have been hit twice, but only part of that overlap (or none) might be inside the target region that required multiple destruction. This problem, when one considered aiming error, size and shape of target, multiplicity of hits required, and so on, stymied us for quite a while.

With modern computers the problem doesn't look very hard because one could readily keep track of the number of times a small unit was struck, but we did not have such a facility at that time. We tried various (perhaps ridiculous) methods to keep track of how often a place had been hit—colors, shadings, little pieces of graph paper stuck onto other pieces; we even considered and tried modeling clay so that a bomb pattern might be represented by a pat of modeling clay, similar to a pat of butter. Stacking these up was not a solution to the problem.

Once we got a plan going on this problem, everyone engaged in the work—secretaries, mathematicians, and so on. And before it was over, we had a report about the size of a small telephone book. We also found need for some of the more esoteric distribution functions treated in mathematics but not often used in applied work: mixtures of continuous and discrete distributions.

As another example of the larger work, I was lent to SRG-Columbia on a project for the Navy with Savage, Wallis, Milton Friedman, and others. John Curtiss (a classmate of Wilks in graduate studies in statistics at the University of Iowa) was the naval officer in charge of receiving the work, which required building tables for sampling lots of material to consider whether they should be accepted or otherwise handled. The idea of acceptance sampling of manufactured material is very general and applied to parts as well as finished products, from items as mundane as soup spoons to trucks or guns. Inevitably, there had to be many substantial tables indicating the sizes of the lots, the sizes of the samples, and the probability of accepting a lot as related to the various qualities of materials. In the end, we published a book on acceptance sampling, one version for the Navy, and after the war, one version for the general public, entitled *Sampling Inspection*.

The work with SRG-Columbia on acceptance sampling had considerable impact on Jimmie and me. We wrote a 100-page report on quality control methods based on ideas I had picked up in the various quality control courses and on Jimmie's natural brilliance. We submitted it to Allen Wallis.

What we were expecting in the way of comments were suggested rearrangements of sections, and perhaps requests for more explanation in the introduction. Wallis turned the paper over to Milton Friedman, later a noted economist, who was second in command at SRG-Columbia, and Milton tore into the paper with gusto. He used a pencil to mark it up, and not a page was unmarked. We could scarcely see the paper for the changes. And he wrote in the margins and on the backs of the pages. It must have taken a great amount of time to make these corrections, all done in one weekend. We had never seen a manuscript that had undergone such an editorial process. We were astonished and prepared to defend everything. We did not yet understand the value of criticism and how hard it is to get good complaints.

After a shock period, it took us a couple of days to go through the paper and consider Friedman's changes. A great many of them were small issues of wording, such as eliminating "of the" from a phrase like "all of the sampled pieces," and generally tightening the writing by eliminating what I now call "waiting words"—words written while waiting for the actual idea to strike the writer, such as "consideration of the possibility that." These are often identifiable by their roundaboutness and by the lengths of the words themselves. At any rate, after a couple of days' work on Friedman's suggestions, we understood most of his changes and went to talk with him about our disagreements.

We probably did not realize that we had accepted about 90 percent of his corrections without argument, even though it may have taken us a while to get the point. Most of the rest we thought were just wrong, and we were going to fight about them. Milton loved that. He is never better than in an argument. He always has a systematic story to tell about every part of his thesis—he outlined his point, such as: 1, 2, 2a, 2b, 2c, 3. Arguing with Milton was very wearing, because he was systematic and often passionless. It was also very discouraging because he won so often.

Later I got to know Milton better, and he talked with me about problems in economics that I was close to; after he gave me his position on a matter, I would ask, "And what do your opponents say?" He would produce their arguments with the same systematic approach, but with occasional side remarks such as, "This is not as important as it sounds," "This doesn't really matter because it doesn't come up," "The real meat of their argument is in this point, and it is very hard to oppose and I have not yet a full answer for it." Like Jimmie and other very strong scholars, he was very capable of putting himself in the other person's shoes in making an argument.

Milton orally beat Jimmie and me to a pulp over our objections, and as we left, totally defeated, he stopped us and said, "You know, you fellows have a lot of good things to say and you ought to learn how to say them. There are some books which will do you a lot of good," and he named a few, including Strunk and White's *Elements of Style* and Fowler's *Modern English Usage*. After that, Jimmie and I spent a lot of time reading such sources. I still enjoy reading freshman English texts, and I often learn something new.

One of the surprises I had in such reading over the years was that sometimes problems in writing are statistical. I had found that metaphors and similes were a lot of trouble. I would put them into something I wrote, but then after reflecting I would gradually find them unsatisfactory for one reason or another and eliminate them. This seemed very inefficient. Finally I found that there was a statistical solution to the problem. Some author pointed out that metaphors are hard to write because they must satisfy a lot of different conditions, and therefore it is difficult to find a good one. The author's solution was to write down ten metaphors and pick the best of these. I tried this and found it a big success.

I began using metaphors again, but they did meet these conditions. As time went on, I again used them less and less, now for a different reason. It is hard to write down a new metaphor if it doesn't look better than the best you have so far. Thus the idea that you are writing down only ten metaphors is illusory from a time point of view. My calculations show that if you have a graded set of metaphors, each with a score of "appropriateness" from zero to one, you have to produce infinitely many, on the average, most of which are never written down, in order to get 10 written. The success of the sample of 10 metaphors comes not so much from the 10 but from the many considered and rejected. And so the reason I rarely use metaphors now is not that I don't have a good method for producing them, but because I found them very costly to produce. Still, it is nice to know that the metaphor problem has a statistical solution.

Returning now to SRGPJr, the opportunity to work with a team on a sequence of problems with deadlines was a valuable experience. I learned some entirely new attitudes toward problems. First, I found that the formulations of the problem were very important and that those early sessions when we discovered what the problem was and volunteered for the tasks deeply guided the further work. This activity also showed that the problem itself was not set in stone because sometimes we were working on several versions of a problem at the same time. That we could have this room to reformulate problems at the office is partly a tribute to Williams's ability to get the problems in the field described in a sufficiently general way.

Thus as a result of these experiences, I was changing from a student to a research scholar. The deadlines and the idea of reframing the problem added much to my training. Finally, learning to write on demand (and doing so in a given period of time as much as I could, and living with the results) all changed me from a person who did not know how to deal with a research job into one who did. As one outcome, when I returned to Princeton to complete my dissertation, it went very well, and I enjoyed doing it.

The other research experiences I had in New York were also very helpful. From the work on sampling inspection, Jimmie and I picked up a problem from Allen Wallis. He wanted to know how to get unbiased estimates for the probability of success when the sampling was done in some complicated way, especially in sequential analysis situations where items are drawn one at a time and stopping depends on the outcomes of the draws.

For example, suppose in quality control that, instead of drawing a sample of size 5 and observing how many of the items are satisfactory and how many are not, you sample one at a time until you find either 3 satisfactory or 3 unsatisfactory and then stop. What would the estimates be for each possible stopping point that could occur? The coordinates of the stopping points for this example have as the first entry the number of satisfactory items found before stopping and as the second entry the number of unsatisfactory items found before stopping: $((3,0),(3,1),(3,2),(0,3),(1,3),(2,3))$. We want the average estimate to give the correct answer, that is, we want an unbiased estimate. We spent a long time on this problem and finally came up with an exact answer to the question. One of Jimmie's insights paid off.

On mathematical issues, it often is hard to give the general reader the precise gist of a problem and its solution, but this particular idea has a good basis in the reader's own experience, and so I will explain in detail in the following box for those who would like to follow the development.

BIAS

In much of everyday life we speak of bias as a subjective matter in a person or an attitude. In mathematical statistics, bias is a very specific measurable quantity. It is the difference between the true value of a quantity and the average value of its estimates. When that difference is zero, the estimation method, or more formally, the estimator is said to be unbiased.

Our research is applied to the proportion of successes or, in baseball, batting averages. If 100 trials lead to 40 successes and 60 failures, the observed proportion of successes is $40/100 = 0.4$. In baseball, a "hit" might be a success and a "trial" a time at bat. In a medical example, a "cure" might be a success, a "non-cure" a failure, and a "trial" an attempt to treat one patient. Because so many processes in life have this two-category or binomial outcome and break naturally into discrete trials, the theory of such binomial processes has wide application.

The first intellectual hump to get over distinguishes the true or long-run rate from the rate observed in a fixed number of trials. It is not hard to believe that a nice smooth coin has a probability of $1/2$ of coming up heads (H) and $1/2$ of tails (T) when tossed. We take that $1/2$ as the long-run or true probability of a head. If we toss the coin twice, four possibilities HH, HT, TH, and TT can occur, each with probability $1/4$. If, based on the outcome of any of these two-trial experiments, we computed the observed proportion of heads, we would find the 4 outcomes listed producing observed proportions $1, 1/2, 1/2$, and 0, respectively. This set of numbers forms the estimator or estimates of the true proportion of heads for samples of size 2. An estimator is a rule for computing estimates following the experiment. An experiment produces a specific outcome and we associate with it a single number, an estimate. The collection of outcome-estimate pairs forms the estimator. Sometimes we speak of an unbiased estimate when we mean an unbiased estimator. In other words, one-quarter of the time we observe HH and apply the familiar formula, regarding heads as a success:

$$ESTIMATOR: estimate = \frac{number\ of\ successes}{number\ of\ trials}$$

and get $2/2 = 1$, or 100 percent. Half the time (HT and TH) the estimate is $1/2$, and one-quarter of the time (TT) it is 0. The average of the four equally likely estimates is $(1 + 1/2 + 1/2 + 0)/4 = 1/2$, which happens to be the true probability. When the average of the estimates exactly equals the true value, we say that the estimator is *unbiased*. Naturally, unbiasedness is a rather attractive property of an estimator. Although it may generate answers that are not correct in individual experiments—here HH and TT lead to 1 and 0—it does do well on the average.

The estimator we are all used to, observed proportion of successes, is unbiased not only for the two-coin problem, but for arbitrary numbers of coins. Better yet, the unbiasedness is not restricted to situations where the probability of success is 1/2, but to arbitrary probabilities of success, and that is why it is useful when we do not know the true probability. For example, consider a 6-sided die with faces colored fuchsia (F) and five other colors labeled A, B, C, D, E. If it is tossed twice, there are 36 possible outcomes

AA	AB	AC	AD	AE	AF
BA	BB	BC	BD	BE	BF
CA	CB	CC	CD	CE	CF
DA	DB	DC	DD	DE	DF
EA	EB	EC	ED	EE	EF
FA	FB	FC	FD	FE	FF

We see 1 outcome FF with two occurrences of fuchsia, 10 outcomes with one F, and 25 outcomes with zero Fs. Only one of the 36 pairs has two Fs and thus an estimate of 1, 10 pairs have one F and thus an estimate of 1/2, and 25 pairs have no Fs and thus an estimate of 0. We want to know if the average estimate is 1/6 because then the estimator would be unbiased for this problem. The average of the 36 estimates is

$$\frac{1(1) + 10(\frac{1}{2}) + 25(0)}{36} = \frac{6}{36} = \frac{1}{6}$$

and so we have found that the estimator is unbiased. Again, this result is not restricted to two trials or the probability 1/6, but works for any fixed number of trials and fixed probability of success on a single trial. That is, the average of all the estimates weighted by their frequency is the true proportion of successes, and that is the definition of unbiasedness for binomial problems.

On the one hand, this is a marvelous result and very appealing. On the other hand, it has some disappointments. For example, when there is only one trial, the only outcomes are 0 and 1, and so at least one of these is as far as it can get from the true value, whatever it is. We might prefer an estimator that managed to be more often closer to the true value, even if it did not average up exactly right. We won't treat that issue here.

Let us continue with the problem of unbiased estimation when we do not have a fixed number of trials. The desire for such estimation can arise in special kinds of practical sampling such as quality control problems or sequential analysis, and also in various sorts of games. For example, some playoffs are settled by "best out of 3" or "best out of 5," and the World Series in baseball and the final championship of basketball by "best out of 7." In these situations the number of trials is not fixed as it was in our examples of the coin and die tosses, and so the calculations such as we made earlier might not apply.

Suppose that I play an unfair game—I have a probability of 0.4 of winning on a given trial, and my opponent a probability of 0.6 of winning—and whoever first wins two trials wins the event, and this stops the series of trials. Then if W stands for my winning a trial and L for my losing, the possible sequences and their associated probabilities are WW (0.160), WLW (0.096), LWW (0.096), WLL (0.144), LWL (0.144), LL (0.360). We want to see if we have an unbiased estimator of the probability of W. If we now compute the observed proportion of wins (Ws) in each of the six series and weight them by their frequencies, we get

$$1(.160) + (2/3)(.192) + (1/3)(.288) + 0(.360) = .384.$$

That .384, though close to .400, the true probability, is not exactly the same implies that we have a biased estimator.

The problem Savage and I worked on for Wallis was to find out whether there were unbiased estimates, and if so, what they were. We found that for these problems an unbiased estimate based on the outcome of a set of trials with a given total of successes and of failures was a simple quotient, though not as simple as the formula for an estimator given earlier. The denominator of the new quotient was the number of different series that produce the given number of wins and losses at a stopping point. For example, if we stopped at 1 win and 2 losses, the denominator would be 2, because both WLL and LWL lead to stopping with 1 win and 2 losses. The numerator of the new quotient is the number of such series starting with a success. In the best-out-of-3 problem with 1 win and 2 losses, the numerator would be 1 based on WLL, the only series with the right totals starting with W. Thus in our example, the proposed estimate would be 1/2 for 1 win and 2 losses.

Carrying this idea out for all four possible end points: 2 wins, 2 losses, gives the four estimates: 1, 1/2, 1/2, 0. When weighted by their probabilities, we find

$$1 \times .16 + \frac{1}{2} \times .48 + 0 \times .36 = .40$$

which is the correct single-trial probability for this example, and thus we have produced an unbiased estimator.

Coming back to the problem of a best-out-of-5 playoff mentioned at the beginning of the discussion, the estimates would be

| (3,0): 1/1; | (3,1): 2/3; | (3,2): 3/6; |
| (0,3): 0/1; | (1,3): 1/3; | (2,3): 3/6. |

I have given the numerator and denominator of the quotient without reducing to lowest terms. I find the fact that the (3,2) and (2,3) outcomes both give 3/6 or 1/2 as the estimate rather attractive. An interpretation is that the players (or teams) were evenly matched at the end of the first 4 trials. One or the other had to win the final point, and so although the final win decides the match, it doesn't prove much about the comparative ability of the teams.

Although it might be hard to figure out the number of series ending with a given pair of counts, that is merely a technical problem. What is the objection to the estimator? One further small example will illustrate the difficulty. Suppose in playing a game with an opponent I win the series if I win the first trial, W, or if I lose the first trial and win the second, LW; and I lose the series if I lose the first two trials, LL. The proposed estimator says that if W occurs, I estimate my success rate per trial as 1—well and good. If I lose both, I estimate my success rate as 0, because no sequences with two Ls start with W—again, well and good. But if I lose the first and win the second, I estimate the success rate as 0, again because no sequences with one W and one L start with W. (Had it started with W, the series would have been over.) And so now, having observed one success W and one failure L in two trials, the estimator tells us to announce our estimate of the probability of success as zero! A good many people find that outrageous, and they blame the trouble on the requirement of unbiasedness.

Might there not be other estimators that produce more intuitively satisfying results? A feature of our paper was to show that in the great variety of practical problems, the estimator we provided was the only—the unique—unbiased estimator, and so unbiasedness was stuck with this anti-intuitive result. Inevitably, unbiasedness lost some of its appeal for statisticians, not just for this problem, but more generally.

In defense of the unbiased estimator, it could be said that the implication of the request is to get a good estimate on the average over repetitions. Consequently, one should be rewarding long-run averages rather than single trial behavior. Once that is agreed, the misbehavior of the unbiased estimator is not so upsetting.

It turned out that Allen had also given this problem to Abe Girshick, though the latter's work went in a different direction. In publishing, Abe, Jimmie, and I combined the results.

Cecil Hastings's virtuosic work on computing, especially for mensuration (finding areas and volumes), led me to hope we could get better information about the properties of order statistics than I had. These quantities were important in my thesis, and so I wanted as a practical matter to have their means, variances, and correlations (or covariances).

What is an order statistic? When you are given a set of measurements randomly drawn from a distribution, their order is random. But we could reorder them according to size. Then the smallest one is the first order statistic, the largest is the nth order statistic in a sample of size n, and as a more familiar example, the median in an odd-sized sample—the middle measurement—is also an order statistic.

Whereas when the observations are sampled from the original distribution, the successive observations are supposed to be statistically independent, this is not true of the order statistics. If you have only two observations, then there must be some correlation between the order statistics because, however large the smaller one is, the larger one must be at least that large. This constraint creates correlation.

I did not have any trouble getting good approximations to the means and the variances of the order statistics by standard numerical approximations. Getting the covariances, or the correlations, was something else entirely, except for the uniform distribution, which rarely comes up in actual measurement problems. For some years this covariance problem for measurements drawn from the normal distribution was hard for numerical analysts. Today it is nothing, but then it was a lot of trouble.

Hastings figured out a way for us to get covariances for the normal up to samples of size 10 to a few decimal places. And in discussion at Princeton with John Tukey and Charles Winsor, I raised the question of whether it would be easy to get this information for some distribution other than the normal and the uniform distributions. Tukey knew how to do it for a certain unusual distribution provided certain mathematical tables were available. Winsor knew where the tables were and how to use them. So we all got together and assembled a four-authored paper on the "Low Moments for Small Samples," illustrated for several distributions.

Jimmie liked to read aloud and be read to. In some evenings we fought our way through Samuel Butler's *The Authoress of the Odyssey*. Butler wanted to show that the *Odyssey* was written by a woman at a particular port in the Mediterranean, Trapani, Sicily, a place in the news during World War II. Butler had such a strong sense of humor that it was hard to take him seriously, because he engaged in so many anachronisms. He was serious though (he made his own translation of the *Odyssey*), and was reasonably convincing to an amateur. Later we heard that scholars didn't believe him on either count. When I read aloud, Jimmie always wanted me to read the Greek passages, but I always said "and then a lot of Greek." He wanted me to sound it out because he claimed he could often make out what it said, "It may spell Merry Christmas!" One night when Virginia and I went to visit the Savages, we found a note on the door written in English transliterated to Greek letters, "The key is over the door. (It would be just our luck to get a Greek burglar.)"

★ ★ ★

Shortly after World War II concluded in August 1945, Virginia and I returned to Princeton. Except for some special mop-up work I did for Mina Rees to help in closing out the work of the Applied Mathematics Panel, I worked on my thesis and on other research papers that had emerged during our stay in New York.

References

Clopper, C. J. and Pearson, E. S. (1934). The use of confidence or fiducial limits illustrated in the case of the binomial. *Biometrika*, 26:404–413.

David, H. T. (1962). The sample mean among the moderate order statistics. *Annals of Mathematical Statistics*, 33:1160–1166.

David, H. T. (1963). The sample mean among the extreme normal order statistics. *Annals of Mathematical Statistics*, 34:33–55.

Fisher, R. A. (1939). The sampling distribution of some statistics obtained from non-linear equations. *Annals of Eugenics*, 9:238–249.

Freeman, H. A., Friedman, M., Mosteller, F., Wallis, W. A., editors, and the Statistical Research Group of Columbia University (1948). *Sampling Inspection*. New York: McGraw-Hill.

Girshick, M. A. (1939). On the sampling theory of the roots of determinantal equations. *Annals of Mathematical Statistics*, 10:203–224.

Girshick, M. A., Mosteller, F., and Savage, L. J. (1946). Unbiased estimates for certain binomial sampling problems with applications. *Annals of Mathematical Statistics*, 17:13–23.

Hastings, C. Jr., Mosteller, F., Tukey, J. W., and Winsor, C. P. (1947). Low moments for small samples: A comparative study of order statistics. *Annals of Mathematical Statistics*, 18:413–426.

Hsu, P. L. (1939). On the distribution of roots of certain determinantal equations. *Annals of Eugenics*, 9:250–258.

Mizuki, M. (1966). *The Number of Generalized Runs in a Markov Chain Sequence of a Fixed Length*. Ph.D. thesis, Harvard University.

Mood, A. M. (1940). The distribution theory of runs. *Annals of Mathematical Statistics*, 11:367–392.

Mood, A. M. (1951). On the distribution of the characteristic roots of normal second-moment matrices. *Annals of Mathematical Statistics*, 22:266–273.

Mosteller, F. (1941). Note on an application of runs to quality control charts. *Annals of Mathematical Statistics*, 12:228–232.

Roy, S. N. (1939). p-statistics, or some generalizations on the analysis of variance appropriate to multivariate problems. *Sankhyā*, 3:341–396.

Stouffer, S. A., Guttman, L., Suchman, E. A., Lazarsfeld, P. F., Star, S. A., and Clausen, J. A. (1950). *Measurement and Prediction. Studies in Social Psychology in World War II*, Vol. IV. Princeton, NJ: Princeton University Press.

Stouffer, S. A., Lumsdaine, A. A., Lumsdaine, M. H., Williams, R. M. Jr., Smith, M. B., Janis, I. L., Star, S. A., and Cottrell, L. S. Jr. (1949). *The American Soldier: Combat and Its Aftermath. Studies in Social Psychology in World War II*, Vol. II. Princeton, NJ: Princeton University Press.

Stouffer, S. A., Suchman, E. A., DeVinney, L. C., Star, S. A., and Williams, R. M. Jr. (1949). *The American Soldier: Adjustment During Army Life. Studies in Social Psychology in World War II*, Vol. I. Princeton, NJ: Princeton University Press.

von Bortkiewicz, L. (1917). *Die Iterationen.* Berlin: Verlag von Julius Springer.

von Neumann, J. and Morgenstern, O. (1944). *Theory of Games and Economic Behavior.* Princeton, NJ: Princeton University Press.

Wald, A. (1950). *Statistical Decision Functions.* New York: Wiley.

Wallis, W. A. (1980). The Statistical Research Group, 1942–1945. *Journal of the American Statistical Association,* 75:320–330.

Wallis, W. A. and Moore, G. H. (1941). *A Significance Test for Time Series and Other Ordered Observations.* New York: National Bureau of Economic Research.

Wolfowitz, J. (1943). On the theory of runs with some applications to quality control. *Annals of Mathematical Statistics,* 14:280–288.

13

Completing the Doctorate

When Virginia and I came back to Princeton after WWII, she again became Merrill Flood's secretary, and I was to write my dissertation. Social life in Princeton burgeoned, and both duplicate bridge and folk dancing were all the rage. Virginia was most pleased to participate in the folk dancing. She had always enjoyed dancing, and the folk dancing had the advantage that it started early in the evening and was over early so that it did not intrude on her resting hours—she was an early riser and had to get to work first thing in the morning. Duplicate bridge started rather late because it did not begin until all players were assembled—and some were always late; and then when playing was over, we were still not finished because it took an endless time to make the calculations required for the scoring. Players did not know how well they had done, or at least not usually because we were not allowed to talk about what had happened at the various tables for fear of giving information to others who had not yet played the hands.

How did she and I learn to play bridge? Although we had often played with Virginia's parents back in Pittsburgh, neither of us had studied the game. Virginia's father was a good player and a pithy critic; it is from him we have the family saying applied to any bungled activity, "Poorly bid and poorly played." By accident, we owned a very small book that gave the elements of a method called the Culbertson system, developed by the bridge expert Ely Culbertson. Although this system was already old-fashioned by the time we began to play, it was the only book we had, and so we tried to use it. I called it the Cumbersome system. When we went to Trenton, New Jersey, and played in a more serious tournament than the local ones we were used to attending, one pair of opponents—to whom we had to announce our system—could not believe that we were playing this system and called the tournament director to complain, and he assured them that this was a legitimate system in the rules of the game and that we did not have to explain it to them. Even so, they sometimes sent us away from the table and asked what certain bids meant, which they were allowed to do.

F. Mosteller, *The Pleasures of Statistics: The Autobiography of Frederick Mosteller*,
DOI 10.1007/978-0-387-77956-0_13,
© Springer Science + Business Media, LLC 2010

At the same time, Merrill Flood, who was a whiz at all sorts of games and sports, decided that he wanted to play duplicate bridge more seriously than he had before and wanted a partner who could be available often. As a graduate student writing a dissertation, he thought I'd have plenty of time and so he asked me to join him in this venture. I explained that we played the Cumbersome system, and asked what he played. He didn't play anything, but he had been reading a book by Charles Goren, *Better Bridge for Better Players*. Because I didn't have any preference, we decided to try to use Goren's system. As a text, the book itself was excellent. It had hard homework problems that taught us a great deal. Shortly, Merrill and I began playing together in local tournaments and then going to more important ones in Atlantic City, The Oranges, New York, and so on. We began to accumulate master points, mostly from local tournaments. Often it was great fun. We were beaten by some of the greatest bridge players in the United States, and we beat a few ourselves. Part of our pride though came from playing against Goren himself, and from playing him and his partner dead even. It was only fair; after all, we were using his book.

One attractive and successful bridge player named Helen Sobel always played with one or another bridge columnist. At each tournament where Merrill and I met her, we were trounced, and he claimed it was because I liked her. Not long after we played with her, she was named U.S. bridge player of the year, and so probably she and her partner were just much better than we were. Toward the end of that year I began to understand something about bridge on a level different from when I had started. I began to feel from looking at my hand and listening to the bidding that I could visualize what the cards in other people's hands were. I suppose that good players do that very well. I also realized that duplicate bridge is a wearing game and that every player wants to reassess every successful and every unsuccessful hand to a fare-thee-well as soon as it is over. When you have been successful, of course, it's a pleasure. At any rate, after I left Princeton and went to Harvard, I never played another game of duplicate bridge, and that left more time for other things.

★ ★ ★

But you didn't want to hear about folk dancing and bridge, but about statistics. Although I was finishing up various statistical papers just then, my fundamental task was to complete my thesis. The training I had at SRGPJr stood me in good stead. I knew how to break the task down into chunks and work on a chunk for a while until it was either finished or a cul-de-sac.

I worked at night. After folk dancing, for example, Virginia and I would come home, and I would settle down to work and she would go to bed. I would work long hours during the night and sleep til midmorning and then go to the library at Fine Hall or to see colleagues. Unfortunately, Sam Wilks, who had suggested the problem I was working on, was still heavily involved with

Washington agencies and so was rarely around to talk with, though when he was there, he was always willing to discuss technical problems. As a result, I would wander around the halls and wind up talking with John Tukey, who was always generous with his time and his ideas. I usually talked with him about situations where I was stuck. He taught me to get out of such a rut and find a new line. New lines come to something even if they don't solve the problem one started out on. And so during the course of the year, pieces of the thesis materialized, and it gradually began to build itself into something substantial. I had one terrible moment when I read essentially the title of one piece of my thesis in the *New Yorker* magazine at the bottom of one of their columns intended to laugh at anyone who would put words together so turgidly. I understood them perfectly. The work in question was indeed tightly related to what I was doing, but I wasn't being ruined by the developments, which happened to be worked on in the Graduate School of Education at Harvard University under the direction of Truman Kelley, an important educational statistician. Although I met him when I went to Harvard, I did not get to know him well.

Most reading I have done about creativity has involved flashes of insight that suddenly lead the writer to solve a hitherto intractable problem, and although I have occasionally had such nice strokes of lightning, it seemed to me during this period and the next few years that my advances were always made in a fit of anger. In many problems, one has a clear notion of what a nice answer will look like, or even exactly how it should look. When on successive derivations or calculations the result does not come out, and yet one believes that it is genuinely hidden in the mess of formulas, frustration builds. One decides to try the same attack one more time but very carefully checking each step as it comes up and writing large and legibly, all this amidst a sort of cold fury that the previous attempts have not delivered the desired answer. This care and anger became part of the final discovery process for me for years. Much of it I brought on myself because of lack of neatness and impatience to get finished when the goal was apparently in sight.

At the same time that I was working on the thesis, I had other papers in process. Tukey and Wilks had formed up a statistics seminar that was extremely active, and I had a chance to deliver the paper on unbiased estimation there. I had expected to be finished with presenting it in one session, but the results were so anti-intuitive that I was asked to return the next week and continue the discussion. In working on something like the thesis, many little offshoots of the work are developed, and some of these I have never published.

One offshoot of my thesis work was substantial interest on my part in what are called nonparametric methods. Some parts of the thesis used nonparametric methods and others did not. One idea I had was to develop a test for slippage. If one had data from several different processes—for example, repeated measurements from several different machines that were manufacturing piece parts, how would we tell whether one or more of these machines were producing parts with a different average diameter from the others? I developed a nonparametric test for such a departure from equality. Later, Tukey and I wrote another paper on the same topic providing more information about the test.

In addition, Hastings, Tukey, Winsor, and I were completing our joint paper on order statistics. And, of course, I was looking around for a job.

I was rather surprised to find one day that I had a thesis in hand, and that it was time to get it typed up. I went over it with Wilks, and then redrafted it. Virginia and her office mate Virginia Santowasso typed it up on Flood's typewriters at their office.

The opportunity came to join Samuel Stouffer at Harvard in the new Department of Social Relations. Although this post would not be in a mathematics department, it did seem to fit well with some of the work I had done during my time at Princeton, and Sam Wilks encouraged me to take that post. I suppose his own work in education and the social sciences made him feel that this was a valuable and growing field.

★ ★ ★

Just as Virginia and I were moving to Cambridge, I was invited to attend a small statistical conference at Lake Junaluska, a retreat for the Methodist Church, in North Carolina. This conference was arranged by Gertrude Cox to follow a set of summer courses given at North Carolina State University at Raleigh. Some of the faculty from those courses, some students, and other people were invited. Gertrude was a tremendous organizer. (After leaving Iowa State College, she built up substantial statistics departments at both North Carolina State University and the University of North Carolina at Chapel Hill and set up the Research Triangle Institute.) The greatest attraction was that R. A. Fisher would attend the conference.

John Tukey invited me to go with him in his station wagon starting from Princeton, and he drove us down. John worked a good deal of the time—as they said when he got an honorary degree at one university, "His work is his fun." After we were nicely started on the road to North Carolina, John said that he thought we ought to try to write a paper on analyzing binomial probabilities. R. A. Fisher had noted that the arc sine transformation had the property of approximately stabilizing the variance of binomial proportions. To visualize this transformation required special graph paper. If you plot on one axis of a graph the square root of the number of successes in a binomial sample and on the other axis the square root of the number of failures, then the point so determined would in repeated samples of the same size from the same distribution (that is, from a process that had a fixed proportion of successes) vary along a circle whose radius is the square root of the sample size. It also meant that we could plot the results of several experiments of even different sizes on the same graph paper and get a vision of their behavior and their unreliability; and because of the constancy of the variance, we would appreciate how the points varied from one experiment to another. John's idea was to have such square-root by square-root paper drawn up and produced commercially. While this was being done, he proposed that we should write a paper explaining the uses of this invention.

I was astonished at how many ideas we got down on paper as we drove. When we stopped for food, we would continue the discussion, and even when we were at Lake Junaluska, we continued to write the paper.

On the way home we did the same, and so when we reached Princeton again we had a substantial sheaf of pages. John got someone to draw up a large model of the graph paper and mount it on the kind of screening used to prevent flies from entering the windows—it was perhaps 4 feet by 7 feet, and, because it was mounted on screening, it could be rolled up.

Because John and I had diverse backgrounds, we had a great many applications to illustrate the uses of this paper. Although we started work in the summer of 1946, the publication finally appeared in 1949. William G. Cochran was the Editor of the *Journal of the American Statistical Association* at this time. He was concerned about the length of the article. He said that although the idea of publishing the graph paper and its uses was a good one, the reader did not have to know every thought Mosteller and Tukey had had about the analysis of binomial data. He was primarily concerned about the total space being given over to the article, which after being shortened from the original still ran 39 pages in the journal. We presented the article at an annual meeting and people expressed considerable interest. Meanwhile, John had persuaded the Codex Book Company of Norwood, Massachusetts, to produce the special square-root graph paper. One sense in which the paper was a great success was that we were asked for a great many reprints through the years. The experience of developing a long manuscript with Tukey was one that I have enjoyed repeatedly through the years.

To get back to the conference at Lake Junaluska, this was a most enjoyable conference. The group was modest in size and the agenda was wide open. At the organizing meeting someone chaired the session, possibly Gertrude Cox, and asked what topics people were prepared to talk about and what topics people would like to hear about. A substantial list of topics was laid out, including Bayesian inference and multiple comparisons, and members of the audience volunteered to give talks on all these topics. Amazingly to me, R. A. Fisher volunteered for the Bayesian inference. I also presented a paper on a Bayesian approach to combining means. Jacob Wolfowitz was at the conference and pointed out an error in the reasoning in my paper, and so I was able to correct it before it was published in the *Journal of the American Statistical Association* in 1948. After the meeting, Fisher questioned me closely about this paper on pooling means; he was neither negative nor positive about it, though he was not enthusiastic about Bayesian inference generally. Earlier I had showed a draft of the pooling paper to Jimmie Savage because he was a bit interested in Bayesian inference, and he gave me a good suggestion. He asked one of his punchy questions, "Freddie, why do you study the question, 'Which of these two dumb methods is better?' Why not find out what the best one is?" With that hint, I returned to the drawing board and strengthened the paper a great deal. Occasionally I have found this a good question to raise with a student or a young scholar. It is easy to become trapped in a comparison—suboptimizing.

Fisher was in an excellent mood all during the conference. Everyone was delighted to meet him, and no one was trying to oppose his work or principles, at least not directly. In later years when I met and talked with him at meetings and socially, he did not seem as happy as at this occasion.

Phillip Rulon, a professor of education from Harvard University, had attended the summer courses at Raleigh and had been invited to the summer conference, and so this was an opportunity to meet a Harvard statistician before I got there, and we had a number of useful conversations. In later years we cooperated in a good bit of teaching. Although we planned to prepare a book together, we never succeeded in completing it, though we had enough pages. I believe we were both too busy at research. He had a private educational research group in addition to his professorship, and the two efforts kept him very busy. At that time, he was very much engaged in thinking about the analysis of variance, a field that I was not then so attracted by, though now in 1990, I am.

Along with all the speeches, we also had a substantial hearts card game. Tukey didn't like bridge, but he did like hearts. At the time, he was taking a substantial interest in analysis of variance and design of experiments. He designed a huge hearts experiment where after each round of deals we had to rearrange our seats so that we had balance about who sat near whom and who was the dealer, and so on. Who played in this game? To the best of my recollection, it was Fred Stephan, David Duncan, Charles Winsor, Tukey, and I. When all was said and done, it turned out that the only "effect" that was significant in the analysis was that of players. To no one's surprise, it turned out that Tukey was the best hearts player.

References

Girshick, M. A., Mosteller, F., and Savage, L. J. (1946). Unbiased estimates for certain binomial sampling problems with applications. *Annals of Mathematical Statistics*, 17:13–23.

Hastings, C. Jr., Mosteller, F., Tukey, J. W., and Winsor, C. P. (1947). Low moments for small samples: A comparative study of order statistics. *Annals of Mathematical Statistics*, 18:413–426.

Mosteller, F. (1948a). A k-sample slippage test for an extreme population. *Annals of Mathematical Statistics*, 19:58–65.

Mosteller, F. (1948b). On pooling data. *Journal of the American Statistical Association*, 43:231–242.

Mosteller, F. and Tukey, J. W. (1949). The uses and usefulness of binomial probability paper. *Journal of the American Statistical Association*, 44:174–212.

Mosteller, F. and Tukey, J. W. (1950). Significance levels for a k-sample slippage test. *Annals of Mathematical Statistics*, 21:120–123.

14

Coming to Harvard University

When I was still discussing the possible move to Harvard on completion of my doctorate at Princeton in 1946, Virginia and I traveled to Cambridge and met Talcott Parsons, the chairman of the new Department of Social Relations. Although he was among the most widely cited sociologists in the world, I brought away no quotation from this visit, but rather an appreciation of him as a man of action. He took us to dinner at a very fine restaurant and ordered wine. Although Virginia and I were familiar with cocktails, wine was new to us. When the sommelier brought the bottle and offered the tasting glass to Talcott, he took a sip and startled us by announcing in his big voice, "It is spoiled, bring another bottle." He was decisive, commanding, not the least embarrassed, and all went as he ordered. Virginia and I didn't run into another spoiled bottle of wine until ten years later, at a wine tasting we were giving in our home.

Talcott made us feel welcome, even though he was a somewhat formal and formidable person, not through stature but through voice and mien. Although he was not quantitatively inclined, he liked theory and mathematical models, and he encouraged work of all kinds in all the social sciences. He understood there were many ways to advance social science. He and Samuel Stouffer worked together most effectively to develop the Department of Social Relations. They used the device of a department and a laboratory. Talcott chaired the Department, and Sam directed the Laboratory. Appointing power was through the Department. The Laboratory at least for several years had funds that could be used to support beginning scholars and innovative research groups. These research funds came from private foundations and from the government. By carefully matching Department funds with Laboratory funds, they could vary assignments flexibly and get both teaching and research done in an effective manner.

Although the Department of Social Relations was established in January 1946, the possibility of such a social science department had been discussed for two or three years by Talcott Parsons (sociologist), Gordon Allport (so-

F. Mosteller, *The Pleasures of Statistics: The Autobiography of Frederick Mosteller*,
DOI 10.1007/978-0-387-77956-0_14,
© Springer Science + Business Media, LLC 2010

cial psychologist), Clyde Kluckhohn (anthropologist), Henry Murray (clinical psychologist), and Hobart Mowrer (education and psychology).

Harvard President James Conant appointed a special committee of experts from outside the university in the spring of 1945 to review the social science situation, but by fall the Departments of Anthropology, Psychology, and Sociology met and voted to appoint a committee to plan a new department. Because of all the previous discussion, the committee was able to make a proposal, have it ratified by the three departments, and get faculty approval in January.

Conant's committee did produce a fine report, *The Place of Psychology in an Ideal University*, that included a department like that of Social Relations among its options, but not as its primary proposal. That committee wanted to draw together psychology from the whole university, not just from the Faculty of Arts and Sciences. Having now worked in several faculties at Harvard, I know that that route is a tough one at this University, even though it works well at some others. Apart from any matters of philosophy or personality, the methods of financing teaching positions in various parts of the University differ substantially. Furthermore, what is regarded as appropriate research often differs from faculty to faculty. In this event, the Department of Social Relations was already established, and the university-wide alternative was no longer feasible.

★ ★ ★

On the third floor of Emerson Hall, my office-mate for the first few years was R. Freed Bales, at first a sociologist (a student of Talcott Parsons) and later a social psychologist. He led the department's research effort for studying the interactions among members of small groups. (In addition, Freed was a talented artist who had studied oil painting. His wife Dorothy is a well-known violinist.) I had a chance to participate in some early research in small groups as a result of our proximity. Among the joys of the department were the great variety of kinds of research going on and the challenge to the statistician to bring fresh quantitative skills to bear for people who needed and wanted them. Most graduate students worked on empirical research as part of their training, and they generated a steady stream of statistical questions running from trivially easy to impossible.

Because the department offered degrees in social anthropology, social psychology, clinical psychology, and sociology, much of the research was interdisciplinary, and I attended seminar after seminar with faculty and students from all the disciplines. Through the years, Clyde Kluckhohn and John Roberts in anthropology; Gordon Allport, Jerome Bruner, Eleanor Maccoby, and Robert Sears in social psychology; Eugenia Hanfmann, Gardner Lindzey, Henry Murray, and Robert White in clinical psychology; and Talcott Parsons, Freed Bales, George Homans, Samuel Stouffer, Florence Kluckhohn, and Peter Rossi in sociology helped with my education in social sciences. Of course, we had a

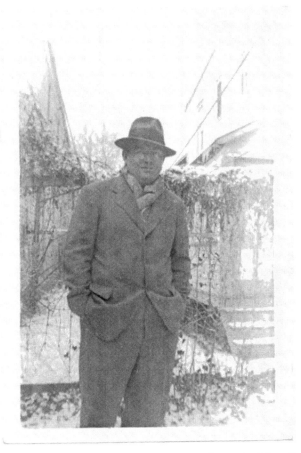

Fig. 14.1. Fred on Dunster Street in Cambridge, where the Mostellers first lived upon his arrival at Harvard, circa 1946.

constant stream of visitors, and I got to know Paul Lazarsfeld, Clyde Coombs, Louis Guttman, William Hill, and Margaret Mead and her husband Gregory Bateson.

The atmosphere and tone of social science discussions in Emerson Hall differed vastly from those in mathematics at Fine Hall in Princeton. At Fine Hall, intellectual disagreements among graduate students led to instant confrontations: "That's wrong because..." and, "You forget the key condition..." combined with attempts to clarify the truth with such kind remarks as, "You'll never get there that way, here's how..." or, "Hand over the chalk, I know a better way." Perhaps faculty were more restrained, but the mathematics students were both brusque and thick-skinned. None of it was personal, or at least not much, and fellow students were most generous when asked for in-

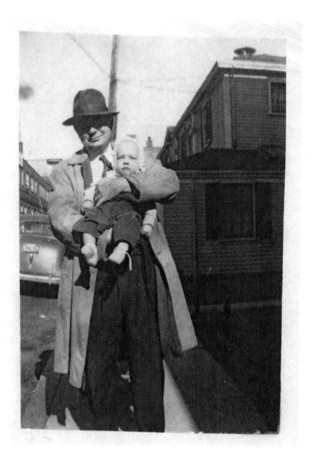

Fig. 14.2. Fred on Dunster Street in Cambridge with his infant son, William (Bill), circa 1947.

formation they had, because they loved to explain to others the mathematics that they knew.

In the seminars at Emerson Hall I found that I was the only one who seemed to be able to come right out and say that I thought someone was mistaken, and it took quite a while to socialize me. I gradually learned some useful phrases, such as "Might there not be another way to look at it?" or "Have you considered such and such?" It was hard, though, because I was impatient to learn and wanted to get right to the point.

Freed Bales and I had some good discussions on extrasensory perception studies, and we designed a new study of our own that we would carry out over a period of months, using each other as transmitters and as subjects. I set up quality-control charts so that we could see how often we had made more or fewer correct guesses than was reasonable according to chance. We checked each other's scoring of each session, and we both kept discovering errors. You'd think it would be easy to line up two columns of one-digit numbers and decide which pairs are alike and which ones are not, but it is easy to make mistakes.

After we got launched, we had regular sessions, and we kept plotting up the outcomes on the charts, but we wouldn't tell anyone what our control chart was about, because even though we wanted to do this experiment, we did not feel it very central to our work. And we knew there would be some friendly put-downs. One trouble with ESP experiments seems to be that one needs a lot of trials. Also, after the first flush of enthusiasm wears off, it is a real bore organizing the materials, carrying out the sessions, and scoring the results. As time went on and our scores showed both statistical regularity and mediocrity of mental receiving, Freed and I became discouraged. Our plan had been to proceed for a given number of sessions decided in advance (a nice design feature); but, about a third of the way through, we let the whole thing lapse. I'm sure we still feel a bit guilty, yet we were not getting anywhere, and we were merely proving that RFB and FM were not sending well to each other. Nevertheless, the experience helped cement a permanent relationship.

At the same time, this experience illustrates a form of publication bias. Because we were finding nothing but chance results, we did not complete the experiment and did not publish our results, whereas someone with more lucky guesses might publish.

Over the years, I have helped a couple of groups set up ESP experiments, because at one time Harvard had some endowment funds to be used for such research. In one instance, the experiment got around the problems of many trials and boredom. A graduate student in physics had read of some results achieved by subjects who wished that dice fairly tossed would come up a certain way. As reported, the data seemed to show success from wishing, but maybe not enough that Las Vegas would crumble. The physicist reasoned that to turn a die so it came up in a favorable way would require some force to be exerted on it. If the brain could send out forces, then physicists had delicate instruments that would respond violently to very tiny forces and so would be enormously more sensitive at detecting the forces than the outcomes of repeated rolling of dice. With the help of a young physics professor and about $50, they set up such a sensitive instrument in the basement of a building. During the summer, groups came in and tried by forceful thinking to push a target. A very tiny force would cause a dot of light to move several feet. Only once all summer did the dot move, although scores of people singly and in groups tried to push the target with their minds. When the professor was brought back to re-inspect the equipment, he said one direction of balancing had not been properly carried out, and so it might have been possible that a group of people all walking out of a classroom at the same time could have caused the movement. We'll never know, but this method did seem like an imaginative research direction.

When Freed was well along with his small-group research, the Laboratory constructed a room for observing small groups so that their actions and interactions could be recorded and observed without disturbing their work.

Freed taught Henry Riecken and me and some others a little about oil painting, and we met regularly in the room and painted one evening about every two weeks. Others, like R. Duncan Luce and Renato Tagiuri, already knew how, and they joined this Buckeye Club too. In origin this name is obscure, but its idea was that we wanted to be skilled enough to paint real world things so that viewers would recognize exactly what the subject was. (This is a genuine boat, not an abstract basket of flowers.)

I was amused to find one day that I did all my painting left-handed in spite of my first-grade teacher.

One delightful consequence of trying to paint has been a much better appreciation of art in galleries and museums, together with the activity of hunting up these places in cities the world over.

$$\star \star \star$$

The 1946 set of first-year graduate students included many men and some women returning to education from wartime experiences. Because they were so mature, intense, and full of purpose, in addition to possessing the usual brilliance one expects of graduate students, this group must have been one of the most outstanding classes in Harvard's history. I became close friends then and for life with Raymond Bauer, Gardner Lindzey, Henry Riecken, and Renato Tagiuri.

Because it's a small world, we have had many connections through the years. All of them have had various faculty appointments at Harvard University. I have done research with some and worked on professional and academic committees with them.

I supervised a few undergraduate honors theses and a few doctoral dissertations during this period. At this time, von Neumann and Morgenstern's book, *Theory of Games and Economic Behavior*, led to much research on ideas of utility, and I thought it would be worth actually trying to measure utility in real people to see what would happen. Among the graduate students in clinical psychology, the late Philip Nogee was very quantitatively inclined and eager to participate in designing and executing such an experiment. For the central experiment our idea was to create a sequence of bets associated with outcomes from a toss of several dice. The bets offered before each roll of the dice were sometimes very favorable to the bettor and sometimes unfavorable. The sense is the mathematical one of expected payoff.

If a coin is flipped, the chance of heads is $1/2$. If you were to receive \$2 when it comes up heads, but nothing if it comes up tails, the average payoff or expected value is the product $\$2 \times \frac{1}{2} + \$0 \times \frac{1}{2} = \$1$. From the point of view of expectations, if you were to pay more than \$1 to play a game based on these outcomes, you would be a loser in the long run. If you paid less than \$1, you would gain on the average. If you paid exactly \$1, we speak of the game as being fair.

It is a bit surprising that many people play unfair games regularly. For example, people buy lottery tickets knowing that the state intends to make a substantial profit. Most people are aware of this and are also aware that the winning numbers are chosen by chance, so that skill in choosing numbers to bet on has little role. (It may have a small role in situations where the size of the award depends on the number of winners. Then avoiding popular numbers could be relatively advantageous, even though there is a loss on the average.)

Why do people play losing games? Although many explanations are given, including the idea that holding a lottery ticket for a future drawing has entertainment value, another explanation might be that some people have different utilities for money. For example, you might be unwilling to pay $1.01 for a 50-50 chance at $2, but you might be willing to pay $1.50 for one chance in a million at $1,000,000, a bet which also has expected value of $1. By knowing how much you would pay for different chances, we could map your utility curve. Nogee and I wanted to base these utilities on actual behavior rather than on paper-and-pencil tests.

By varying the payoff and the probabilities of winning, it was possible to calculate for each participant in such a game the utility of money. Some people might stick to odds that were exactly determined by mathematics, taking bets that were more favorable than the average gain, rejecting those with less. Others might value big gains as more or less than their mathematical expectations. From the behavior of the individuals during a sequence of sessions where dice were rolled after choices were made for a variety of bets, we were able to plot their utility curves.

Along with this information, Nogee had attached a mechanism that timed the responses—that is, the time taken by a subject in the experiment to decide whether to take or refuse the bet. On the basis of this information he hoped to write a dissertation relating the personal utility information to the information about time to decision. Considering all the ways things can go wrong, I'm pleased to say that both aspects of the investigation worked out well, and Nogee did complete his dissertation. Although he and I published together the results of the primary study, except for depositing his thesis, he never published his decision-time results. My recollection is that the findings were instructive. Because we had the utility curve for each individual, we knew what any bet was worth to that individual as assessed by the utility theory. Consequently, we knew whether a proposed bet was favorable to the person on his or her own terms. One way to interpret the behavior, then, is to determine whether the individual behaves correctly as a rational person on the basis of his or her own utility curve. (Rationality means greed in this setting.) If a person declines a favorable bet or accepts an unfavorable one, we might say the person made a mistake. If we had not had the personal utility curves, we could give the explanation that the person did not have the same utility for money that simple mathematical theory would suggest, but we could take care of this objection using the curves.

For me, the memorable thing that Nogee found out was that on average, the subjects took longer to come to what, for them, were mistaken decisions than to correct ones when their preferences were taken into account (the utilities). Furthermore, the worse the mistake, the longer the decision time on average. Some of the effect probably comes from very favorable or very unfavorable gambles being quickly recognized as old friends or enemies with nearly evenly balanced gambles requiring more thought.

That year the annual meeting of the statistical societies was to be held in Chicago, and I was invited to present our paper on measuring utility. By chance, Freed Bales was speaking there too on his contributions to group interaction. We splurged and took a bedroom sleeper from South Station. The Pullman car seemed brand new and the accommodations roomy, and we went to sleep planning to arrive in Chicago early in the morning. At about 2 A.M. a terrible hammering on the door woke us, and the conductor told us the car had a hotbox and we were to move to another car. It had begun to snow. The other car seemed old enough to have been used by Abraham Lincoln and was noisy, bumpy, and cold. Although we had expected to arrive about 8 A.M., we awoke at 10 A.M. in some consternation, but the porter explained that snow as well as the car trouble had made us very late. My talk was scheduled for about 4 P.M.

Snow continued, and the train finally arrived in Chicago somewhat after 4 P.M. Freed and I rushed to the auditorium and arrived just before the close of my session, chaired by Jacob Marschak. One of the discussants, Armen Alchian, an economist, had kindly delivered my talk, some said better than I could have done. I was allowed to answer a couple of questions. I was very disappointed, because I had looked forward to this talk more than others I had made up to that time, and perhaps more than any in my whole career except the one on the authorship of *The Federalist* papers. Nevertheless, the paper may have had better treatment by being presented in absentia, because certain infelicities in the economic remarks were handled by the discussants, and Nogee and I were able to take good advantage of their criticisms in preparing the paper for publication. Later, Ward Edwards, a graduate student in the Department of Psychology, wrote a thesis with me on probabilistic matters related to utility theory. He also joined with Harold Lindman and Jimmie Savage in writing a fine paper on applied Bayesian inference when they were together on the faculty of the University of Michigan.

Between the work on measuring utility and stochastic learning models, my office had lots of nearly ready-made projects suitable for honors theses in Social Relations. Judith Slepian Berger reviewed several suggestions and chose what I regarded as a hard one. She planned to organize an experiment on verbal learning by small children at several schools. Almost overnight she made the arrangements and designed the protocol for the study. She had no difficulty analyzing her data and writing up the thesis.

In the utility field, David Carver also carried out a rather technical investigation the same year. It was somewhat mathematically oriented but required experimentation. The next year he entered medical school.

While teaching in Social Relations, I also taught some courses for the Department of Mathematics and had the opportunity to direct several honors theses and a couple of doctoral theses. Among the honors students in mathematics were Leonard Baum and Peter Duren. For the doctorate, Robert Kozelka was a young mathematician with interests in social science. While working with me he began helping others with statistical problems and became close friends with John Roberts, an anthropologist I knew well in Social Relations and with whom Robert Bush also worked. As a result, Kozelka has continued his career as a mathematical statistician with applied work in the social sciences, and he sometimes chaired the Department of Mathematics at Williams College.

Reed Dawson, Jr., with whom I had played a Japanese board game called Gomoku (like tic-tac-toe, except played on a large board requiring 5 in a row to win) in Fine Hall at Princeton, wrote a thesis in statistics with me at Harvard. I believe he went into private consulting on the West Coast.

In Social Relations itself, I had relatively few doctoral students, though Elaine Cumming wrote with me about the problem of educating communities about mental illness. Harold Garfinkel wrote a joint thesis with Talcott Parsons and me. David Hays worked with me and Robert Bush in the learning area and also with Freed Bales in the study of small groups before he went to the RAND Corporation.

★ ★ ★

After Talcott Parsons had chaired the department for about seven years, he wanted to take a sabbatical for the academic year 1953–54. I had been reading C. P. Snow's book *The Masters*. Snow's discussion of the Two Cultures fitted my experience as well, but his exploration of the struggle for head of the college had no reality for me. Although Talcott had chaired the department far longer than usual, not one of the permanent members had stepped forward, offering to be the acting chair for the sabbatical year. The department had several distinguished social scientists with tenure—Allport, Bruner, Homans, C. Kluckhohn, Murray, Solomon, Sorokin, Stouffer, White, and Zimmerman— and nobody wanted to be the chair. Talcott called me in and told me that the department wanted me to be acting chair for the year. When I mentioned the people listed above, each had found some excuse; apparently I was the only one unimaginative enough to be trapped. Needless to say, it was a strange year for me, because I had no experience running anything, let alone a large department. In some ways I was fortunate that it was a large department, because size of necessity leads to some efficiencies. Many tasks a chair might have to face were already in the hands of faculty leaders, administrators, and secretaries—there were separate offices for undergraduate and for graduate

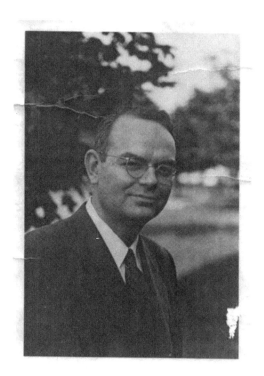

Fig. 14.3. Fred, circa 1950.

teaching, and a separate laboratory for the research side of things. I learned something about how Harvard worked. It's not so easy. Fifteen years later I was puzzled how to handle an administrative issue and after several phone calls found a woman who knew. She said, "It's surprising you don't know this. How long have you been here?" I said, "Twenty years." She said, "Oh, well, you're new here." Over the year, I learned about department meetings, how to get faculty appointed, budgets, annual reports, and even about going to meetings of the Faculty of Arts and Sciences, which I had been avoiding. It turned out that department chairs had a special responsibility to attend. Later on, these experiences helped me in chairing other Harvard departments.

An important activity of the year was a self-survey of the behavioral sciences at Harvard, one of five universities (with Chicago, Michigan, North Carolina, and Stanford) supported by the Ford Foundation for such a study. My recollection is that Francis Sutton and Eleanor Maccoby, with support from Sam Stouffer, led the part of the self-survey dealing with Social Relations and contributed to the more general report. I had met both Frank and Eleanor at Princeton. Sutton, like me, was a graduate student in mathematics there before he won a Junior Fellowship and came to Harvard, where he took a doctorate in sociology.

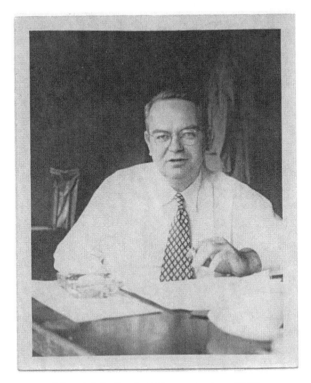

Fig. 14.4. Fred at Harvard, circa 1952.

Eleanor and her husband Nathan, like many others on their way to an annual meeting of the American Psychological Association, had stopped in Princeton to visit Launor Carter, a psychologist, during the summer of 1940, when Launor and I had an apartment. I had also seen something of them in Washington, D.C., during World War II.

Frank and Eleanor put together an impressive report with many findings that were astonishing, at least to me. For example, in some departments the graduate students could never see their professors, and the teaching was poorly done. I tried to learn from the observations in my dealing with students and in my classroom teaching.

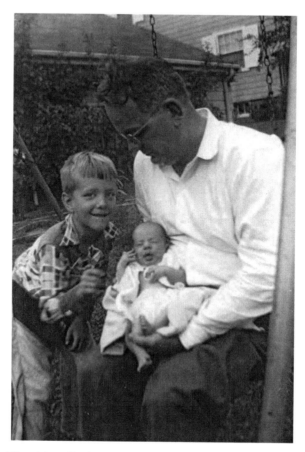

Fig. 14.5. Fred and his children Bill and Gale in 1953.

References

Edwards, W. D. (1952). *Probability Preferences in Gambling Behavior*. Ph.D. thesis, Harvard University.

Edwards, W., Lindman, H., and Savage, L. J. (1963). Bayesian statistical inference for psychological research. *Psychological Review*, 70:193–242.

Gregg, A. et al. (1947). *The place of psychology in an ideal university: The report of the University Commission to advise on the future of psychology at Harvard*. Cambridge, MA: Harvard University Press.

Mosteller, F. and Nogee, P. (1951). An experimental measurement of utility. *The Journal of Political Economy*, 59:371–404. (Reprinted P-524 in The Bobbs-Merrill Reprint Series in the Social Sciences.)

Snow, C. P. (1951). *The Masters*. New York: Macmillan.

von Neumann, J. and Morgenstern, O. (1944). *Theory of Games and Economic Behavior*. Princeton, NJ: Princeton University Press.

15

Organizing Statistics

How can one persuade an old university to create a new department? Universities are usually organized along disciplinary lines, but at Harvard and many others, statistics has been an exception. Before 1946, few universities in the United States had departments of statistics. When I came to Harvard, statistics, just as today, was taught in various departments throughout the University. Let me list a few teachers and places in 1946: William Leonard Crum and Edwin Frickey in Economics; Saunders MacLane in Mathematics; Richard von Mises in Applied Mathematics; Harold Thomas, Jr., in Engineering (his father had taught me engineering drawing at Carnegie when I was a freshman); Truman Kelley, David Tiedeman, and others in the Graduate School of Education; and Hugo Muench in the Department of Biostatistics, which he chaired beginning in 1947; I taught mathematical statistics for the Department of Mathematics and quantitative methods for Social Relations. The list could readily be lengthened.

Even though many courses in statistics were being taught, I found few people to talk with about the contemporary state of statistics because the faculty were dealing primarily with applications in subject matter areas, just as I was in my teaching and advising in Social Relations. I needed, and thought Harvard needed, more contribution from the growing edge of the field. And so, after talks with Sam Stouffer and Talcott Parsons, I initiated further discussions with people in the Department of Mathematics and with applied mathematicians in Engineering. In Mathematics, Garrett Birkhoff and Lars Ahlfors (chairing Mathematics) were most encouraging; and Harold Thomas (sanitary engineering and flood problems), Raymond Redheffer (special probability problems), David Middleton (signal detection), and I in 1947 discussed developing a Department of Statistics in the Faculty of Arts and Sciences at Harvard. I presented the resulting proposal to the Department of Mathematics, who in turn approved it. In the time I have been at Harvard, Mathematics has been enthusiastic about developing new areas of mathematics, usually applied, in the University, as long as Mathematics was not responsible for applied work. They feel that they have a broad but circumscribed mission in the center

F. Mosteller, *The Pleasures of Statistics: The Autobiography of Frederick Mosteller,*
DOI 10.1007/978-0-387-77956-0_15,
© Springer Science + Business Media, LLC 2010

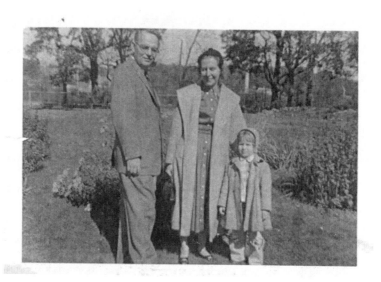

Fig. 15.1. Fred and Virginia with Gale, circa late 1950s.

of the discipline of mathematics, and that they must stick to that. Inevitably, the mission widens with the years. We statisticians have had nothing but encouragement and generous treatment from Mathematics at Harvard. At some institutions matters are much less agreeable.

As a result of these meetings and recommendations, Stouffer and I met with the provost, Paul Buck, near the turn of the year 1949 and proposed the new department to him. In April 1950, I heard from Dean Buck. He felt that the field of statistics was too narrow for a department. It is wise not to take the reasons for refusals very seriously unless they point to opportunities to remedy a defect or omission. Otherwise, one would waste a lot of time, as in this case, trying to argue that a discipline taught in ten departments and used in scores could not be narrow. Years later, another dean of Arts and Sciences, Henry Rosovsky, argued essentially the opposite. He told me that the future would bring full-time experts in statistics to each discipline separately and that people like me who enjoyed working in several fields of application were dinosaurs, soon to be extinct. In essence, he felt that the field was too broad. In economics, Rosovsky's theory was already in operation, because at least two kinds of economic statisticians worked full-time in their respective subjects. Some worked on national accounts and followed numerical series to appreciate what was changing in the economy. Others worked in the methodology of measurement—econometrics—and tried to tease information out of non-experimental data. Indeed, many fields today do have full-time statisticians, as he described.

Dean Buck's negative message did not depress me a great deal, because I still had a man-in-the-street mentality that believed bureaucracies require major movements to change them. The reason for not going forward—too narrow a field—reinforced that view. Perhaps I would have done better to go directly to President Conant; still, one purpose of a provost is to be a buffer for the president. President Bok has always made it clear that he is available to see individual faculty members, and I have found it true with only modest advance notice.[1]

Until the self-study program in 1953–54 (described in Chapter 14), I did not think hard again about the possibility of a Department of Statistics. The self-study program, with W. Allen Wallis as a special coordinator for the committees at all five universities, naturally included statistics in the behavioral sciences being studied, because statistics offers key support for that work. I served as a member of the Visiting Committee for the University of Michigan, which did not have a department of statistics. For various reasons most self-study committee members visited all five schools at one time or another, and I could see that statistics as a discipline fared better and advanced faster at the schools with departments: the University of Chicago, the University of North Carolina, and Stanford University. A major recommendation emerging from the self-study program was that departments of statistics should be set up at the University of Michigan and at Harvard.

Although this flurry of discussion started me thinking again about a department, I was about to go on a sabbatical visit to the statistics department

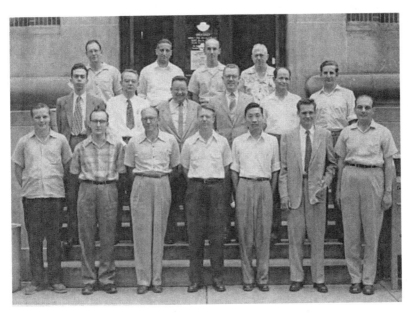

Fig. 15.2. Fred at the University of Michigan Conference on Multidimensional Models in 1954.

at the University of Chicago, and so I would not be at home to press immediately for this development.

My year at Chicago (1954–55) made me very enthusiastic about being related to a department of statistics because of the faculty's warmth, variety of interests, participation in many activities, and interrelation with other departments. People in psychology, sociology, education, economics, mathematics, and business all made me welcome. I was even asked to be a reader of Gary Becker's thesis, a marvelously innovative economics investigation assessing the financial costs of prejudice and discrimination.

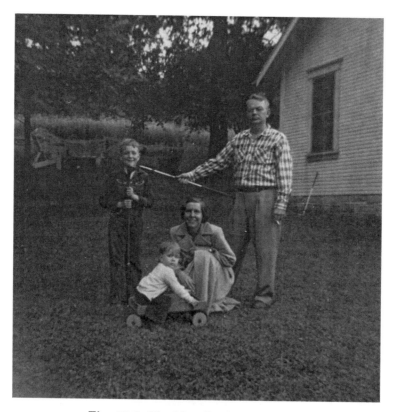

Fig. 15.3. The Mosteller family in 1955.

All this led me to think that the proposal for a department at Harvard was not so out of the question. We had a new dean, McGeorge Bundy (Mac), who had been a mathematics major as an undergraduate at Yale, and we had the recommendation of an all-star Visiting Committee explaining the need for a department, and even suggesting that I should organize it.[2]

Mac Bundy took many initiatives. For example, he led the plan to bring Advanced Placement in Mathematics and in other fields to Harvard under-

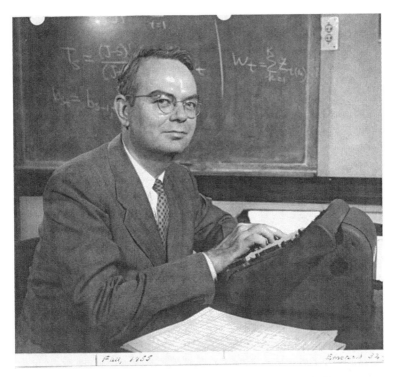

Fig. 15.4. Fred working with a calculator in 1955.

graduates. Over the years this has had impressive consequences. Once taking more mathematics in secondary school could pay off in colleges and universities, strong students went out of their way to prepare themselves. In turn, that preparation saved a student a year or two in moving to the frontier of his or her field. Professor Andrew Gleason of Mathematics and I had served on a lot of committees for mathematical organizations dealing with such encouragement for young people, and so we were delighted that Bundy was able to move the legislation through the faculty. The gains went well beyond Harvard because, when a few major universities take such steps successfully, others are reassured and follow. The secondary schools then upgrade their curriculum so that their graduates can take advantage of the new opportunities. In my own family this movement made it possible for my daughter to have two more years of mathematics in secondary school than I had had, even though I had taken all the mathematics offered in a strong program in the Pittsburgh public schools.

Of course, the Home Committee of the self-study program had also recommended the establishment of a department. Because I was on the Home Committee and chairing Social Relations, this recommendation was not likely to carry as much weight as that of the Visiting Committee.

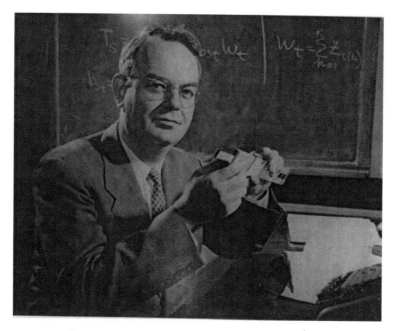

Fig. 15.5. Fred working with a slide rule in 1955

In May 1955, while I was still visiting the University of Chicago, Dean Bundy invited me to serve on a Committee on Applied Mathematics and Statistics[3] to advise the administration on the course that studies in applied mathematics and statistics should take. Dean J. H. Van Vleck, later a Nobel Prize winner, was to chair the Committee composed of many distinguished scholars, among them Wassily Leontief of input-output analysis fame, who also received a Nobel award.

The Committee decided it should consider 1) the undergraduate curriculum and 2) the graduate curriculum in applied mathematics, 3) plans for statistics, and 4) the next computing machine to bring to Harvard. Naturally, a subcommittee dealt with each item.

I chaired the statistics subcommittee, and it included G. Birkhoff, R. C. Minnick, G. Orcutt, and H. A. Thomas, Jr. By mid-March of 1956, all the subcommittee reports were in, and Mac Bundy responded to the recommendation for a statistics department with concern for the source of the funds needed for the new appointments. As I knew nothing about raising funds for professorships, this sounded like the end of the new statistics initiative, though this time for a reason I understood. Still, the letter did not say "No" absolutely.

By fall I had received a most attractive offer to chair an expanding department of statistics at another university, and Virginia and I concluded that if Harvard did not want a department, I should move, much as we had enjoyed

Harvard. Mac decided in December 1956 to go ahead with the department, provided the Faculty approved, and asked me to begin making arrangements for recruiting an outstanding senior and junior faculty. To help with the search and the preparations for the Faculty presentation, he asked Guy Orcutt and Garrett Birkhoff to serve on the committee.

On the search effort we fortunately recruited William G. Cochran, who was then head of Biostatistics at Johns Hopkins and contributing vigorously to the literature in statistical methodology. He had experience with doctoral students at Iowa State, University of North Carolina, and Johns Hopkins, and had unusually broad interests. He agreed to come if the department was created.

We also were fortunate in getting John W. Pratt to join us. He had been an undergraduate at Princeton and had taken his doctorate at Stanford.

We tried too to get Arthur P. Dempster, who had finished his doctorate at Princeton, but he preferred to go to Bell Laboratories for a while. He joined us a year later.

At the same time that we worked on the recruiting, we worked on the presentation to the Faculty. To help this along, I visited department meetings and explained the idea of a Department of Statistics to each of Mathematics, Economics, Psychology, Social Relations, and the Division of Engineering and Applied Physics.

On February 12, 1957 (Lincoln's birthday), I gave a short speech proposing a Department of Statistics, my first speech at a meeting of the Faculty of Arts and Sciences; Van Vleck moved the establishment of the Department, Lynn Loomis of Mathematics seconded it, Robert White supported it for Social Relations, Seymour Harris of Economics spoke for it (he spoke at nearly every faculty meeting), and Edwin Newman and Arthur Smithies raised questions. Bundy said that initially only graduate degrees would be given. The total time on the floor of the faculty meeting before approval was 14 minutes.

Howard Raiffa agreed on November 26 to come to the Harvard Business School with part time in Statistics. Later we established the undergraduate program, and the *Harvard Crimson* carried that announcement on Lincoln's birthday, 1963.

To come back to the original question—How do you establish a new department at an old university? Very slowly.

During the first year, the department was housed over a bank on Dunster Street among dentists, attorneys, and insurance people. In the fall of 1958, we moved into attractive quarters in a building called Geographic Explorations at 2 Divinity Avenue, near the Busch-Reisinger Museum and beside the not-yet-built William James Hall. The first floor was taken by the Harvard-Yenching Institute and the second by Mathematics, and we got much of the third floor in an addition for offices, though the space was intended ultimately to be further stacks for the Harvard-Yenching Library. For years their personnel would ask us wistfully when we were leaving. But that did not occur until the Science Center was completed in 1972.

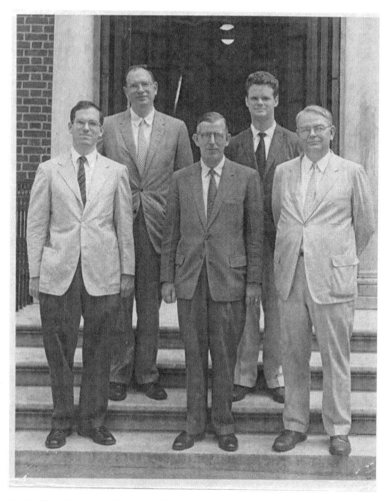

Fig. 15.6. The Harvard Statistics Department in May of 1959. Front row, left to right: John Pratt, William Cochran, and Fred Mosteller. Back row, left to right: Howard Raiffa and Arthur Dempster.

In the third of a century after its founding, the Department granted 103 doctorates in statistics. At the beginning, the distribution of graduate students was about one-third women and two-thirds men. For a long while, no women completed their doctorates, and the faculty had long discussions about what to do. What was happening could not be explained by differential ability. The women students were at least as strong as the men, but they would leave to get married and apparently not follow up as professional statisticians. We were up against a cultural phenomenon. The day eventually came though when some women began completing their degrees.

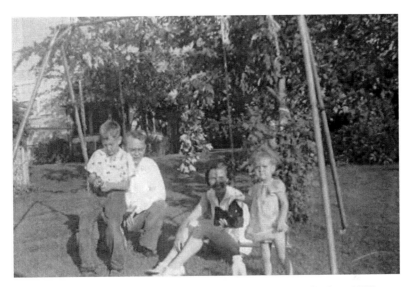

Fig. 15.7. The Mostellers in their Belmont backyard, circa 1957.

The first woman to complete her doctorate was one of my students, Janet Dixon Elashoff, whose father, Wilfrid Dixon, was in my graduate class in statistics at Princeton and is famous for his contributions to statistical computing, especially the biomedical programs BMDP. Janet finished in 1966 and has gone into work in medical statistics. She married Robert Elashoff, another of my thesis students, who also went into medical statistics. Janet was followed in the same year by Margaret Drolette, a faculty member at Harvard in the Department of Biostatistics. She had taken some reading courses with me before the Department of Statistics was formed. She wrote her thesis with William G. Cochran.

In 1967, Yvonne Bishop completed her dissertation on large-scale contingency tables using examples from the National Halothane Study (see Chapter 5), where she had contributed so much. To round out the 1960s, Asha Seth Kapadia completed her doctorate in 1969. I had not noted until writing this summary that all four women went initially into the health and medicine arena. Through 1989, over a fifth of the doctorates in statistics have been completed by women. Society changed.[4]

All the statistics faculty were directing graduate student theses, and our small department had nearly as many doctorates per year as the large departments at Berkeley and Stanford. Students were supported partly through fellowships, through teaching, and through the projects in the department from the Ford Foundation, the National Science Foundation, and the Office of Naval Research. Some students found remunerative and exciting work in research centers throughout the University. In some of these efforts the students occasionally found dissertations. The variety of topics chosen for these was very broad.

Students in Statistics who worked with me on their theses (many worked with me on projects and wrote their theses with other professors) mainly made contributions to methods of data analysis, though some worked on special probability problems that ultimately contributed to data analysis.

Among the data analysis problems is that of handling results that seem very different from other results in the same study or collection. For an example from sports, if almost all batting averages of regular players are recorded from .200 to .350 and then you come across an item like .420 (George Sisler, 1922), that is an outlier and you wonder how to handle it in the analysis of batting averages. One way is to have what are called robust methods of analysis. They are designed to defend themselves against outliers and yet to use the data very efficiently when the simplifying assumptions we use for theory are not badly broken. Michael L. Brown and Richard W. Hill both wrote about methods of handling such data when one is using values of several variables

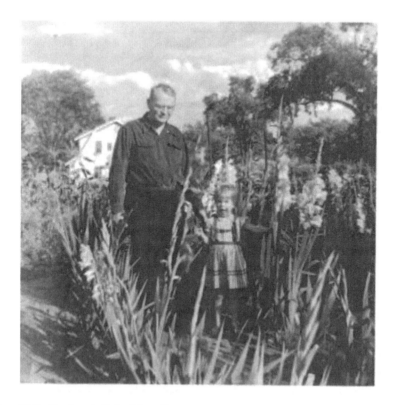

Fig. 15.8. Fred and Gale Mosteller in 1957, in the gladiola garden Fred liked to plant each year with the help of his family.

to predict some outcome on another variable and when any of the variables may produce outliers.

Sometimes an analysis can be more informative when carried out on a scale of measurement different from that of the raw data. Fluctuations in stock market prices, for example, seem to act in a multiplicative rather than an additive way. When that sort of behavior occurs, we usually analyze the logarithms of the data rather than the raw data. At the end, however, people usually want to know their answers in the original scale—banks work in dollars, not logarithms or square roots of dollars. Going back to the original scale has some complications, and Farhad Mehran compared methods for taking such steps back. He later worked for the International Labour Organization and for the World Bank.

In addition to Yvonne Bishop, several students worked on problems where the variables are not measured, but categorical, such as sex, region of the country, type of workplace, or occupation. Robert Elashoff studied situations where the data involved simultaneously both categorical and continuous variables.

Stephen Fienberg worked on the estimation of cell proportions in contingency tables in his thesis and also wrote with John Gilbert on the geometry of contingency tables. Sometimes we do not have the joint data required for estimation such as Bishop and Fienberg worked on, but we may have partial information. For example, we might know in a 3-variable problem with categories young-old, male-female, and east-west, the number who have at least one child. Someone may be able to provide these numbers for pairs of variables such as young and male, young and east, and male and east, but not for the three simultaneously young and male and east. Gudmund Iversen worked on estimation when data are missing as they are in this example. Similarly, David Lax studied how to make inferences in policy problems when some variables are unobserved.

When you were in secondary school, you may have had to solve quadratic or cubic equations. Usually these were set up to produce fairly nice answers by using methods of factoring. These polynomial equations—polynomials set equal to zero—have as many roots as the highest power of the variable entering the equation. Thus $x^6 - 2x^2 + 1 = 0$ has six roots, not all of which need be real. In some areas of work such as economics, the coefficients of the powers of x and the constant term may be drawn at random from a distribution. It turns out that some problems having to do with interest rates depend on the roots of the resulting polynomial equation. What sort of sizes do the roots of such random polynomials have? Considerable work has been done on such problems by mathematicians. One of my students, William Fairley, worked on the distribution of roots in some special situations. One well-known finding is that the real roots of these random equations tend to pile up around $x = 1$ and $x = -1$, which to me was quite a surprise.

In many circumstances in the world we worry about multiple events. For example, there is a saying that bad news comes in threes. Joseph Naus has studied, both in his thesis and in his later scholarly work, how often we can expect clusters of events to occur in a short time interval. For example, suppose we have random events like accidents occurring on the average once a month (30 days) over a 10-year period. What is the chance that some period of length 30 days has at least 4 events? The 30 days can start anywhere, not necessarily at the beginning of a calendar month. Naus's work helps us answer such questions about clustering.

Thomas Lehrer, who has considerable fame for his songs, sometimes worked on such statistical problems and has continued his strong interest in mathematics. His musical activities often drew him away from such work. He spends much of his time teaching mathematics at the University of California at Santa Cruz.

It seems that my students have gone in many successful, and interesting, directions.

Notes

1. Derek Bok served as President of Harvard University from 1971 to 1991, including the time during which Mosteller wrote this chapter.
2. The Visiting Committee: Dean A. Clark, Taylor Cole, Ernest R. Hilgard, William A. Makintosh, Robert K. Merton, George P. Murdock, Chairman.
3. The Committee on Applied Mathematics and Statistics: J. H. Van Vleck, Chairman; H. H. Aiken, G. Birkhoff, G. F. Carrier, S. Goldstein, E. C. Kemble, W. Leontief, D. H. Menzel, W.E. Moffitt, C. F. Mosteller, G. H. Orcutt, H. A. Thomas, Jr.
4. Earlier, in the 1920s, women had pursued advanced studies—the generation that produced Margaret Mead and Dorothy Swain Thomas, for example. The Great Depression may have set that movement back for a third of a century.

Part III

Continuing Activities

16

Evaluation

A graduate student, Robert Goodnow, in Social Relations had a substantial impact on my life shortly after I came to Harvard, an impact that has rippled through the years. Bob, like many social psychologists, was quantitatively inclined and had good training in statistics and its applications before he became a graduate student. He used his statistical training to help support himself in graduate school by working on projects in the Department of Anesthesia directed by Henry K. Beecher at Massachusetts General Hospital in Boston. Beecher was an organizer and a researcher, and his anesthesia department was among the first to be formed in the U.S.A.

Beecher had many bright physicians carrying out research, either evaluating drugs and medications, especially analgesics, or studying the physiology of the upper respiratory system. These many investigations naturally created the need for special statistical designs and analyses. So many projects required statistical assistance that Goodnow suggested to Beecher that he ask me to help, not only because of the size of the research effort but also because some of the problems being treated required new statistical or mathematical developments.

By working with Beecher's group, I got to know many young anesthesiologists and through them worked on many medical problems. Several became heads of departments of anesthesia or other medical departments throughout the country. Among those I have maintained relations with are John Hedley-Whyte from Beth Israel Hospital. We have worked together intermittently through the years, usually on a seminar basis with us often jointly heading a group. As I write, we have been studying the treatment of back-pain in Massachusetts through claims data to see who prescribes what operations and whether hospitals differ in their treatment. I coauthored a paper on placebo reactors with Beecher, Arthur Keats, and Louis Lasagna, formerly at the University of Rochester and currently at Tufts University Medical School. Lasagna in particular has made special studies of the Food and Drug Administration's drug approval process. In Chapter 5, I discuss work with John Bunker of Stanford Medical School, who led the National Halothane Study and developed the study of institutional differences, which had an advisory committee that I served on. Later, we worked together at Harvard in a Faculty Seminar and edited a book entitled *Costs, Risks, and Benefits of Surgery* with the surgeon Benjamin Barnes. Formerly in Beecher's department, Henrik H. Bendixen helped us with this same book by writing about the cost of intensive care after he had gone to the Columbia University College of Physicians and Surgeons. Probably the anesthesiologist I coauthored the most papers with was Bucknam McPeek of the Department of Anesthesia at Massachusetts General Hospital. These were by no means the only young anesthesiologists I advised, but I have worked more with them than with some of the others such as A. S. Keats, who worked with Beecher, Lasagna, and me on oral analgesics, and who worked on coughing, for example. Gene Smith also worked with Beecher. Gene studied special groups of people, such as nurses and their attitudes toward one another (for example, smokers were regarded rather negatively compared with non-smokers long before the current bans came into being). He studied the problems that part-time college students face. In addition, he worked with Beecher on quantifying pain in humans. Needless to say, the variety of these problems together with those in Social Relations widened my perspective about applications of statistics.

Beecher wrote beautifully, I thought, and he delivered his papers at conferences by reading them, but with feeling. He had a curious view and habit. When giving a scientific paper, unlike many of us, he did not like to speak extemporaneously. Instead he prepared for questions by thinking of what someone might ask and having responses typed up on small slips of paper. When someone asked a question, he fanned through his prepared responses and read the appropriate one. But if the question asked was not one he had prepared for, he would, I think, read the one he had not yet used that would do the audience the most good. When the answer was totally unrelated to the question, this often left the inquirer with a very puzzled expression.

Among the many important contributions made by Beecher and his colleagues were those with Donald P. Todd to try to assess the contribution to the total death rate made by anesthesia in surgery—about 1 in 1500 administrations at that time.

Beecher's group was interested in assessing the size of the placebo response to various ailments such as postoperative pain, seasickness, headache, and other undesirable troubles—averaging up to about 35 percent relief—he called it "the powerful placebo." Because the average size of the placebo effect is so large, it is very important in medicine to compare the response of patients to a new treatment with that of others who act as controls, either by receiving a standard treatment or a placebo. If we merely compare the patient's responses before and after treatment, a worthless treatment would be credited with the positive response associated with placebos, and be erroneously judged therefore to be valuable. This same study of placebos happens also to be an early example of meta-analysis in the field of medicine. In meta-analysis, we combine quantitative information from several comparable studies to get stronger and more generalizable results than the individual investigations can provide. Usually the studies are oriented to the same treatment and disease, but in Beecher's study, he had a variety of sources of illnesses and was making the point that in medical studies generally the investigator can readily be misled about efficacy of a treatment unless suitable controls are used. My work with Lasagna, J. M. von Felsinger, and Beecher was oriented to the question of whether some people were placebo responders while others were not and, if so, how they might be distinguished.

Beecher also headed a commission that came to an agreement on brain death when medicine became so successful that it could keep human organisms that would never recover consciousness alive indefinitely. I advised on the statistics of the first two of these, but not the third. Beecher came from a tradition where scientific controversies led to vigorous written and oral confrontations, a tradition that I was familiar with from statistics early in the century, where R. A. Fisher and Karl Pearson wrote about one another's work in a vein I found embarrassing. Because I was asked to read many papers in preparation, I was sometimes able to dissuade Harry from making his point in a way that would infuriate the person whose work was being discussed.

Although Beecher was a leader in applying methods of controlled experimentation in research in medicine both for the evaluation of medical technologies and for more basic research in medical science, he was much concerned about the ethics of investigation. He wrote a provocative and controversial paper describing a number of investigations that others had carried out that he regarded as inappropriate. The paper had considerable influence and probably encouraged the creation of institutional review boards in institutions carrying out research. Even though this process puts more friction in the system of investigation, society benefits in several ways.

The boards are usually composed of people from many walks of life as well as medical scientists, and these members can represent societal interests from several points of view. Of course, they disallow some investigations.

In addition, in a good board the actual process of investigation is reviewed to make sure that the study is efficiently designed so that fewer subjects may be needed and that investigators are more certain to be able to evaluate beneficial effects when they are present. Thus, ethics demands that research be well designed.

After we established a Department of Statistics, my colleague William G. Cochran sometimes also helped with the work at the Department of Anesthesia.

In the end, my experience with Beecher, which was primarily oriented to the assessment of medical technologies, connected me to many studies and people working in that field, and my work in it increased later in my life, starting about 1975.

★ ★ ★

The studies of the Kinsey Report, the 1948 Pre-election Polls, and the Coleman Report all dealt with evaluation or technology assessment laced heavily with statistical methods. Two other early experiences sharpened both my interest and that of John Gilbert in this field. One was our work in the field of education, the other a report written for the President's Commission on Federal Statistics.

Our work on the issue of the need for experimentation in the field of education (growing from the Coleman Report) already had made us attentive to the problems of field work. John and I were also working on the National Assessment of Educational Progress, a continuing national survey of achievement of school children at various grades. At that time the work was done in Denver under the organization of the Education Commission of the States. Later the assessment continued under the Educational Testing Service at Princeton, New Jersey.

By asking the same questions of children of the same ages in different years, one could find out whether the educational performance of the children of the United States was rising or falling. This information was available on a regional basis and not for specific school districts or states or cities, though information about urban and rural areas could be produced.

Each state and school district would have preferred to know how its children were performing, but that was beyond the capabilities of the survey. In various years, the survey dealt with different topics, such as mathematics, writing, literature, citizenship, and art.

Naturally, school districts also wanted to know how they could improve the performance of their pupils. Gilbert and I worked with the program for several years along with John Tukey and others. Our experience with the seminar on equality of educational opportunity stimulated us to want experiments carried out in the field of education in addition to the survey. What the surveys could do was tell which disciplinary topics were showing improvement or loss in performance, but they did not tell what to do about it, except insofar as particular age, ethnic, regional, or urban-rural groups were identified as having trouble or improving.

The approach, through repeated surveys, had advantages over a one-shot sample survey such as the Coleman Report because it made possible assessment of changes in performance. The National Assessment program also was set up to aid school districts that wanted to make surveys of their own.

A second additional stimulus for our attention to evaluation came from the President's Commission on Federal Statistics. Allen Wallis chaired the Commission (he had become acquainted with Nixon when Nixon was vice-president), and I served as vice-chairman. As we worked through the statistical methods being used to gather information for policy, I saw again that experimentation was rarely used, even when what was desired was to find the effect of introducing a change. Richard Light, Herbert Winokur, and I wrote a special piece for the Commission's second volume (which had many papers on special topics) discussing the merits and difficulties of field studies.

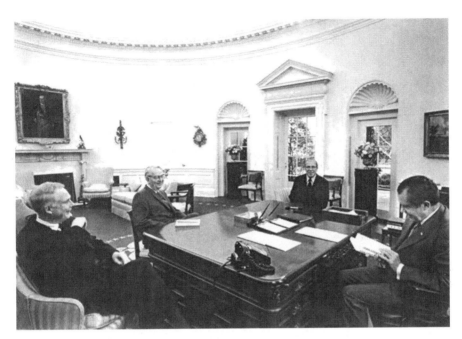

Fig. 16.1. W. Allen Wallis, Fred, George Schultz (Director of the Office of Management and Budget), and President Richard Nixon in the Oval Office for the presentation of the report of the President's Commission on Federal Statistics, 1971.

We illustrated the idea with several examples of important programs that had used randomized studies to assess the effects of the treatments being administered. We especially emphasized that an evaluation of a treatment that turned out to produce "no effect" was a valuable result because it showed that the program did not do what was hoped and allowed the funds for it to be used for other ideas. For example, in a nursing-home study the hope was that with special physical training the patients could improve their self-care capabilities compared to the patients in similar conditions without training. Success would be beneficial in at least two ways. First, patient morale would be improved because most patients prefer to do things for themselves and often even resent the need for help; furthermore, their ability to function might improve. Second, less staff effort spent in these hands-on activities would free time for other tasks.

More than 2,000 patients took part in the study, which randomized patients into two groups, the training group and the control group. As it turned out, the rehabilitation training for improved self-care had practically no effect on the patient's ability to function and did not reduce the number or length of hospitalizations, nor the mortality. It was valuable to know such results before the program was implemented in that form in hundreds of nursing homes

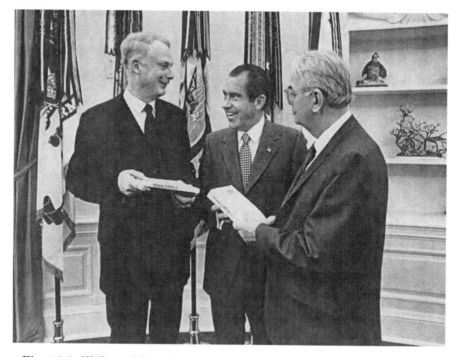

Fig. 16.2. Wallis and Mosteller with President Nixon in the Oval Office, 1971.

throughout the country. The program was well evaluated, and that was a success.

People often wonder whether we cannot do better than randomizing patients to studies. In a study of schools, they may say, "Why don't we put the new teaching program in the Jones School and the usual teaching program in the Smith School and compare the results?" Part of the difficulty flows from the myriad ways that the Jones School differs from the Smith School. The Jones School may have more families with traditions of education and learning, and thus more home support for the work, probably leading to better performance. Or weird things can happen: if the material being studied is French literature, it is possible that one of the schools has many more children of French descent, with corresponding intensity of interest.

Once one begins to worry about these difficulties, the suggestion is often made that we use methods of matching. For example, in comparing two exercise programs intended to prepare men for some ordeal, we might try to make sure that the groups start out with comparable numbers at each weight in pounds—perhaps counting the numbers in each 10-pound interval, such as 140–149. As soon as this suggestion is made, someone will want to match for both height and weight. If we had about 10 categories for weight and 10 for height, now we have 100 categories matching weight and height simultaneously. Next, someone will suggest that an even better variable to match for would be initial physical condition, and without worrying about all the ways this might be assessed, we can imagine 5 categories for it, and now we have 500 weight-height-physical condition categories. As the variables for matching increase in number, the number of categories continues to multiply. Soon most categories will have 0 or 1 person.

This matching approach can do much to improve the reliability of the comparison, but it often leaves a residual difficulty. One group may tend to be high on all the unmatched variables favorable to the exercise program; and so, even though the categories have comparable numbers, one group may still have a bias favoring one of the programs.

To get around this, we can take a pair of people who are "matched" as nearly as we decide to match, and then randomly assign one to program A and one to program B, keeping track of the fact that this group of two was matched as a pair. If we do this, then a later analysis can take advantage of the stratifications induced by the matching and avoid any residual bias by the randomization of the assignment. Thus the matching idea is a good one; but it has no end, because one can always think of another variable or attribute that may be important in a comparison—for example, attitudes may be more important than physical condition. I helped design and carry out such a matching study for comparing exercise programs in World War II. As I recall, the army was troubled that one of their programs for putting new soldiers in good physical shape left them slower, though stronger, than they were when they started.

Many studies do not use matching, but assign items or people to treatments at random as they enter the study. This step takes account of the biases at the moment of entry. (Other biases may arise later.) It does not give the benefit of matching that may be useful in the analysis for improving the precision of the estimates of effects found in the experiment.

To return to the President's Commission on Federal Statistics, our paper made two main recommendations: first, "Controlled field studies [randomized trials] should be used more frequently to improve both new and continuing social, health, and welfare programs." And second, "Steps in several areas should be taken to create a more suitable climate for doing controlled field studies." To execute the first recommendation, organizations needed to be developed that could carry out such studies, and Congress could write controlled field studies into enabling legislation for program evaluations. Long-term funding would be required if controlled field studies were to be integrated into program design.

For the second recommendation, we pointed out the need to better inform the public about the problems new social programs have and the role of evaluation in their evolution. We noted that effective field studies needed cooperation and understanding at several levels, and that political experts would often be needed to aid in implementation. Finally, legal problems arise that might need untangling in some instances, as when a federal program makes one arrangement and the state government finds itself in conflict, and a program manager is caught legally in the middle.

Although our paper appeared in the second volume of *Federal Statistics: Report of the President's Commission*, which had no official standing, the official Commission Report recommended that, for evaluation, "the procedures set forth in the paper in Volume II, Chapter 6, by Light, Mosteller and Winokur relating to the use of controlled field studies for improving public policy, should be followed in setting forth evaluation plans."[1]

★ ★ ★

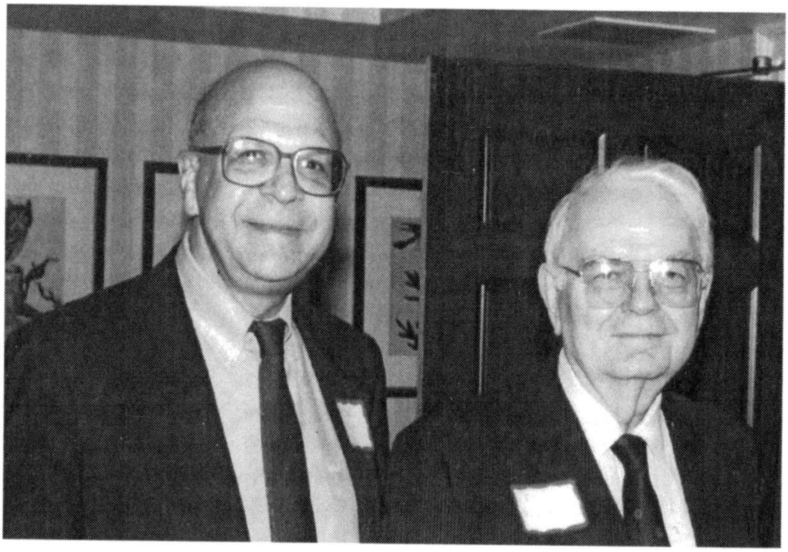

Fig. 16.3. Richard Light and Fred at Mosteller's 80th birthday celebration in 1996.

One never knows how effective such recommendations and such commissions are. My own attitude has been that, when opportunities to participate in such ventures come up, one should try to participate. Just like social programs, most won't accomplish much, but now and again one gets a winner. One has also to recognize that one is involved in a large social process and that things that seem hopeless at one moment may suddenly become urgent and relevant when an issue galvanizes society.

Carl Bennett, a statistician with Battelle Memorial Institute in Seattle, and Arthur Lumsdaine, a psychologist I had known first at Princeton in graduate school and later in Washington during World War II and then again through the Social Science Research Council, invited Gilbert and me to attend a conference on social research methods in Seattle. The plans for this

meeting were laid long in advance, and so we had perhaps a year to prepare our paper. The time seemed ripe to consider our attitude toward various
methods of evaluation. Gilbert and I asked Richard Light, a statistician who
wrote his dissertation with me, and a professor in both the Harvard School
of Education and the John F. Kennedy School of Government, to join us in
preparing the paper for the Seattle conference.

The mists of memory and the vagaries of my files do not supply the charge
required of the paper for Seattle, but it included the idea of assessing social
innovations. For a substantial period we three could not find a way to get
started on the paper. Although we had regular meetings, nothing came of
them. It was not because of disagreement. For the most part we tried to
explain to one another why it was important that we do something about
evaluation, but then someone would say, "Well, just what is it that we are
trying to do?" By then, all of us had learned that time on task really mattered.
(Some research by David Wiley and his colleagues was very compelling on the
value of time on task.) You might think that spending time on a task when
you don't know what to do will not pay off, but original work does develop
by sticking to the area and trying to shake ideas loose. Because of the time-
on-task principle, we decided that we would meet on Saturday mornings and,
instead of discussing what it was we wanted to do, we would start to write
about what needed to be done in the social field. Each of us had a typewriter
or a pencil or pen, and we kept writing. After two Saturdays of what seemed
to be the ultimate in frustration, we assembled all the pieces of paper that
had been written.

We analyzed these chaotic writings and decided that we first needed a
review of the outcomes of innovations in the social and medical fields. Then
from that review we would decide what to do next. Taking this empirical
case-study approach was not entirely natural for us.

It might seem that statisticians would grab for a list of concrete examples from the start, but that would be a misunderstanding. In statistics, case
studies do not have a very good reputation. Some reasons are that one example arbitrarily drawn from a population of studies may be misleading, bias in
reporting may distort the findings, case studies often turn out to be extreme
examples, and selection of aspects of the study by the reader may lead to
mistaken generalizations. (Robert K. Yin in his book *Case Study Research:
Design and Methods* explains how to use the case study as a research tool.)
When we statisticians do collect cases, we like to have a definite population
from which we sample, so that we know what population we are trying to
make an inference to. We had none. Furthermore, our own bent was rather
to formulate a methodological question that could be answered by creating
formulas and tables.

We did want to look at more than one study. We gathered, on the basis of our knowledge of several important innovations in the social field and
medicine, what some actual findings were from the evaluations. The sample
of studies we gathered was not drawn from any well-defined population, but

the sample consisted of studies that had been well enough evaluated that we had clear views about the success of the innovations. Today, I might be less believing, but at the time we were learning.

Where did we get our lists of innovations that had been evaluated? We had three main sources: we had come across a list of social studies compiled by Jack Elinson and Cyrille Gell of Columbia University. (I had worked with Jack on sample surveys in the Research Branch of the War Department during World War II.) The list was very informative. Also we recalled that Robert Boruch of Northwestern University had a list, Light had a list from the field of education, and I had one from law and social science. Bucknam McPeek helped us develop a list of 10 surgical studies that used randomization. This sounds like a great bundle; but because our lists overlapped, the total count was 28, including 8 social innovations, 8 socio-medical, and 12 medical innovations.

We rated the performance of each innovation on a 5-point scale: $--$ harmful, $-$ slightly harmful, 0 neutral, $+$ slightly beneficial, $++$ very beneficial. Table 16.1 shows the results stratified by type of innovation.

Table 16.1. Ratings of 28 Innovations

Type of Innovation

Rating	Social	Socio-medical	Medical	Total
$++$	3	1	2	6
$+$	2	2	2	6
0	3	4	6	13
$-$	0	1	1	2
$--$	0	0	1	1
Total	8	8	12	28

Although others might change our ratings slightly, the overall picture shown by the table would not change much. Six innovations or 21 percent got $++$ ratings. We thought that, because of the way we collected the sample, the proportion of $++$'s here was larger than would appear in a sample from the total population of trials evaluated by randomized investigations. Most innovations did not work, though few were actually harmful.

As an example of a neutral innovation, we illustrate with a study of potentially delinquent girls. The investigators hoped to reduce the numbers of delinquent girls by predicting which girls in a school were likely to become delinquent, and then giving both individual and group treatment to girls who exhibited potential problem behavior. The girls with potential problem behavior were randomly assigned to two groups; one group received the preventive treatment, and the other got no treatment. It turned out that, although the investigators were able to identify potentially delinquent girls, none of the measures of success of treatment showed an effect. Although the identification method was a success and might be useful again, the preventive therapy did not work, and that is why we rated it 0.

For an innovation receiving a ++ rating, the Salk vaccine experiment offers an illustration. The children vaccinated with the Salk vaccine got paralytic poliomyelitis at a rate less than half that of those not treated.[2]

Once this factual material was available, we were able to think about the general problem of evaluation of innovations. What should we say about social experimentation? The more we looked into it, the more we seemed to need experiments, as opposed to sample surveys or demonstration programs. When a treatment has been proved to be effective, demonstration programs help practitioners learn how to put the treatment in place in a wise manner. But first you have to have an effective treatment.

Once we acquired these materials, we did not find writing so hard after all. We tried to put together a substantial statement about the need for, and benefits of, controlled field trials. At the close, we contrasted the idea of a controlled field trial with the common method of trying this and that without the ability to find out whether the innovation offered benefits. We admitted that in some instances that method could work. When the effects were huge, what some call slam-bang effects, then the big improvement would be detected. The effectiveness of antibiotics is an example of a slam-bang effect. But for modest improvements, such an approach cannot be expected to work. We wrote, "We do one thing here, another there in an unplanned way. The result is that we spend our money, often put people at risk, and learn little. This haphazard approach is not 'experimenting' with people; instead, it is *fooling around with people*." In conclusion, we said that this haphazard approach was the principal alternative to randomized controlled field trials.

At milestones in the work we rewarded ourselves by going to Locke-Ober's restaurant for lunch on Saturday. It is a convenient subway ride from Harvard Square. We went when the first draft was completed and again when we had made the changes suggested by Bennett and Lumsdaine after they had reviewed the papers for the conference.

Because Light and I were teaching part-time at the Kennedy School of Government, our economist friend Richard Zeckhauser found out about this paper. He was editing, with others, *Benefit-Cost and Policy Analysis 1974* for Aldine Publishing Company, and he thought that a part of our paper would fit into it. He got permission from Bennett and Lumsdaine to use parts of it. The latter were far behind in their publication plans because, as usual, some conference participants had not met their deadlines. And so the Zeckhauser book actually appeared before the Bennett and Lumsdaine work. Through the two publications, the paper received considerable publicity.

Preparing this paper gave us some new ideas about how to think about practical problems, especially that a concrete set of cases might be instructive even if they were not drawn from a known population. And this had consequences for us later. Light says that since that time he has much more often started on a new topic with an attempt to make a collection of concrete cases.

Similarly, in my later work with Gilbert and McPeek and also still later with John Bailar III, I found this approach not only stimulating for the writer but also for the readers. Journalists understand this very well.

★ ★ ★

At Harvard in 1972, I became dissatisfied with the small amount of interplay between the graduate students in the Department of Statistics and groups carrying out empirical work. I knew that Howard H. Hiatt, then Dean of the School of Public Health, was organizing a center for the analysis of health practices. He and I, with others, had several discussions about ways we could do more about both issues. We discussed the possibility of a seminar something like the one that Moynihan and Pettigrew arranged for the Coleman Report. Although we had no Coleman Report in health, we did have many statistical problems of medical evaluation, and the idea of setting up the seminar seemed viable. With the blessing of the Departments of Biostatistics (in the School of Public Health) and Statistics (in the Faculty of Arts and Sciences) and of the newly formed Center for the Analysis of Health Practices, led by Howard Frazier, we started a seminar under my chairmanship. We invited anyone who wished to join. The seminar met at the School of Public Health. We had regular speakers much of the time, and we also had groups dedicated to certain kinds of problems. For example, I participated for many years in the Surgery group, chaired at first by John Bunker, who was visiting Harvard from 1973–75. Other groups were studying such areas as Child Health, Protocols for Surgical Experiments, and Mental Health. All told, I think about 100 people participated in the seminar at some time.

The format of the Faculty Seminar in Health and Medicine was similar to that of the Moynihan-Pettigrew seminar in that we had a light supper, speakers, and then meetings of the subgroups addressing special problems. Sometimes we did not have speakers and had only subgroup meetings. This seminar differed from the earlier one in that many members initially seemed rather at sea about why they were there. "What are we going to do?" they asked. I wanted to be non-directive about this, and so I said we would do whatever they wanted to do, but that being professors we would probably profess, which implied activities such as writing articles and books for publication, holding conferences on special topics, and writing legislation in some instances.

In some ways the problems of the seminar on equality of educational opportunity were different from the one on medical practices, because on the surface the equality seminar dealt with a report and its critique. The real issue, though, was elementary and secondary education and how to improve it. In medical practices we had no report, but the agenda was to improve health and medical practices by evaluation.

Probably, in starting up such a general venture, having a report to criticize or a book to read offers a helpful start. People who are unused to interdisciplinary work and have a clear path in their own professional activity may need some entering wedge to help them move into the cooperative mode.

I chaired the seminar the first year, John Bunker did it the second year when I was in California on sabbatical, and John Hedley-Whyte chaired it the third year. The Surgery Group continued throughout this period and long after.[3] I chaired that group along with Hedley-Whyte after Bunker returned to Stanford. After the seminar ended, we moved the Surgery Group meetings to the Department of Statistics. We concluded the Surgery Group in 1982 when David Hamburg came to Harvard to head the Division of Health Policy Research and Education. With his encouragement we formed a new working group on Health Science Policy.[4]

It was not surprising that some of these interdisciplinary groups were unable to work up enthusiasm for this approach, and they quit meeting. In one or two instances, the group formulated problems they could handle better within their regular research programs; in others they did not find a suitable problem that had mutual attraction for the members. Others continued in one form or another for a long period and produced papers and books. For example, one group started out with students from statistics and a couple of professors and gradually wrote a strong book about the design and analysis of observational studies as distinct from experiments.[5] At first this group on observational studies met regularly with the seminar, but then it broke off and met separately at regular times more convenient for the members. Nevertheless, they received some modest support from the seminar to complete their volume, and some members of the seminar offered critiques of parts of their manuscript.

Central to the seminar's mission was learning to evaluate and learning why to evaluate procedures and methods in health and medicine. At that time, it was still not widely realized that much of what is done in medicine and health had not been evaluated, an exception being the safety and efficacy of drugs, supervised by the Food and Drug Administration.

As for the Surgery Group, Bunker and I had no doubts from the beginning about what the product of our work should be. We planned a book, though its shape took a while to develop. Our group gradually laid out a program to write a series of papers describing and illustrating the problems of evaluation of surgical practices. The advice to prepare an outline, while easy to give, may not be so easy to execute. Our plan did not emerge in just one thoughtful meeting but took a long time to formulate.

Once organized, a book tends to sound like a very natural way of thinking. The purpose of the whole book was summed up in the question "How can we get the most from the resources we allocate to surgical care?" Our book, entitled *Costs, Risks, and Benefits of Surgery*, ultimately had that feature with parts on background and general principles of cost-benefit and decision analysis, the evaluation of surgical innovations, and the assessment of costs, risks, and benefits of established procedures with a similar treatment of new procedures.

We were fortunate in getting the cooperation of economists and policy analysts to write treatments of the economic and decision theory chapters. The seminar met at the School of Public Health. We had contributions to the volume of papers by some people who were not members of the Surgery Group or even of the seminar. In some instances we knew of people who had written on special topics, and we were able to get them to prepare a paper directed toward the goal of the book. For example, the anesthesiologist Henrik H. Bendixen spoke to the Surgery Group on costs of intensive care and the comparative value of intensive care for various kinds of patients. At the time, no work on cost-benefit analysis had adequate medical examples illustrating both the methods and the needs for their use.

I shall not try to list all the examples, but there were 22 papers in all, of which at least 14 dealt with the evaluation of specific diseases or treatments or procedures.

At this time, the work of John E. Wennberg, now of Dartmouth, and his colleagues on small-area variation helped to illustrate the need for evaluation in surgery and in other areas of medicine. When comparable populations of patients have vastly different frequencies of treatment for a disease, something is troubling the medical system. For example, Gittelsohn and Wennberg found that, in 1969–71 for 13 hospital service areas of Vermont, rather homogeneous in their populations, the age-adjusted rates for tonsillectomies and adenoidectomies varied from 4 to 41 per 1,000 children per year. Put another way, by the age of 20 years, a child in one of the low service areas had a 9 percent chance of having such organs removed, whereas in an extreme service area, the child had a 60 percent chance of losing them. It seemed very unlikely that differences in the children's populations would create this difference in rates of removal. Instead, it seemed that differing attitudes of the physicians led to these differences in rates. It was not obvious that removing more tonsils was either better or worse medicine. Rather, the data showed that medicine did not have agreement about what should be done. Gittelsohn and Wennberg also reviewed the costs associated with the procedures being carried out.

Separately they reviewed the rates at which these and other procedures were being carried out in Vermont, Saskatchewan, U.S.A., England and Wales, and with U.S. Government employees in different insurance plans (Blue Cross/Blue Shield and Group). Tonsillectomy and adenoidectomy rates varied from 20 per 10,000 of all ages for U. S. Employees in group insurance to 87 per 10,000 for citizens of Saskatchewan. BC/BS U.S. Employees had 75 per 10,000.

To take another illustration, hysterectomy had a low rate of 21 in England and Wales and a high rate of 63 in Saskatchewan. Looking again at the 13 Vermont service areas, they varied from 30 to 60.

Similar big variations were found for appendectomy, prostatectomy, and cholecystectomy (gall bladder operations). Wennberg and his colleagues have continued to write on this idea of variation by area and to do research on it with similar findings on many topics. Thus, they have developed a substantial list of operations and medical procedures that have large unexplained variations in rates of use. Because they feel that this means that medicine has not been able to decide what to do about the particular disease or able to settle on which of these procedures is appropriate, they have encouraged the Congress to allocate funds for the deeper examination of some of these procedures. In 1989 and 1990, the National Center for Health Services Research and Health Care Technology Assessment was given funds especially for research on problems whose treatments had substantial areal variation. Very possibly, careful study over a period of years will lead to solid conclusions. It should be noted, though, that randomized trials were not among the methods that the legislation funded, and so the best comparisons are not yet being made more available. Much can be learned, but medicine, Congress, and probably physicians and the general public still do not adequately appreciate the need for trials. This work on areal variation then continues to be a valuable basis for further research as we come to the close of the twentieth century.

Bunker and I persuaded one of the surgeons in the Surgery Group, Benjamin A. Barnes, to join us in editing the book for the group. I had known him at the time of my work with Beecher. Barnes at that earlier time had been working on a problem of survival after burns and the relation of age and the amount of body burned to survival. This special type of dosage-response relation had not been much studied in the biostatistical literature, and we worked out a plan that was satisfactory for the problem. At that time of my life, I often worked up methods without following through to proper publication in my own professional statistical journals. It was not that I did not want to do it or did not have time, though perhaps I did not, but that I often did not appreciate that some problems had not been solved and that generalizations would be useful to the professions involved—both statistics and, in this instance, medicine.

⋆ ⋆ ⋆

As a result of my work with him in the National Halothane Study, Charles G. Child III asked me to prepare a paper for the Study on Surgical Services for the United States (known as the SOSSUS report). John Gilbert and Bucknam McPeek joined me in preparing this paper, published in 1976. Its essential message was that, in treatments for cancer, it was important to assess quality of life associated with the treatment. One reason for this importance was that not many treatments have the desired life-extending effects and therefore in choosing among treatments, it was important to assess the quality of life rather than the quantity.

Some investigators did not understand this need because they felt that they already knew that many cancer treatments led to undesirable side effects, but that these were nothing compared with the life-saving possibilities. The side of this argument that is right is that the side effects are not important compared to life-saving, but the weak part overlooks the unhappy fact that many treatments do not have firm life-saving effects but still do have side effects, whatever their beneficial aspects. We explained, then, why it is useful to be sure to measure quality of life in these circumstances. We reiterated this idea in a revision of this paper for *Costs, Risks, and Benefits of Surgery*.

Although health services researchers have developed tools for measuring quality of life, the wide use of such measures has been slow in coming, especially in research on medical technology assessment. To help encourage more frequent use of these methods, Jennifer Falotico-Taylor and I edited a book published in 1989 for the Institute of Medicine entitled *Quality of Life and Technology Assessment.*

Why do we need quality of life measures? Partly because medicine has advanced so much and been so successful. With the defeat of so many killing infectious diseases, much of medicine is no longer devoted to life saving, but to comfort and convenience. Once we realize that these are the goals, we need to be able to assess them. Can people deal with their jobs, friends, relatives? Can individuals care for themselves? Are they able to walk, enjoy leisure activities, and think clearly? If all we measure are death rates and hospitalizations, we miss out on the main goals of modern medicine, producing a better life.

For our major contribution to *Costs, Risks, and Benefits of Surgery*, Gilbert, McPeek, and I tried to assess what happens in surgery and anesthesia when innovations are appraised. This effort was prompted in part by previous work at the Bennett-Lumsdaine conference in Seattle. Recall that there we did not have a solid sample from a defined population, but merely collected papers we could find on lists. To improve on that approach, we hoped to get a sample from a known population. For surgery we had the possibility of using the lists created by the National Library of Medicine, called MEDLARS, which started in 1964. From this bibliographic listing, we got information about titles and authors of surgery papers produced from 1964 to 1972. At the National Library of Medicine, Charlotte Kenton was most helpful, and at the Francis A. Countway Library of Medicine at Harvard, Katherine Binderup helped us with the searches. Finally, Mary B. Ettling, then a student at Radcliffe, screened the material for this search and made it possible for us to concentrate on 107 clinical trials of surgery and anesthesia in the period 1964–1972. We wanted to see how well these innovations made out when they were tested.

We needed to read the papers and find out what they concluded about each innovation. It looked like a difficult problem, because I was going to go to California on sabbatical just at this time. Sometimes family preferences help work things out. My wife Virginia likes to drive, or at least enjoys it more than she does my driving, and so she volunteered to do as much of the driving as seemed appropriate. I was able to sit in the back seat of the car and read the papers on the way west and make notes on them. By the time we got to California, I had a summary of the 107 papers, and we coauthors were able to focus our attention on the 32 among these that included randomized controlled trials.

Table 16.2. Summary for Innovations in Randomized Clinical Trials[6]

	Primary	Secondary	Total
Innovation highly preferred	1	4[a]	5
Innovation preferred	5	2	7
About equal, innovation a success	2	2	4
About equal, innovation a disappoint- ment	7[a]	3	10
Standard preferred	3	3	6
Standard highly preferred	1	3	4
TOTALS: Comparisons	19	17	36
Papers	18[c]	14[b]	32

[a]One paper provided 2 such comparisons.
[b]Three papers provided 2 comparisons.
[c]One paper provided 2 comparisons.

The ratings we assigned (Table 16.2) are similar to those we used in the Bennett-Lumsdaine book. In the medical studies we could be more confident about the ratings because their authors usually produced a pithy conclusion that left little doubt about the appropriate rating, and we were usually able to give a one-sentence quotation or summary that led to the rating. For example, in summarizing an operation (for duodenal ulcer) called selective vagotomy compared with the standard truncal vagotomy, the authors said, "The main reason for adopting selective vagotomy has been the hope that diarrhea...would be eliminated....There was no significant difference in the incidence of diarrhea one year after operation."

We found it useful to separate the innovations that were about equal to the standard into two classes: (1) those which were regarded as a success because they were equally good and offered the physician an additional method of treatment, and (2) those regarded as a disappointment because, although equal in performance, they did not seem to be a practical substitute, perhaps because of costs or training or personnel requirements.

An additional distinction between kinds of innovations seemed useful. Some innovations were intended to treat the condition the patient suffered from—we called these primary treatments. Other treatments were intended to speed or smooth the course of recovery from the operation, for example, by preventing infections or other complications—we called these secondary treatments.

What we found was somewhat similar to our findings in the social science investigation. Note that among 36 comparisons between pairs of treatments in randomized trials, an innovation versus a standard therapy, in only 5 was the innovation highly favored. In 12 it was preferred or highly preferred, and in 16

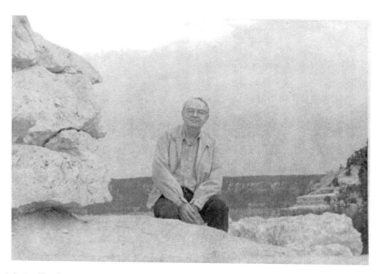

Fig. 16.4. Fred at the edge of the Grand Canyon (en route to Belmont after a sabbatical in Berkeley, CA), 1975.

it could be regarded as a success even though sometimes it was not actually better than the standard except that it gave the physician an additional tool. So the general message is similar to that of the social science paper (Table 16.1), but this time on a stronger methodological base because we had a population that we had sampled from, and we found that innovations do not often turn out extremely well. Once one sees this, one has explanations for it. Medicine has been going a long time, and we would be very upset if every time someone came up with an innovation it was better than what we had been doing. It would suggest that medical research had not been doing its job. At the same time the finding shows that it is very important that evaluations be carried out, for otherwise we will not know advances from retreats, especially when retreats are frequent. Table 16.2 shows that the standard was preferred to the innovation in 20 of 36 comparisons, probably because the standard itself was fairly effective.

People always want other methods than randomized trials for evaluating new therapies. When we reviewed 11 observational studies (containing 12 comparisons), we found that they tended to make innovations look good. Using the same notion of success for them as we used before, 5 of 12 comparisons found the innovation highly preferred, 7 of 12 preferred or better, and 8 of 12 regarded as at least a success. That's a success rate of two-thirds for observational studies as compared with 44 percent for randomized trials. We interpret this to mean that the innovation seems to be favored by the observational study more than by the randomized trial, and therefore we do not trust the observational study as much. In later years I have tried to follow up this problem, as have others.

Although William G. Cochran, from the Department of Statistics at Harvard, first declined to come to the seminar (he had had some health problems) and then declined to lead a group, somehow the graduate students persuaded him first to come to the seminar and then to lead a group after all. His group wrote an impressive paper for *Costs, Risks, and Benefits of Surgery* reviewing the designs of experiments in the surgical treatment of duodenal ulcer.

For the common operation for surgical treatment of suspected acute appendicitis, Raymond Neutra wrote an instructive paper. Generally speaking, surgeons prefer not to operate if the patient is not diseased. Thus, if a patient does not have appendicitis, it seems better not to take out the appendix. (An exception occurs when some other abdominal operation is carried out. As preventive medicine, surgeons then often snatch the appendix on the way by, so as to avoid having to do another operation later just for appendicitis.)

The question still remains, though, what should be the appropriate conditions leading to appendectomy. If we think of a person as having a severity score for the disease running from, say, 1 to 24, then by modeling the process of disease, operation, and death, Neutra was able to consider various outcomes: deaths, hospital costs, and convalescent days. Suppose that a program was created that did not operate on anyone with a score less than x but did operate on everyone with a score as great as, or greater than, x. Then for each value of x Neutra estimated the numbers of deaths, the hospital costs in millions of dollars, and the numbers of convalescent days. To minimize the number of deaths, one would operate at score 5; to minimize the hospital costs, one would operate at score 16; and to minimize number of convalescent days, one would operate at 14. There is a conflict between minimizing deaths and minimizing either hospital costs or convalescent days. This is a forceful example of a sort that occurs frequently in cost-benefit analysis, namely that different criteria lead to different "best" things to do. To reduce deaths to a minimum may produce hundreds of extra years of convalescence.

The issue of choice of endpoint for optimization has great importance for society, because we cannot hope to do all the "best" things at the same time. If we minimize the deaths, then we will produce many more wasted hospital days, and when saving one additional life means many lifetimes of needless convalescence plus associated societal costs from medical expenditures and lifetimes of absences from productive work, we begin to see the need for studying trade-offs.

Probably the most famous aphorism dealing with multiple endpoints is the goal "to do the greatest good for the greatest number." This is a great motto and a good campaign slogan, but it is not ordinarily an available option. The "greatest good" would give all resources or as much as he or she could use to one person, whereas helping the "greatest number" would give a little to as many as possible. It is a rare accident when the optimum occurs for several possible variables simultaneously.

The book made four main recommendations. First, that more studies of the effectiveness of surgical treatments be carried out, especially where there is professional disagreement (as indicated, for example, by small-area variation). Second, that we need to improve our grasp of the components of cost-benefit analysis, of the merits of the various data-gathering techniques, and of the ethics of data gathering.

One problem that continues is the tendency of experts to believe that they know more than they do, just as laymen do. Physicians have the obligation to do the best for their patients. This obligation seems to conflict with the idea of allowing their patients to participate in investigations needed to find out the effectiveness of a therapy. The question is, should a physician have to have documentable evidence before believing some treatment is wise?

We have a strange double standard now. As long as a physician treats a patient intending to cure, the treatment is admissible. When the object is to find out whether the treatment has value, the physician is immediately subject to many constraints. By just believing, the physician justifies action. By being agnostic, and willing to find out the truth, the physician stirs up a hornet's nest.

In the area of drugs, though, we have gone past this idea and require at least initially that drugs be safe and beneficial. (We are weakening, though, and in dread diseases we may now allow untried drugs to be used, and this seems likely ultimately to undermine the whole Food and Drug Administration system of regulation.)

The third recommendation suggested training in cost-benefit analysis for medical schools and its introduction into practice. In the field of continuing education, this is happening, and some medical schools do train in cost-benefit analysis. Probably the major effect here, though, will come from the various economic crunches created by rising costs and fiscal failures. Both public and private organizations have a common interest in trying to reduce expenditures, and so this sort of training will be enforced, and also some effects of cost-benefit work will spill over through regulation or reimbursement activities.

Fourth, we recommended that information on outcomes and costs of medical care be made available in a manner suitable for presentation to the public. Some moves in this direction have been made. For example, the Health Care Financing Administration has been presenting information about adjusted death rates for hospitals across the nation for various conditions. The system of Diagnosis-Related Groups does make available some information about costs.

In a more clinical matter, the problem is not easy. Physicians have always tried to explain to their patients, when they have options in care, what the likelihood of various outcomes may be. Delivering such information is hard to do. The patient may be sitting there scared and almost deranged, and now has to consider rational choices when it is hard even to listen to what the physician is saying. Wennberg has been using films to try to help the physician and patient get past these barriers. The films illustrate, through short talks by people who have or have not had treatment, what the outcomes have been like, to help patients consider whether they should have the treatment.

Wennberg's first work has been in the treatment of the prostate and the decision whether to have a prostatectomy. The outcomes of the surgery differ a great deal from patient to patient, and so the patients' preferences matter in considering whether to have the operation at a given time or to engage in watchful waiting. These developments are pathbreaking efforts at improving both patients' choices and the quality of their informed consent.

★ ★ ★

After Dean Hiatt completed his term as dean of the School of Public Health, he introduced the Program in Clinical Effectiveness at the teaching hospitals of the Harvard Medical School. His general idea was that introducing basic biology into medicine in mid-century had made a big difference to medical knowledge and practice. In its turn, he felt training in evaluation would make a difference in a similar way in clinical programs. At the close of our century, so many good technologies are being invented and marketed that it is important for practicing physicians to know how to do evaluation and how to act on the results in practice. Such simple ideas as choosing between two equivalent therapies on the basis of their cost has not traditionally been part of the medical education. Naturally, the new program is much more sophisticated than this, and physicians holding important posts all over the country have been learning about decision theory, cost-effectiveness analysis, and generally how to appraise medical procedures and even programs. As these leaders carry the program back to their own institutions, the approach will be more widely disseminated, and we can expect gradually improved health care. If we waste less and use the more effective techniques, the nation can afford more and will get better care.

I would not like to leave the impression that I think technology can fix everything in society or that simple economics is preferable to compassion. I do want society to have the opportunity to make its choices, when it is forced to choose, as it must, on the basis of solid information on the performance and the costs of technologies modulated by ethics and law.

Notes

1. Recommendation 5-10, Vol. I, p. 5.
2. Francis et al. (1955) and Meier (1957, 1972).
3. Membership of Surgery Group

Walter H. Abelmann (1974–75)
Clark C. Abt (1974–75)
Ernest M. Barsamian (1974–75)
Benjamin A. Barnes (1973–76)
David Berengut (1974–75)
John P. Bunker (1973–75)
Joan Chmiel (1975–76)
Jean Dunegan (1973–74)
Mary Ettling (1975–76)
Garry F. Fitzpatrick (1973–75)
Floyd J. Fowler, Jr. (1974–75)
Maurice S. Fox (1973–75)
Miriam Gasko-Green (1975–76)
John P. Gilbert (1973–76)
Alan Gittelsohn (1973–74)
Jerry R. Green (1974–75)
John Hedley-Whyte (1975–76)
Nan Laird (1975–76)
John J. Lamberti (1973–74)
Frederick C. Lane (1974–75)
Robert Lew (1975–76)
Willard G. Manning, Jr. (1974–75)
William V. McDermott, Jr. (1974–75)
Barbara J. McNeil (1973–76)

Bucknam McPeek (1973–76)
Klim McPherson (1973–74)
Lillian Miao (1973–75)
Alfred P. Morgan, Jr. (1973–75)
Frederick Mosteller (1973–76)
Duncan Neuhauser (1973–75)
Raymond R. Neutra (1973–75)
John Petkau (1975–76)
Joseph S. Pliskin (1973–75)
Nava Pliskin (1973–75)
John Raker (1975–76)
Mark Rogers (1973–74)
Donald Shepard (1974–75)
Richard Singer (1974–75)
Keith Soper (1975–76)
Michael Stoto (1975–76)
Judith Strenio (1975–76)
Amy K. Taylor (1973–75)
Kenneth Wachter (1974–75)
Peter Walker (1973–74)
John E. Wennberg (1973–75)
David A. Wise (1974–75)
Jane Worcester (1974–75)

4. Chapter 22 discusses the Health Science Policy Working Group.
5. Anderson et al. (1980).
6. Gilbert, McPeek, and Mosteller (1977), p. 128.

References

Anderson, S., Auquier, A., Hauck, W. W., Oakes, D., Vandaele, W. A., and Weisberg, H. I., with contributions from A. S. Bryk and J. Kleinman (1980). *Statistical Methods for Comparative Studies: Techniques for Bias Reduction.* New York: Wiley.

Barnes, B. A. (1977). Discarded operations: Surgical innovation by trial and error. Chapter 8 in J. P. Bunker, B. A. Barnes, and F. Mosteller, editors, *Costs, Risks, and Benefits of Surgery.* New York: Oxford University Press. 109–123.

Barsamian, E. M. (1977). The rise and fall of internal mammary artery ligation in the treatment of angina pectoris and the lessons learned. Chapter 13 in J. P. Bunker, B. A. Barnes, and F. Mosteller, editors, *Costs, Risks, and Benefits of Surgery.* New York: Oxford University Press. 212–220.

Beecher, H. K. (1955). The powerful placebo. *Journal of the American Medical Association,* 159(17):1602–1606.

Beecher, H. K. (1966). Ethics and clinical research. *The New England Journal of Medicine,* 274(24):1354–1360.

Beecher, H. K., Keats, A. S., Mosteller, F., and Lasagna, L. (1953). The effectiveness of oral analgesics (morphine, codeine, acetylsalicylic acid) and the problem of placebo "reactors" and "non-reactors." *Journal of Pharmacology and Experimental Therapeutics,* 109(4):393–400.

Beecher, H. K. and Todd, D. P. (1954). A study of the deaths associated with anesthesia and surgery. *Annals of Surgery,* 140:2–34.

Bennett, C. A. and Lumsdaine, Arthur A., editors. (1975). *Evaluation and Experiment: Some Critical Issues in Assessing Social Programs.* New York: Academic Press.

Boruch, R. F. (1972). Abstracts of randomized experiments for planning and evaluating social programs. Compiled for the Social Science Research Council's Committee on Experimentation for Planning and Evaluating Social Programs and for the Project on Measurement and Experimentation in Social Settings at Northwestern University. Unpublished.

Boruch, R. F. with Davis, S. (1974). Appendix: Abstracts of controlled experiments for planning and evaluating social programs. In H. W. Riecken and R. F. Boruch, *Social Experimentation as a Method for Planning and Evaluating Social Intervention.* New York: Academic Press.

Bunker, J. P., Barnes, B. A., and Mosteller, F., editors. (1977). *Costs, Risks, and Benefits of Surgery.* New York: Oxford University Press.

Cochran, W. G., Diaconis, P., Donner, A. P., Hoaglin, D. C., O'Connor, N. E., Peterson, O. L., and Rosenoer, V. M. (1977). Experiments in surgical treatment of duodenal ulcer. Chapter 11 in J. P. Bunker, B. A. Barnes, and F. Mosteller, editors, *Costs, Risks, and Benefits of Surgery.* New York: Oxford University Press. 176–197.

Elinson, J., with abstracts prepared by C. Gell, and the School of Public Health, Columbia University (March 15–17, 1967). The effectiveness of social action programs in health and welfare. Working paper, Ross Conference on Pediatric Research: Problems of assessing the effectiveness of child health services.

Francis, T., Jr., Korns, R. F., Voight, R. B., Boisen, M., Hemphill, F. M., Napier, J. A., and Tolchinsky, E. (1955). An evaluation of the 1954 poliomyelitis vaccine trials: Summary report. *American Journal of Public Health*, 45(5, Part 2):1–51.

Gilbert, J. P., Light, R. J., and Mosteller, F. (1975a). Assessing social innovations: An empirical base for policy. In R. Zeckhauser, A. Harberger, R. Haveman, L. Lynn, Jr., W. Niskanen, and A. Williams, editors, *Benefit-Cost and Policy Analysis 1974: An Aldine Annual on Forecasting, Decision-making, and Evaluation*. Chicago: Aldine Publishing Company. 3–65.

Gilbert, J. P., Light, R. J., and Mosteller, F. (1975b). Assessing social innovations: An empirical base for policy. In C. A. Bennett and A. A. Lumsdaine, editors, *Evaluation and Experiment: Some Critical Issues in Assessing Social Programs*. New York: Academic Press. 39–193.

Gilbert, J. P., McPeek, B., and Mosteller, F. (1977). Progress in surgery and anesthesia: Benefits and risks of innovative therapy. Chapter 9 in J. P. Bunker, B. A. Barnes, and F. Mosteller, editors, *Costs, Risks, and Benefits of Surgery*. New York: Oxford University Press. 124–169.

Gittelsohn, A. M. and Wennberg, J. E. (1977). On the incidence of tonsillectomy and other common surgical procedures. Chapter 7 in J. P. Bunker, B. A. Barnes and F. Mosteller, editors, *Costs, Risks, and Benefits of Surgery*. New York: Oxford University Press. 91–106.

Kelman, H. R. (1962). An experiment in the rehabilitation of nursing home patients. *Public Health Reports*, 77(4):356–367.

Lasagna, L., Mosteller, F., von Felsinger, J. M., and Beecher, H. K. (1954). A study of the placebo response. *American Journal of Medicine*, 16:770–779.

Light, R. J., Mosteller, F., and Winokur, H. S. Jr. (1971). Using controlled field studies to improve public policy. Chapter 6 in *Federal Statistics: Report of the President's Commission*, Vol II. Washington, D.C.: U. S. Government Printing Office. 367–398.

McPeek, B., Gilbert, J. P., and Mosteller, F. (1977). The end result: Quality of life. Chapter 10 in J. P. Bunker, B. A. Barnes, and F. Mosteller, editors, *Costs, Risks, and Benefits of Surgery*. New York: Oxford University Press. 170–175.

McPeek, B., McPeek, C., and Mosteller, F. (1982). In memoriam: John Parker Gilbert (1926–1980). *The American Statistician*, 36:37.

Meier, P. (1957). Safety of the poliomyelitis vaccine. *Science*, 125:1067–1071.

Meier, P. (1972). The biggest public health experiment ever: The 1954 field trial of the salk poliomyelitis vaccine. In J. M. Tanur, F. Mosteller, W. H. Kruskal, R. F. Link, R. S. Pieters, and G. R. Rising, editors, *Statistics: A Guide to the Unknown*. San Francisco: Holden-Day. 3–14.

Meyer, H. J., Borgatta, E. F., and Jones, W. C. (1975). *Girls at Vocational High: An Experiment in Social Work Intervention.* New York: Russell Sage Foundation.

Miao, L. L. (1977). Gastric freezing: An example of the evaluation of medical therapy by randomized clinical trials. Chapter 12 in J. P. Bunker, B. A. Barnes, and F. Mosteller, editors, *Costs, Risks, and Benefits of Surgery.* New York: Oxford University Press. 198–211.

Mosteller, F. and Falotico-Taylor, J., editors (1989). *Quality of Life and Technology Assessment,* monograph of the Council on Health Care Technology, Institute of Medicine. Washington, D.C.: National Academy Press.

Mosteller, F., Gilbert, J. P., and McPeek, B. (1976). Measuring the quality of life. In *Surgery in the United States: A Summary Report of the Study on Surgical Services for the United States,* sponsored jointly by the American College of Surgeons and The American Surgical Association, Vol. III. 2283–2299.

Neutra, R. (1977). Indications for the surgical treatment of suspected acute appendicitis: A cost-effectiveness approach. Chapter 18 in J. P. Bunker, B. A. Barnes, and F. Mosteller, editors, *Costs, Risks, and Benefits of Surgery.* New York: Oxford University Press. 277–307.

The President's Commission on Federal Statistics (1971). *Federal Statistics: Report of the President's Commission* (2 volumes). Washington, D.C.: U.S. Government Printing Office.

Yin, R. K. (1984). *Case Study Research: Design and Methods.* Applied Social Research Methods Series, Vol. V. Beverly Hills, CA: Sage Publications.

Zeckhauser, R., Harberger, A. C., Haveman, R. H., Lynn, L. E. Jr., Niskanen, W. A., and Williams, A., editors (1975). *Benefit-Cost and Policy Analysis 1974: An Aldine Annual on Forecasting, Decision-making, and Evaluation.* Chicago: Aldine Publishing Company.

17

Teaching

After a talk I gave at a scientific meeting when I was middle-aged, a very elderly man introduced himself afterward as one of my former students. I thought he meant that he had been a student in our statistical television course on Continental Classroom, but he denied it. No, it was back at Carnegie Institute of Technology. I had almost forgotten that in my senior year there I had taught a night-school course.

The distribution of ages of participants in night-school courses is much different from that in daytime. I had taught this gentleman one course in algebra and trigonometry, and happily with that training he went on to become head of a large corporation in the steel industry. He did not actually claim that that experience was the main reason for his success, but I was willing to assume it.

I had taken a practice-teaching course under the direction of E. G. Olds, because at that time I was hoping to be a mathematics teacher in a secondary school. To qualify for a teaching certificate, one had to take a certain number of college courses related to teaching. Olds was most conscientious about attending the practice-teaching course and listening to the lecture and responses to questions, and based on his notes, he gave me much good advice. Some of it no longer applies, because architecture has changed. For example, in winter a key point in the old days was to notice when the room got too warm, because then it was time to open the windows and wake up the students; today many public buildings do not have windows that open.

I learned other important things. For example, I learned to rehearse the lecture. Olds emphasized getting an outline of the lecture firmly in hand, including the examples. Whether from him or from myself, I soon discovered that I might drastically underestimate the time it takes to give an example. (Even my mother used to ask me, "Is this a long story?") This is especially true when examples have to work out right, for sometimes there are glitches. At first in arrogance, a teacher may grab an example out of the air and work through it off the cuff in the classroom. The pitfalls can be ghastly. The example may be ill chosen in that it produces all sorts of algebraic complications one did

F. Mosteller, *The Pleasures of Statistics: The Autobiography of Frederick Mosteller*,
DOI 10.1007/978-0-387-77956-0_17,
© Springer Science + Business Media, LLC 2010

not wish to emphasize, or it may involve nasty arithmetic when it is important that the result be exactly rather than approximately correct. The instructor may make mistakes and not be able to locate the difficulty. Students then go off in wrong directions, and the disarrayed class becomes a disaster.

When used with control and great skill, however, such seeming mistakes can form part of an effective teaching style that I call the stumblebum technique. A friend of mine at the Massachusetts Institute of Technology used the stumblebum technique regularly and to good effect. He would start on an easy development where he had explained clearly what he hoped to do, and after a step or two toward the goal, he would stand back from the board with a puzzled look and say that he couldn't seem to see what to do next. The students (bright, eager MITers) would go after it like their beaver mascot, and he would say, "Oh, yes, that's a good suggestion," and, "Maybe that will work," with the result that the students participated in the development of the theorem, or at least many did. (We teachers tend to overestimate the numbers in the class who actually participate in such efforts, and I believe most students are frozen out of the discussion. A teacher using this technique can increase the participation by encouraging the quiet class members.) This is a top-notch educational device when you can bring it off.

I once watched a grade-school teacher—he taught children from first through third grade in an Iron Curtain country, Hungary as I recall—use the stumblebum technique by making obvious mistakes, and the children would learn by leading this kindly, helpless old man through the task. He was so good an actor that at an international meeting of mathematics teachers, he had about 100 adults standing up and shouting at him to help him fix up what he was doing. I could scarcely control my laughter, because he was so experienced at this device and so gently pleased and happily surprised with the suggestions. The lecture itself was on a probabilistic topic, and I stole it for use in Harvard classes by telling the students that this is how they teach probability to children in Hungary. It treated a topic that I always had difficulty explaining very well—the exact distribution of the sum of two independent random numbers, such as occur when two dice are tossed and we add the numbers of dots on their top faces—and the Harvard students liked it and learned quickly, I think, because they were no longer threatened by the material and had an amusing story of children being educated through play. The same example, rather abstract without the story of the children, had little interest for most of the students in my earlier teaching years.

Unfortunately, the stumblebum approach is time-consuming, because one has to walk up blind alleys to get the most out of the method, and so although occasionally it is practical, we have to recognize that we cannot expect to teach the mathematics that it has taken societies millennia to develop by making young people invent the whole thing for themselves. Sometimes this approach is called the Socratic Method. We have to move along at a faster pace most of the time.

Uncertainty about the amount of time needed to carry out a lecture and proof from bad experiences about what could be covered in an hour led me to work out the lecture as Olds suggested, including the details of the examples. Even so, I found that I still didn't know how long it all would take. Listing the material in a good outline and even giving the steps still didn't tell how long the lesson would take, even when uninterrupted by the students' questions. To get timing, I would go to an empty classroom and deliver the lecture aloud. I found that it wasn't adequate to tell myself sotto voce what I was going to say, because one has a tendency to cheat and not actually deliver the whole message and to pretend that whole pages worth of material have been said that have not been delivered. Some chunks went on forever with little progress or content and included sentences I floundered on because they were such tongue twisters. Straightening these out and eliminating excessive illustrations helped a great deal. I didn't memorize the lectures. I did sometimes learn to start certain sentences in a special way so that they led smoothly to a conclusion. Thus I had to practice a lecture several times, and consequently preparing a one-hour lecture was very time-consuming. The advantage was that, when I got to class, my effort could go into the delivery with attention to the class and its responses instead of having to worry about the content of the lecture and how I was moving along. (Utter silence in a class is as big a clue about the lecture as the curious incident of the dog that did nothing in the night in the Sherlock Holmes story.) This doesn't mean that all problems have been solved, but it takes a great burden off the beginning teacher.

In spite of all the effort, problems still arise—for example, when the same notation is mistakenly used for two or three different things. "But, sir, I thought k was to be used for...." I still had not understood the value of students' questions, and I had not yet come to want examples that have stature. Later in my life I wanted the examples used in lectures to have some importance if possible. I distinguish this from interest for the student. I like an example to have historical importance if possible—for instance, the example used the first time a method was put forward, or a problem that formerly could not be solved without the method, or a central question that was resolved by the method—central because it had either social or intellectual significance.

Unfortunately, what I call stature and what I call student interest have little relation to each other. I do not have trouble picking out problems that have stature, intellectual or social, but finding out which problems have student interest must come from experience.

The problem of airplanes with several engines has usually attracted attention. When a plane can fly if it has more than half its engines working, but crashes otherwise, and engines fail independently with the same probability, is it better to be on a 1-, 2-, 3-, or 4-engine plane? Because college people often travel in planes, some personal threat may stimulate attention.

Another example of a problem that challenges students is the isolates problem, which on the face of it seems rather dry and uninteresting, and is very difficult to solve for people who are not well prepared in the mathematics of combinatorics. The problem's story is that in a class of, say, 10 people, each student is asked independently to choose two other class members as companions. If the students do their choosing at random, what is the probability that at least one person is not chosen? It is easy to simulate the answer to this question by carrying out the assignment of choices repeatedly using random numbers. It is not easy to carry out the algebra. Students in elementary statistics classes regarded this problem as a serious challenge and worked hard on it. I suppose that the threat of being an isolate personally piques them. How often could not being chosen be just a matter of chance, rather than a consequence of an unattractive personality?

Using Random Numbers

A few words about random numbers and their uses in simulations and sampling may help to clarify their use and value. In straightforward uses of random numbers, each member of a set of categories has equal probability. For example, the one-digit random numbers can be regarded as drawn from the set of 10 equally likely digits $0, 1, 2, \ldots, 9$. Thus each has probability $1/10$ of occurring in each position in a random number table. In any finite number of random numbers, say 100, we do not expect each of the digits 0 through 9 to occur exactly 10 times, but we do not expect their proportions to vary far from 0.1. Of course, once you have picked a digit, say 4, from a table, there is nothing random about it. The randomness refers to the process that led to the table of digits.

From Table 17.1 let us enumerate the numbers of 0's, 1's, and so on in the 100 random digits in the first two rows. We then find for this first hundred the counts:

Digit:	0	1	2	3	4	5	6	7	8	9
Occurrences:	12	16	12	6	7	10	7	9	11	10

For the second 100 digits and the third 100 digits in this table we find:

Digit:	0	1	2	3	4	5	6	7	8	9
Occurrences:										
Second 100:	8	11	5	12	15	13	6	12	11	7
Third 100:	6	7	15	13	7	7	14	11	12	8

These outcomes of sampling 100 digits three times illustrate the kind of variability that occurs in such sampling. Although we should get 10 occurrences on the average for each digit in each set of 100, we see that that exact count occurred only twice in 30 opportunities. The counts for the digits varied from

Table **17.1.** 1000 Random Digits †

Line Number	Column Number				
	00-09	10-19	20-29	30-39	40-49
00	15544 80712	97742 21500	97081 42451	50623 56071	28882 28739
01	01011 21285	04729 39986	73150 31548	30168 76189	56996 19210
02	47435 53308	40718 29050	74858 64517	93573 51058	68501 42723
03	91312 75137	86274 59834	69844 19853	06917 17413	44474 86530
04	12775 08768	80791 16298	22934 09630	98862 39746	64623 32768
05	31466 43761	94872 92230	52367 13205	38634 55882	77518 36252
06	09300 43847	40881 51243	97810 18903	53914 31688	06220 40422
07	73582 13810	57784 72454	68997 72229	30340 08844	53924 89630
08	11092 81392	58189 22697	41063 09451	09789 00637	06450 85990
09	93322 98567	00116 35605	66790 52965	62877 21740	56476 49296
10	80134 12484	67089 08674	70753 90959	45842 59844	45214 36505
11	97888 31797	95037 84400	76041 96668	75920 68482	56855 97417
12	92612 27084	59459 69380	98654 20407	88151 56263	27126 63797
13	72744 45586	43279 44218	83638 05422	00995 70217	78925 39097
14	96256 70653	45285 26293	78305 80252	03625 40159	68760 84716
15	07851 47452	66742 83331	54701 06573	98169 37499	67756 68301
16	25594 41552	96475 56151	02089 33748	65239 89956	89559 33687
17	65358 15155	59374 80940	03411 94656	69440 47156	77115 99463
18	09402 31008	53424 21928	02198 61201	02457 87214	59750 51330
19	97424 90765	01634 37328	41243 33564	17884 94747	93650 77668

†A good source of random digits and random normal deviates is *A Million Random Digits with 100,000 Normal Deviates*, The RAND Corporation. Glencoe, Ill.: Free Press of Glencoe, 1955.

5 to 16 in these three sets of 100. Thus when we say 10 are "expected," it does not mean that the occurrence necessarily has high frequency.

We can also use the digits for larger sets of categories. For example, if we use 2-digit numbers, then the 100 numbers 00, 01, 02, ..., 98, 99 each have probability .01 of occurring in a given position. If we want to sample, say, 5 items from among 100, we first number the items from 00 to 99. Then we take 5 successive non-overlapping 2-digit random numbers from the table and choose the items with those numbers to get a random sample of 5. If the same 2-digit number occurs more than once, it is ignored after its first occurrence. In our table, we might decide in advance before looking at the table to use the first 2 digits in successive rows to choose our sample of 5, and therefore the items numbered 15, 01, 47, 91, and 12 would be chosen for the sample.

If we wanted to choose from a population of items with a count different from an even power of 10, then one way to sample would just waste some of the random digits. If the population had 65 items, we could use 2-digit numbers after assigning the items the numbers 01, 02, through 65. When a 2-digit random number exceeds 65, or is 00, we ignore it. In our example of drawing a random sample of 5 from the 65 items, using the random numbers in the first 2 digits in each row will give the sample 15, 01, 47, 12, and 31 because we must omit the number 91.

If the number of items is just larger than a power of 10, for example 1001, we would have to use an additional digit in the random numbers (here, 4 digits) and waste nearly nine-tenths of the drawings. Mathematicians have ways around this, but I would be telling most people more than they wish to know if I went into it. Random numbers are comparatively cheap, and so wasting them usually does not have a high cost.

These methods can help with sampling of items. Another very important use is for simulation. Let me illustrate with the example of the isolates problem. The general idea is to carry the process through to completion many times. In each trial, the final answer might be the number of students out of 10 who are not chosen. That number is then recorded, and the process is repeated many times so as to find (approximately) the probability that 0, 1, 2, and so on are not chosen.

Let us run through one simulation. Number our students from 0 through 9. We use the first two digits in each row of our random number table to choose the students, going on to the next digit in that row if either the choosing student's own number or a number previously chosen in that line occurs. For the choosing student 0, the random numbers are 1 and 5 in the first line of our random number table; for the choosing student 1, the random numbers in the second line are 0 and 1, but 1 is the choosing student's own number, and a flurry of 0s and 1s are bypassed until we get to a useful 2. Continuing in this manner, we get the pattern shown in Table 17.2 for our first simulation.

Table 17.2. One simulation of the isolates problem using random numbers in a class of 10 students, each choosing two others.

					Chosen					
Chooser	0	1	2	3	4	5	6	7	8	9
0	—	x				x				
1	x	—	x							
2			—		x			x		
3		x		—						x
4		x	x		—					
5		x		x		—				
6	x						—			x
7				x		x		—		
8	x	x							—	
9			x	x						—
Times chosen	3	5	3	3	1	2	0	1	0	2

Table 17.2 shows one complete execution or simulation of the process described in the isolates problem. It shows that 2 students were not chosen. It also shows that by chance one student was chosen by half the class and thus seems very popular. When Cleo Youtz carried out the simulation 1000 times, she found the results given in Table 17.3.

Table 17.3. Outcomes for 1000 simulations of the isolates problem compared with theoretical frequencies.

Number chosen	Number of isolates	Simulation frequency	Theoretical frequency
10	0	289	274
9	1	441	456
8	2	229	226
7	3	37	41
6	4	4	3
5	5	0	0
4	6	0	0
3	7	0	0
		1000	1000

Estimated from the simulation, the probability that we get no isolates is .289, which means that the estimated probability that one or more would be isolates by chance is $1 - .289 = .711$. Thus in the preponderance of cases, some people will be isolates with 10 people and 2 choices each. Rarely would four or more isolates occur.

The theoretical problem has been solved by Leo Katz, and the correct probabilities to three places have been multiplied by 1000 to compare the true values with the findings from the simulations. The two sets of counts shown in the table are very similar. On the basis of information not given here, we can say that this set of 1000 simulations is closer to the true probabilities than two-thirds of such sets of 1000 simulations would be. Thus, the agreement for our example is a little better than average.

As this example illustrates, by carrying out the process with a computer many times, we often can get an accurate, though usually not exact, answer to the problem.

In scientific work in statistics, instead of uniformly distributed random numbers like ours, we often need random numbers having a special mound-shaped distribution called the normal distribution (also called Gaussian). William S. Gossett, an important statistician who worked for the Guinness Brewery and published under the pseudonym Student, did not have normal random numbers back in 1908 when he was working on a statistical problem, so he approximated them by using the lengths of left middle fingers of criminals from the identification system in use in England at that time (the Bertillon system). He sampled from these by writing them on cards, and then shuffling them. Then he used the information from the samples to solve a mathematical problem in statistics that had plagued practitioners for years. The problem was one of finding out how likely a sample mean was to differ by any given amount from a population mean when the variability of the sample observations had to be estimated from the sample. By a combination of mathematical work and simulations using the samples of lengths of criminals' fingers as random numbers together with a system of curves developed by Karl Pearson, Student found the correct answer. That he might have found a good useful answer is not so surprising, but that he found exactly the correct answer is partly brilliance and partly luck. Other systems of curves were also available; and had he used these, which were more popular than Pearson's on the European Continent, he probably would not have found exactly the correct answer. That was one of the most successful simulations in history. The distribution he found is called Student's t distribution, and it is in wide use today, especially in problems where sample means need to be compared to decide, considering sampling fluctuations, whether they come from populations with essentially identical true means.

Teaching at Carnegie and Princeton

In my extra year at Carnegie, I taught a section in a regular course in analytic geometry. It was a rather routine experience, because I was handed a text, told what the lessons were for the semester, and what the assignments were. Then I went to class and taught with examples, explained the problems and material people had queries about, graded the papers, helped make up the examinations, and graded them.

The contrast was impressive when I went to Princeton and was to be a teaching assistant in a course under the direction of Luther Pfahler Eisenhart, Dean of the Graduate School and former Chairman of the Department of Mathematics. A note in my mailbox informed me that the organizational meeting for the course was to be on a certain day at a certain time in the Professors' Room—a place I had never been. I appeared in good time, but Dean Eisenhart was already there, so I seemed to be late. Two people meeting in an enormous room was also threatening. My only acquaintance with him was through the Graduate School. With his wife and family, he lived in a residence beside the Graduate School dormitories, which was just a nice walk from Fine Hall, the then exquisite mathematics building on the campus. (When the new Fine Hall was built, about 1968, the original Fine Hall was remodeled, losing some of its charm, and renamed Jones Hall.) The Dean and his wife held weekly teas for graduate students on Sunday afternoons, and my roommate and I had feared to attend them until one day we got a special call advising us that we had not attended and that we were expected the following Sunday or else. We came. At another such tea we had the fun of meeting Bertrand Russell.

Eisenhart was a geometer, and he had written books on differential geometry and Riemannian geometry. In addition, though I did not know it then, he had taken a strong interest in having statistics developed at Princeton, and had been central in bringing my mentor S. S. Wilks to Princeton. Furthermore, I later learned that his son, Churchill Eisenhart, had studied some with Wilks, and then gone on after further study in England to become a distinguished statistician. He worked at the National Bureau of Standards. Churchill and I became good friends several years later when I worked in New York toward the close of World War II.

Dean Eisenhart was a very gruff person and possibly hard of hearing. He had a most upsetting habit of asking a question and then, just as you had grasped it and were about to respond with your first word, he would say, "WHAT?" Then, after you had gathered your wits and were again about to follow up his question, he would say, "WHAT?" Perhaps he felt he was asking rhetorical questions, and did not expect or desire answers. At any rate, between his distinction, deanship, and idiosyncrasy, he had me at a considerable disadvantage.

He then explained the purpose of the meeting. He told me that at Princeton University, by tradition, each instructor chose the text he thought best for the course. (At that time the mathematics department had no women faculty.) He then announced that he himself had chosen Luther Pfahler Eisenhart's *Coordinate Geometry* as the text for his section, and asked what I had planned for mine. Instead of bravely standing up for the book I used at Carnegie, or admitting that I had no idea I was to be asked to choose a text and requesting more time, I bowed to fate and said I would use the same text. Probably that was a wise decision. Anyway it taught me a painful lesson. Never choose a text you have not seen.

The difference between the text Eisenhart wrote and the text I had taught from before is intimately related to an important distinction—applications versus mathematics. The book I had taught from at Carnegie was busy teaching students how to solve problems, whereas in the preface to *Coordinate Geometry*, Eisenhart said that the aim of his book "is to encourage the reader to *think* mathematically."

What had happened, according to my psychoanalysis, was that Eisenhart had written several texts on advanced geometry. These texts leaned a little on more elementary mathematics from analytical geometry, and standard texts on that subject did not teach analytical geometry from such a rigorous point of view. Therefore Eisenhart had decided to fill this omission by writing an elementary text with a fairly advanced viewpoint. The problems were very formal and abstract. The reader was not always warned that a statement was a theorem, the clue being that the number of a theorem was enclosed in brackets, whereas equation numbers were enclosed in parentheses. I learned not to like the decimal notation for reference. I also learned to memorize the theorems associated with the numbers and the equations with their equation numbers because they were used repeatedly. Without memory work, the thumbing coefficient became very large.

Once I realized that this book was totally abstract and that a few mathematically inclined students were going to learn a lot from it, and many less inclined were going to hate mathematics for the rest of their lives, I decided that my job was to make this abstract work come alive in the classroom. And so I worked hard to bring seemingly practical problems to class to help the students appreciate what they were learning, and see that it had applied as well as theoretical merits. I say "seemingly" because a good deal of analytic geometry is a helpmate for calculus and deals with problems not lost in antiquity, but found there. I've often wondered how Dean Eisenhart engaged his class's interest, but I never found out. I know that my class scored better on both the midterm and the final than his did. But maybe I taught them problem solving and he taught them deeper mathematics.

Eisenhart was very fussy about language in geometry. For example, when anyone tried to speak of "the equation of a straight line," he always corrected to "*an* equation of a straight line." Such an emphasis on lack of uniqueness, although it seems academic, can sometimes make a big difference in mathematics about what is possible and what is not.

Over the years Dean Eisenhart treated me very well, and my initial feelings of apprehension were not justified. He liked to know what was going on in statistics and was very proud that he had established such a unit in the Department of Mathematics. I came to realize that he felt the statistics students were in a sense his own, even though he rarely taught them and even though they seemed different from the other mathematics students.

★ ★ ★

My next teaching was of two sorts: some statistics in a course Wilks had written a text for (and had not published) and some trigonometry and navigation for marines and naval officers. World War II had come, and some of the officer candidates were being trained at Princeton.

The opening wonder in the primary mathematics course for officers was that the textbook was written by three authors, one of whom was a member of the class. My recollection is that he was assigned to Professor Albert W. Tucker's class. The author was a very quiet person, and as far as I know, just collected his royalties and never asked an embarrassing question. I did not get to know him. My recollection is that his name was Bland (of Lyman M. Kells, Willis F. Kern, and James R. Bland). This is the first time that I had taught spherical trigonometry. The justification was that navigation for long distances, both on the sea and in the air, was based on spherical geometry.

A few of the students were there against their will. They felt they had signed up to go to war, and had, without understanding the consequences, scored high on some academic types of tests, and had been ordered to Princeton. I can still recall two students who did not want to attend this school. They decided to fail the final examination, even though they had done well throughout the course. Both were good students. And so when, on the final examination, they failed all the questions miserably (as often happens on an Ivy League final when the student has decided not to attend a course), the instructor in charge of the course complained to the commandant. Soon there came out an *order* stated somewhat as follows: Candidates Smith and Jones will *pass* the makeup examination in Mathematics xxx on Tuesday, January 21, 0800–1100.

I do not know who explained what to whom, but we provided a makeup examination. Both young men produced good finals in the B+ to A− range, whereupon they were shipped out as they wanted to be. We later had cheerful postcards from them from far away.

Teaching the beginning statistics course was a great deal of fun for me, because it was the first time that I had had a chance to teach in my own subject. I had worked hard on Wilks's book—actually typed it, though I was not a touch typist then and am not now.

I had worked over all the problems and learned a lot from them. It was a little embarrassing to have such professionals as E. W. Barankin and Henry Scheffé sitting in my course for sophomores. They had no business attending, but they were hunting around for some place to visit. Both were already far beyond me in their training and accomplishments. Once in a while Scheffé would ask me a question, but it was just for fear I knew something that he did not know, not to embarrass me.

In the long run this course produced a lot of trouble for me. It was a course based on a year of calculus, and I believed that perhaps even less calculus could also be the basis of a very good elementary course in probability and statistics using continuous measurements. But that is a story I'll return to.

⋆ ⋆ ⋆

While I was at Princeton during the war, the notion of training practical people in quality control was developed by some of the war agencies, especially the Office of Scientific Research and Development. I had already met Walter A. Shewhart. E. G. Olds, Holbrook Working, Paul Peach, Martin A. Brumbaugh, and Paul Clifford (perhaps along with others) had a traveling team teaching quality control to American industry. This training effort was part of a national movement for disseminating quality control methods that had been pioneered at AT&T and Bell Telephone Laboratories by Shewhart and his colleagues Paul Olmstead, Harold F. Dodge, and Harry G. Romig, among others. To take advantage of this methodology for the war effort, they developed short quality control courses. These courses, in addition to a traveling faculty, usually employed at least one statistician from the local arena, but trained him or her at a course given elsewhere shortly before the course was held at a local institution.

Wilks asked me to go to Kent State University to be trained in delivering parts of this quality control course when it was to be held at Princeton University. At Princeton, this was a most successful event. Most students stayed at the Princeton Graduate School dormitories and enjoyed the course and the experience enormously. The relations between the students and the teachers were very close. The students, engineers from industry, were outstanding people, raising the level of the course with good questions and comments from their own experiences. When the course was over, the students petitioned Wilks to make a reunion an annual event, and so he did. It may possibly continue to the present day under the auspices of the Central New Jersey Chapter of the American Statistical Association.

This sequence of courses, together with parallel courses taught at colleges and universities in the evenings, led to the national quality control movement and to the establishment of the American Society for Quality Control. I taught several courses at night in Newark and in Philadelphia. All this was going on both while I was teaching the marines and naval officers at Princeton, and later when I was working at the Statistical Research Group of Princeton in New York. I even helped teach a course in Hershey, Pennsylvania, as I recall, at the corner of Chocolate Avenue and Cocoa Street. It was exciting to see and participate in the spread of statistics, and to get to know so many professional leaders.

W. Edwards Deming had something to do with this movement, but I knew him personally from some other experiences, and not through the quality control route. Today he is famed for quality control both in the United States and in Japan, where there is even an annual school day celebrating statistics, with pupils writing papers on special statistical topics from the earliest grades. They produce amazing graphs and quantitative stories suited to the pupil's age and activities.

As a result of the quality control courses, I attended various meetings related to the development of the American Society for Quality Control, and was a founding member, though not one who was high in its councils.

At a tea in Princeton, I met Jimmie Savage, a mathematician from the University of Michigan, who had the very great honor of being John von Neumann's assistant at the Institute for Advanced Study in Princeton and the severe disappointment that the great man was almost never around. Jimmie was not only nearsighted but also had nystagmus, and so when he tried to read things he brought them very close to his eyes, often looking at them sideways. He was a very humorous person with a sort of sarcastic or cynical bent. I invited him to visit our Missouri Club—the equivalent of office hours for students in mathematics courses who had questions—which met one evening a week. He came and helped students who had queries in more advanced courses.

We ultimately taught in a course together under the leadership of Albert W. Tucker, the topologist and later game-theory expert. Again we were involved in algebra and trigonometry. This time, John W. Tukey had suggested to Tucker that in this beginning course in college mathematics, we should define the trigonometric functions in terms of complex variables. Although this sounds a bit crazy for a beginning course, it had some impressive advantages.

Using the Tukey approach made proofs of many relations that were ordinarily difficult to carry out merely an easy algebraic argument, though sometimes lengthy, and all carried out in an exponent. Jimmie, finding it very hard to see when he was at the blackboard, was somewhat impatient with the method, and so when he came to carry out the algebra, he would set up the program and then say, "Now you carry out this e to the i garbage, and then you find the answer easily to be...." (The base of the natural logarithms is represented by e, and the imaginary unit, square root of -1, is called i.) The result was that the language "e to the i garbage" diffused through the student population very rapidly, but teachers in the other sections were startled and didn't understand what students meant when they asked about the garbage. Soon we all learned this language and found it a useful shortcut, however irreverent.

I was extremely skeptical of the approach, but found that it mechanized the proofs so smoothly that I was more than won over by the end of the semester. We all were surprised at how easily the students took to it. Most of us thought that such an advanced viewpoint would stall them at the opening of the course, and that we would not get the course off the ground. The answer seemed to be that they did not resist the opening idea any harder than what they would have had to swallow as an alternative, and so it was just we young fogies who saw difficulties where few existed. After leaving Princeton, I never taught algebra, trigonometry, or analytic geometry again.

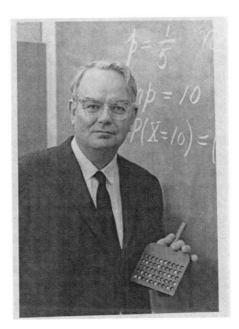

Fig. 17.1. Fred with a mechanical urn sampler, 1964.

Teaching at Harvard

When I went to Harvard University in the fall of 1946, I joined the Department of Social Relations. There I was expected to teach statistics to social scientists and to participate in consulting with research scholars, and, of course, to do my own research. During the first semester, however, Samuel Stouffer, a sociologist who had had statistical training from Karl Pearson, knew his son Egon, and had also studied with Ronald A. Fisher, taught the beginning course in statistics, and I taught the second-semester course. This gave me a marvelous chance to learn about the newly formed Department of Social Relations, its students, and curriculum. I attended courses and seminars, read assigned books, and also participated by consulting on statistical problems and attending department and research meetings.

At the same time, I was welcomed by the mathematics community—for example, by Joseph Walsh and Garrett Birkhoff, and especially by the algebraist Saunders MacLane, whom I had known in New York City when I was working at SRGPJr. He was also part of the Mathematics Panel during World War II under the leadership of Warren Weaver and Mina Rees. At Harvard, MacLane taught an elementary probability and statistics course. He wanted me to take it over and teach such a course for the mathematics department. This was something I very much wanted to do. Teaching courses in one's field strengthens one's professional skills. You get into the nooks and crannies of your work and begin to understand it from many points of view instead of merely fighting your way through the problems by main strength. And so I did often teach mathematical statistics courses in the mathematics department. That did not make me a member of the department, but I had many friends and acquaintances there, including Andrew M. Gleason, Lynn Loomis (who was also a neighbor of George B. Thomas, Jr., of MIT, whom I worked with later), and George Mackey.

Lars Ahlfors, a mathematician from Finland, lived on the second floor of the three-story apartment building on Dunster Street where Virginia and I lived on the third floor, just a block from Harvard Square in Cambridge. We knew many people who lived in these apartments—Edna and Sidney Alexander, John and Dorothy Monro, and Andreas Georgios Papandreou (at that time teaching in the Department of Economics, more recently prime minister of Greece) and his wife. It was very convenient, living only a block from Harvard Yard and about three blocks from the office. My office was in Emerson Hall, third floor.

When I first taught at Harvard, classes met Monday, Wednesday, and Friday or Tuesday, Thursday, and Saturday, aside from courses that met once or twice a week. I don't recall just when it was that Saturday morning was essentially abandoned.

At that time the women at Radcliffe usually had classes separate from the Harvard men. This approach was often inefficient, and so when too few Radcliffe students were available to produce a regular sized section, they were allowed to attend the Harvard classes. One awkwardness emerged. Radcliffe women, at that time, took their examinations under an honor system, whereas Harvard men did not.

I had become acquainted with the honor system at Princeton University. Whatever its faults and abuses may be, an honor system offers flexibility and conveniences for both students and faculty. Problems of conflicts of scheduling are readily resolved. The students can take their examinations in surroundings they find most beneficial to their performance. Students with short illnesses can be examined on recovery without new examinations being created. Fresh examinations may take an instructor several days to prepare. Special requests can be accommodated ("My mother will be visiting Tuesday. Can't I take it Monday or Wednesday?") After a while separate classes for Radcliffe were given up, and I believe years later Radcliffe gave up the honor system. Unfortunately, I fear there is cheating both with and without an honor system.

★ ★ ★

In addition to courses taught for the mathematics department, I sometimes taught also for the Division of Engineering and Applied Physics. There I met Howard Aiken, who built high-speed computers. His electromechanical machines took up a great deal of space, about the size of a small house. With each machine operation the building would shake. One time when George W. Brown, a statistician who also got his doctorate at Princeton, visited Harvard, his alma mater, we watched the huge machine work for a while, and then it fell silent. Two people handling the machine came out, and one said to the other, "Where is the go tape?" This was quickly found and installed, whereupon the machine resumed its noisy ways.

George inquired what a go tape was, because he was in the computing business but had not known of this development. It turned out that, whenever the machine stopped working, Aiken would rush out of his office and hurry the people working on the machine to fix it, and they found they could do that same work faster without his support. They found that it was possible to put an instruction into the machine that said "Go one step more"—essentially nothing more than advancing the tape one notch, like hitting the space bar or carriage return on a typewriter. This kept the machine shaking the building and left Aiken productively working in his office.

★ ★ ★

Once we founded the Department of Statistics in 1957, we developed courses for both undergraduates and graduates. Thinking back on my teaching at Princeton, I knew that a reasonable number of students at Harvard who had a two-semester mathematics requirement would appreciate a semester of statistics and probability after having taken one semester of calculus. Therefore I decided to develop such a course. I was correct that it attracted a sizable enrollment. I gradually prepared a text that delivered the mathematical side of the work at this level and taught the course several times. Not every idea works to perfection. The difficulties were a combination of selection factors and expecting too much from a preparation of one semester of calculus.

In mathematics teaching, we often say that we learn in the second course what the first course was all about. The truth of this comes in part because the second course may use the work of the first course so extensively and repeatedly that one becomes thoroughly trained—essentially one memorizes the steps and activities taught in the first course. In my situation, the students had had the first-semester course and had not had a chance to exercise their skills the way they would have had to do in a second semester of calculus. Thus my students were not prepared at the end of the first semester in the sense of mastery of the material, as opposed to having been merely exposed to it. I was hoping for students who had mastered their first-semester course.

In addition, we had a selection effect—students who do not take the second semester of a two-semester sequence are often, though not always, those who are not doing well in that first semester. Therefore, I fear I was skimming off a fair number of students who neither were much engaged in mathematics nor found themselves strong in that direction, though many genuinely wanted the statistics. After teaching this for several years and revising the materials, and having other people teach from the same materials, I concluded that the course was not as strong an entry in the curriculum as I had hoped, and I abandoned it.

In brief, from the point of view of content, in order to take advantage of the calculus that the students brought with them, one had to amplify it with further calculus material to achieve the techniques needed for the statistical material. What this tended to do, then, was to produce a statistics course with considerable calculus, oriented toward a specific set of goals. One found oneself teaching a weak calculus course while trying to teach a statistics course.

This is not to say that a good course couldn't be constructed, for example, by limiting oneself to finite mathematics rather than insisting on using continuous methods requiring calculus. That has been done successfully by a number of groups, including me and my colleagues. Another route is to abandon the rigorous side of the approach and try to teach students what is important about their research methods without emphasizing the mathematics. That can be most useful, but it does not make an honest contribution toward meeting a mathematics requirement.

Continental Classroom

Because of our work on the Commission on Mathematics for the College Entrance Examination Board, we (many scholars) prepared a book for secondary schools on probability and statistics. This book was successful and was revised and it sold very widely, so much so that the College Entrance Examination Board found it an embarrassment to their non-profit status, or so they said. It was translated into Spanish for use in some Latin-American countries.

Robert E. K. Rourke, George B. Thomas, Jr., and I decided to prepare a new text ourselves using the finite mathematics approach. About the time we were finishing it, the leaders of a series of television courses called Continental Classroom being presented on NBC's national television network asked me if I would like to be considered for giving a course in Probability and Statistics. I found this an attractive idea. I liked to teach, and here was an opportunity to reach many more people than I otherwise could. Our book was going to be ready in time. Addison-Wesley prepared three versions of it. One was prepared especially for the television series, a little shorter than the full book, but longer than the one-semester book we had prepared for secondary schools.

Although I used some visual approaches to presenting my statistics course in class at Harvard (such as sampling beads from a box of beads, some red and some white, to show the sort of variation that occurs in actual sampling), most of these visuals were developed during the quality control courses. For the quality control course given at Princeton, I got the engineering department to create small paddles with holes drilled halfway through, so that one swish of the paddle through a bead box could collect a sample of beads. We asked for paddles with 5, 10, and 50 holes so that samples of each size could be drawn. They insisted on an engineering drawing with tolerances. The 5- and 50-hole paddles were fine, but the 10-hole turned out to have only 8. They redid it, whereupon it had 12 holes. I kept that one and covered the extra two holes. These mistakes show again that counting is hard for us.

Paul Clifford, of Montclair State College, had been asked to give the second half of this Continental Classroom program. I lectured on Monday, Wednesday, and Friday, and he gave further exemplary material and explanations about the problems on Tuesday and Thursday. He had gone to a great deal

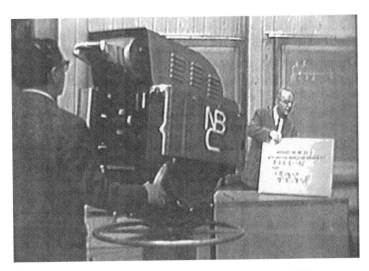

Fig. 17.2. Fred on Continental Classroom, 1961.

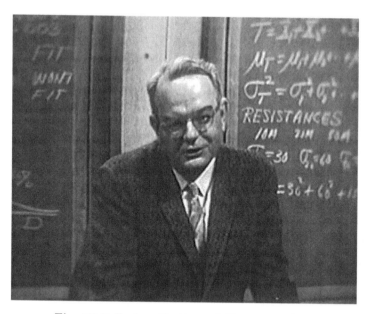

Fig. 17.3. Fred on Continental Classroom, 1961.

of trouble to find and perfect methods of presenting statistics and probability visually to large groups in public. We had enjoyed each other's company in several quality control courses, and so we confidently expected to be able to work well together in the course. We did, though the effort was much more separate than anticipated, because hours when one was not working toward a filming were used gathering and trying out new materials. I lived at home in Belmont, Massachusetts, and came down to New York by train or plane.

One reason for presenting a mathematics course was that the organization running the courses thought correctly that a mathematics course would be much less expensive than a course that required more outside sorts of filming and preparation. Thus, our course had no assistants who thought up new presentations. Instead, we did have assistants who made signs summarizing what the lesson was about or what should have been learned, who gathered or tried to gather material one desired, or went to the library or typed up materials; but we did not have a team who tried to think of original ways to present these mathematical materials to the students in the course—except, of course, Clifford and me.

The Continental Classroom plan for the 1960–61 season included two mathematics courses, one for the fall in modern algebra given by John L. Kelley, then chair of the Department of Mathematics at the University of California at Berkeley, and one for the spring in statistics. John and I knew each other slightly from our work with secondary schools and with committees in professional mathematics organizations. Although I looked forward to getting to know him, we both found ourselves very busy, and also our schedules for taping tended to keep us apart. We did have a few social occasions and some discussions of how to handle special problems in presentations.

After the original contract negotiations were completed, I was put in the charge of Dorothy Culbertson, the widow of Ely Culbertson, the great contract bridge expert. She was a statuesque blond with a take-charge approach that swept all before her. In the midst of total disaster, she was always cheery as could be and knew what to do next. Her fundamental theory was never upset "the star," who was the central figure in a program. The star should never know there was any trouble at all.

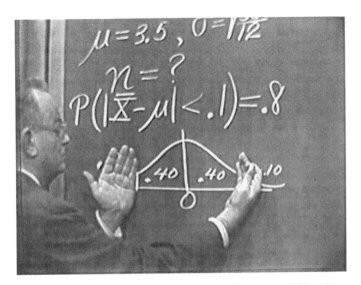

Fig. 17.4. Fred on Continental Classroom, 1961.

Our producer-director, Marvin Einhorn, was a very experienced person. I saw a good bit of him around 5 or 6 A.M. The favorite filming time was 12 noon for one-half hour. To meet that schedule, endless rehearsals and preparation of materials occurred during that morning.

I would, of course, have already made the cue cards for myself. These cards were long white cardboards about a foot or so wide and about three feet high. One wrote the prompts, essentially an outline of the program, on these cards. I often used the start of a sentence rather than the subject matter of the material. I also planned how to move around the set. Putting the start of material that would appear on a chalkboard such as a title, also helped remind me what I was to do next. There were several places for a camera to view usually two chalkboards (these could be turned over during the presentation without the viewers being aware of the change), a place where one could sit and write on a large table, another table where materials and devices were shown, and a position where large cards with statements about what was going to be learned or what had already been presented were shown. These cards were prepared by the person who lettered the signs.

The course was organized on a national basis. The Continental Classroom people had set up a course throughout the nation in secondary schools, colleges, and universities, including teachers' colleges. Each school had a teacher for the course on the home grounds and had regular meetings that I would call section meetings about once a week. At Harvard, the University Extension Course persuaded Gottfried Noether, who helped with the preparation of the course, to be the local person. At that time, he was teaching at Boston University. His interest in nonparametric methods was closely related to the possible content of an elementary non-calculus-based course.

When we decided to do the course, it was necessary to produce a syllabus for it. This syllabus was intended to include what material in the book was going to be covered, what the assignment was, what was the point of the lesson in each instance, some remarks about how to do certain kinds of problems, and some supplementary material for the teacher who wanted more or different material from that in the text. Gottfried took on this task and executed it with speed and depth of understanding. We had a chance to get better acquainted at this time. I appreciated his support and understanding.

As I mentioned, we began rehearsals very early, around 5 or 6 A.M. First, I would go through the lecture myself with my own cue cards and with what materials were ready for the day's program. Then, I would go over it with Marvin Einhorn, the producer, and he would decide where on the set various things would take place. At this early hour, we were not on the stage where the filming would be done, but in a very large office space with room for several people with desks and easels.

After a couple of run-throughs, we separated, and I worked some more on the next few lectures until time to go to the set. At the set, one found a beehive because the light-men, the sound-men, and the crew who prepared the set were calling and shouting to one another. We then ran through another rehearsal on the set—preparing the blackboards and tablets and making sure everyone knew what happened in what order. And finally, the music for the introduction of the program came on, and at its close I began the lecture, just after noon.

In the main, these presentations went like clockwork because they had been heavily rehearsed, perhaps also because no one examined them very critically. I say this because when I did a program for the BBC in England, they had a criticism that kept coming up. I kept saying inches when I was supposed to say centimeters, and they would start the program over. They were troubled with my inability to remember that. I didn't have an appropriate cue card.

Most people supposed that the filming was done in little stretches or that when errors were found, they were edited out and replaced by additional filming. Far from it, every one of the 48 half-hour lessons was filmed once and only once from start to finish. The material was set up so that at the end of a lesson one could add or drop material to make the time fit. One of the men

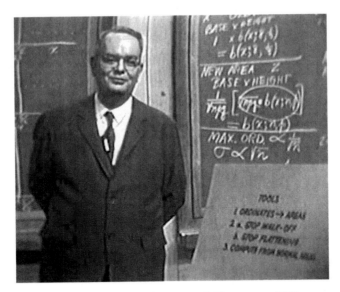

Fig. 17.5. Fred on Continental Classroom, 1961.

working on stage would signal whether to lengthen the lesson or shorten it as the last two minutes drew near. He also carried around the cue cards, which the camera did not see.

Needless to say, there were occasional mistakes. But I had a strong lesson from John L. Kelley when he had a difficulty and had to redo a scene from one of his lectures. He was involved in a very complicated geometric situation with several labeled points and lines. He was then supposed to step up to this complicated figure and draw in one more line, which would illustrate something marvelous. I watched him do the original program, and it was going beautifully until the very last step, when after drawing the line John said some nasty things that I was sure were not going to be in the lesson. What had happened was that at the last minute he had confidently stepped up to the complicated figure and placed the straightedge on it ever so carefully and drawn in entirely the wrong line—thus his discomfort. And so the scene had to be done over, because this line was the major payoff for the lesson.

So a time and set were arranged for a few days after, and then I began to realize the trouble involved. First, it wasn't the same day, and so one had to plan ahead and be sure to wear exactly the same clothes. Second, the exact placement of the person on the stage for the start of the patch had to be marked on the floor. The diagram had to be redrawn and set up. And so when the great day arrived, with, by chance, visitors from important mathematical organizations on the set, John stood in the right clothes, in the right footprints, with the straightedge, and said so beautifully what he was about to do. He then stepped forward and placed the straightedge on the drawing, and again drew a wrong line. I didn't attend the re-remake.

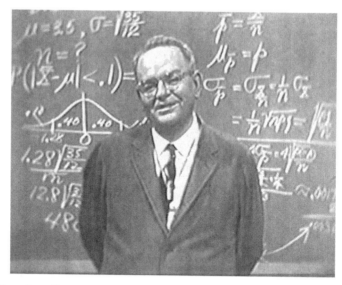

Fig. 17.6. Fred on the final episode of Continental Classroom, 1961.

This experience persuaded me that it would be well not to have retakes, and so if a film had some minor language problem, like saying orally "variance" when I should have said "standard deviation," I did not try to fix it. Instead, I told Paul Clifford about it, and he would mention this when he was doing the problems and examples in his next lecture following my lesson. We did not have complaints about this, and so it apparently worked well. We did sometimes get complaints and sometimes compliments on other matters.

I closed the last lesson with a Latin quotation from my secondary school days. It had the translation "Learn as if you would live forever, live as if you would die tomorrow." Quite a few people wrote in for the exact Latin phrasing. My teacher in Caesar's Gallic Wars would have been pleased.

Through the years, I have met many people who took the course, many of whom viewed it at 6:30 A.M. as I did. Because it appeared on about 195 stations the first year it ran, and then was later repeated, their numbers are large even at that time of the morning. In addition, some schools and other institutions later used the films to teach the course.

Teaching Statistics to Non-Statisticians

Why do people who are not and do not intend to be statisticians study statistics? Their reasons are various, and so one has to distinguish different groups. Those who take courses in mathematical statistics are fairly easy to appreciate. Usually they expect to do advanced work that requires statistics. They think that they will need a solid knowledge of probability and of statistics, and they want to be able to handle minor variations on standard problems without having to ask others for help.

Furthermore, an understanding of probability and its main ideas benefits students as well. In the physical sciences and in technology, some theories of some processes require probability theory. This same mathematics usually can also contribute much to one's understanding of statistical inference. Even though these people do not exactly plan to be statisticians, some of their life is going to be spent on problems that are dealt with by statistics and by statisticians.

In a sense, all of us are statisticians from morning to night, as we move through the uncertain process of going to work, carrying out tasks, and looking out for the weather. We make dozens of statistical decisions a day. Still, we do most of that on a very informal basis.

The students of social science are taking courses in statistics as professionals. They are planning on lifetimes of research, and at least at present, many areas use a great deal of statistics. They need to understand the general idea, and they have to know how to design and implement experiments and other kinds of investigations. Finally, they have to analyze and write up their work in a manner that meets professional standards. For many, this amounts to a good deal of statistics. These people are planning to use various ideas of statistics in very practical ways, and part of their lives will be as statisticians, whether they work in such occupations as sociologists, psychologists, educators, or economists.

They do differ somewhat in their statistical interests. Psychologists, more than sociologists or economists, do experiments. The key feature of an experiment is that the experimenter imposes treatments on the subjects of the investigation. Occasionally sociologists do experiments as well, but they are more likely to carry out observational studies or sample surveys. With a few very notable exceptions, economists rarely carry out experiments; they depend upon observational studies to carry the ball. Exceptions include the negative income tax experiments and the RAND health insurance experiments. These investigations were huge.

The psychologists tend to want to know more about experimentation, and for them, although statistical experimentation evolved largely from agriculture, the ideas carry over well to many other sorts of experimentation. Engineers interested in industrial technology also have interests in these same directions because they have many needs in experimentation. When several chemicals are combined in order to produce a product, the question is how to combine them so as to make the most money for the effort and financing given to the input side. Someone once said that in a chemical plant wherever you see a valve, you know that someone didn't know the answer. The chemical plant is often already set up so that sequences of experiments can be carried out—so many shifts on one formula and process, so many on another, and then the outputs from the different recipes can be evaluated and something very close to optimum chosen.

At any rate, all these groups want to learn statistics from the point of view of design of investigations, and of course their analysis as well. Thus these students plan to be practitioners. It is relatively easy to plan courses for them because, after a field like design of experiments has been studied for a long time, a hierarchy of methods gets developed so that one learns gradually from easy to hard by piling on complications, and we produce special courses in each topic. It was because of heavy training in design and execution of studies that so many of our clinical psychology graduates were named research director in their first position after receiving their doctorate.

For those who will be working heavily using survey methods, we have courses in sample surveys and their analysis. Economists are heavily into methods of predicting the values of some variables from those of others, and we have methods for doing this called "regression"; they lap that up.

Some other groups have a very different attitude toward their statistical education. For example, research physicians want to know what the ideas are in the field and what they need to keep their eyes open for. They do not especially want to learn how to do this work themselves. They do, however, want to be sure that they have the ideas that are important, and understand why they matter. Most of them, though, even if they are researchers in health and medicine, expect to enlist the services of a professional statistician. They do not expect to have to be their own statistician in the design or analysis of their data. Thus they are very oriented to what Arnold S. Relman, editor of the *New England Journal of Medicine*, calls the state of the art. They want to know what is going on in statistics for medicine, how it is being used in practice for the clinician and the researcher, and why it may or may not matter to the researcher. If possible, physicians want to learn this without having to learn how to do it. Although sometimes this is impossible, by trying hard and getting advice from physicians about what they want to know, one can develop special kinds of courses for them that teach what it is all about and why it matters, without insisting that the student learn to solve the kinds of problems we expect the groups mentioned earlier to carry out. For a long time, I thought this approach was not possible, but I now believe that if one gives enough effort to it and has confidence in the idea that a strong statistician will actually be doing the implementation, then many details can be dropped in favor of the big ideas and their consequences. We are learning this kind of teaching. With Relman's cooperation, John C. Bailar III and I produced a book on the state of the art of statistics for medical researchers entitled *Medical Uses of Statistics*.

Some medical students do want to learn about statistical methods, and they prefer to do this by applying the methods to current medical issues. For the teacher, this means being up-to-date on a disease, its diagnoses, and treatments. To supply a course of this nature took Joseph Ingelfinger, Lawrence Thibodeau, James Ware, and me several years to prepare. We had been much encouraged by Dean Howard Hiatt. In the end, we did produce a book, *Biostatistics in Clinical Medicine*. It has been translated into Italian and French.

In the law schools we are still not doing much statistical training, though several useful textbooks have now appeared. These orient themselves primarily toward the statistical legal problems of the day, such as problems of racial or sexual discrimination in the job market, and issues of regulation. Most lawyers count on hiring professional advisers in whatever field they are needed. And so they, like physicians, want to know what sorts of things matter and need to be taken into account.

Team research has become so extensive in medicine that the contributions of experts from several fields are most common. The specialties in medicine, chemistry, biology, computing, statistics, and laboratory work that contribute to medical research have become so extensive and deep, I see no way of returning to the old state where some one author is always responsible for everything in each research paper, and even less possibility that all the coauthors can be responsible for the entire paper.

Discussions of fraud and how these unfortunate events are to be handled usually do not face up to the impossibility of both getting the research done and learning every facet of the work, as well as washing every beaker. We will have to have many more discussions of this poisonous topic because academics do not know how to handle problems of fraud. Still, the impossibility of mastering all facets does not relieve each coauthor from actually reading the manuscript and checking whatever he or she can, as well as aiding the exposition! We do understand at least the idea of checking those aspects of another's work that one can grasp. We do not do it, though, out of a sense of suspicion that something is fraudulent, but because everyone misspells, all papers may have typographical errors, and mistakes in arithmetic are common. We have no systematic approach for detecting fraud. Instead, we depend on one another to tell the truth.

In public policy, the situation differs because some of the students in early stages of their work are required to have hands-on experience with research, whereas in the longer pull, the policy person is likely to be in charge of an agency that purchases statistical work and services. Then the problem for the policy person is more like that of the physician. One difference, though, is that the policy person planning to purchase a study has to be able to appreciate in advance whether the proposed study, if well done, will answer questions the agency needs help on and whether doing the study may lead to embarrassment for the agency in case the information seems to imply policies very different from those currently being supported by the administration further up the line. Thus these people have problems at both ends. On the one hand, when they are young they need to know how to do studies, but when older they need to have some feeling for how the study will come out and what its consequences may be for the agency. This takes more vision and training in the statistics of public policy than most agency heads ever get.

In later years at Harvard, I had a chance to help Howard Raiffa and Don K. Price, at the John F. Kennedy School of Government, develop their quantitative methods course for policy students, and over a period of a few years participated in the teaching. In this way, I began to develop an understanding of the policy side of the work. As a statistician, one is essentially engaged in gathering information, or at least learning how to develop information effectively. A weakness is that one tends to emphasize parts of the work that may in the end not be essential. For example, we statisticians are very concerned about the efficiency of our sampling schemes and our methods of analysis. We want to be able to milk the data for all its information. But other aspects need to be considered too. It is not just whether the information is correct or reliable; it also is a matter of how it is used. Can it and will it be used, and will it be used correctly? And, for that matter, what does "correctly" mean? In many instances the same data are used by both sides in adversary situations. Thus when one thinks of quantitative methods in the realm of public policy, although the students need to know something about the basis for the information being produced, they also need to worry about how it can be used for policy work. For this area, the statistician with ordinary training comes largely unprepared.

References

Bailar, J. C. III and Mosteller, F., editors (1986). *Medical Uses of Statistics.* Waltham, MA: NEJM Books.

Eisenhart, L. P. (1939). *Coordinate Geometry.* Boston: Ginn and Company.

Fairley, W. B. and Mosteller, F., editors (1977). *Statistics and Public Policy.* Reading, MA: Addison-Wesley.

Finkelstein, M. O. (1979). *Quantitative Methods in Law.* New York: The Free Press.

Finkelstein, M. O. and Levin, B. (1990). *Statistics for Lawyers.* New York: Springer-Verlag. 2nd edition, 2001.

Gastwirth, J. L. (1988). *Statistical Reasoning in Law and Public Policy.* Boston: Academic Press.

Gosset, W. S. (1908). The probable error of a mean. *Biometrika,* 6:1–25.

Ingelfinger, J. A., Mosteller, F., Thibodeau, L. A., and Ware, J. H. (1983). *Biostatistics in Clinical Medicine.* New York: Macmillan. 2nd edition, 1987.

Katz, L. (1952). The distribution of the number of isolates in a special group. *Annals of Mathematical Statistics,* 23:271–276.

Kells, L. M., Kern, W. F., and Bland, J. R. (1940). *Plane and Spherical Trigonometry.* New York: McGraw-Hill.

Kershaw, D. and Fair, J., editors (1976). *The New Jersey Income-Maintenance Experiment. Volume I: Operations, Surveys, and Administration.* New York: Academic Press.

Mosteller, F. (1959). *Introductory Probability and Statistical Inference: An Experimental Course.* Revised preliminary edition. New York: College Entrance Examination Board.

Mosteller, F. and Rourke, R. E. K. (1973). *Sturdy Statistics: Nonparametrics and Order Statistics.* Reading, MA: Addison-Wesley.

Mosteller, F., Rourke, R. E. K., and Thomas, G. B. Jr. (1961a). *Probability: A First Course.* Derived from *Probability with Statistical Applications.* Reading, MA: Addison-Wesley.

Mosteller, F., Rourke, R. E. K., and Thomas, G. B. Jr. (1961b). *Probability and Statistics.* Official Textbook for Continental Classroom. Derived from *Probability with Statistical Applications.* Reading, MA: Addison-Wesley.

Mosteller, F., Rourke, R. E. K., and Thomas, G. B. Jr. (1961c). *Probability with Statistical Applications.* Reading, MA: Addison-Wesley.

Mosteller, F., with a group of the Commission on Mathematics of the College Examination Board (1957). *Introductory Probability and Statistical Inference for Secondary Schools.* New York: College Entrance Examination Board

Newhouse, J. P. (1993). *Free for All? Lessons from the RAND Health Insurance Experiment.* Cambridge, MA: Harvard University Press.

Watts, H. W. and Rees, A., editors (1977). *The New Jersey Income-Maintenance Experiment. Volume II: Labor-supply Responses.* New York: Academic Press.

18

Group Writing

One of the lucky moments in my life occurred in August 1955, when I became acquainted with Robert E. K. Rourke, who served with me and others on the Commission on Mathematics of the College Entrance Examination Board under the chairmanship of Professor Albert Tucker of the Department of Mathematics of Princeton University.[1] The Commission was preparing innovative material for the secondary-school mathematics curriculum. The reason was that the College Entrance Examination Board was sensitive to the criticism that standardized examinations tended to freeze the mathematics curriculum of the schools. The Board did not want to be a roadblock in the path of progress. Rourke was head of mathematics and science at the Kent School in Kent, Connecticut.

Bob was a marvelous raconteur and no respecter of persons. Indeed, Father Patterson, then headmaster of the Kent School, once said that nothing was so sacred but what Rourke could degrade it, and yet with Rourke somehow it was always good clean fun. Often the Commission met at the Kent School, as well as in Princeton, New Jersey. Because of muggy heat in the day and mosquitoes at night, Princeton is not the best place for a summer meeting. Kent School is just about at the border between Connecticut and New York and about 85 miles north of New York City; it was a good place for summer group writing. I also met George B. Thomas Jr., from the Massachusetts Institute of Technology, the author of one of the world's most successful calculus books. Joining these people and others has had great consequences for me.

Father Patterson said to me, "What can you say to a mother who comes to you with this query: 'Father Patterson, I just discussed my son's work with Master Rourke. He says my son is just fine except that he has pigeons on his aerial. What does he mean?'" As an experienced teacher, I knew well what Rourke meant. Her son was bright but didn't concentrate long enough at a time on one thing to be nearly as effective as he could be.

At the same time that Bob was a humorist, he was also a deep thinker and a seriously religious man. He regarded the education of the young in mathematics and science as important business. He saw humor in the human condition

F. Mosteller, *The Pleasures of Statistics: The Autobiography of Frederick Mosteller*, DOI 10.1007/978-0-387-77956-0_18, © Springer Science + Business Media, LLC 2010

and made no bones about it, and yet he saw his role of training young people as a major contribution to the growing edge of the nation's citizenry. And why not? How many secondary-school students get to study mathematics with someone who has studied at Harvard under George Birkhoff, Marston Morse, William C. Graustein, William Osgood, and Marshall Stone—absolutely outstanding mathematicians of the first part of the 20th century? Bob had studied graduate mathematics under this faculty but had to leave graduate work because of family economic reverses during the depression of the 1930s. He began teaching mathematics at a private secondary-school in Canada. He was born and raised in Canada and once coauthored a book with a title like "Algebra for Canadians." I did not meet him until after he had come to teach at Kent School, though Albert Tucker, also a Canadian, had often mentioned him.

When his students complained that they should be allowed to take examinations using open books because that was more like what went on in real life, Rourke replied, "Taking mathematics examinations at Kent School *is* real life."

He had a great eye for art and, for modest sums, purchased art from the Canadian Seven[2] early in their careers, and so when I first knew him he had a remarkable art collection.

Alice, Bob's long-suffering wife, was also one of his helpful critics. He would often remind her on these occasions that she could be replaced, but they both knew she couldn't be. And he liked to be curbed just enough so that he was regarded as a devil though he wasn't at all.

On the Commission, we had to do a lot of elementary mathematical writing and criticize it. I learned in working with Bob and George how it should go. It was a great education for me. Bob knew that you couldn't tell people how to improve their writing until you had reassured them that their work was good and worth improving. And so he would take a few minutes at the beginning of a discussion to tell you how wonderful your material was. By the time he finished, one knew that the material under discussion would be most important. And so one was panting to hear whether there was any way to improve it, though this surely seemed doubtful in view of the remarks made so far. All the same, it would finally turn out that there were a few things that could be improved, several, quite a few, actually a lot; indeed, the whole thing needed a complete body-and-fender job—one of Bob's expressions. But by the time Bob got around to helping you in this way, you were eager to revise.

Ever since then I have dinned into my graduate students, "When a colleague gives you a paper to read, he or she wants to hear how wonderful it is. After you have told that and established yourself as a person of taste, discrimination, and intelligence, the author will be happy to hear your suggestions for improvement, no matter how extensive." It works. And if you forget to tell people what you like, they won't listen to your complaints.

All this was most important to me at the time, because I was a professional statistician trying to write for secondary-school teachers who, for the most part, had little training in my field. The Commission did have one secondary-school man who had had some statistical training, Richard S. Pieters, then from Phillips Andover Academy. He and I have worked on joint projects ever since.

Perhaps, dealing with young people, Bob and Richard understood the value of praise, just as Skinner understood the value of reinforcement in the training of rats and pigeons. At any rate, several generations of graduate students and other professionals working with me have benefited from this good information.

In dealing with material people asked him to read, Bob developed what he called "the Rourke Stupidity Test." Because he was often asked to read mathematical material and criticize it, he argued that he would read through carefully with his best effort twice. If then he still did not understand it, he declared that the material was not properly written because it had not passed "the Rourke Stupidity Test." He said that if he was to be a reader to test the clarity of the presentation, then his understanding had to be the criterion by which the material was to be judged. Students often do not understand this idea when they are asked to review an exposition. They tackle the task as if their degree of understanding was to be a judgment of them rather than of the readability of the material.

Bob used to talk about young mathematically talented boys snooping in the library and coming to their teachers with questions from the back of the book. He spoke of these snoops so proudly that you knew he loved it, even though these children were probably destined already for more outstandingly original mathematical careers than his own. He understood that that was his job as a teacher—to produce better trained citizens than those of his own generation.

He wanted teachers he supervised to teach mathematics. He once wrote in the following vein, "Dear X: You are an outstanding teacher, and no one recognizes this more than I. The only difficulty is that you do not know any mathematics and so have nothing to teach. We can remedy this over the next few years...."

His device was to replace department meetings with seminars in mathematics, which he sustained over years, thus giving these good teachers a mathematical education.

He had dreams of glory. He always had good ideas for trying to bring exciting ideas to the students, and he would say, "Do you think we can do this?" And sometimes the Commission could.

Since probability and mathematical statistics were clearly not areas where secondary-school teachers were well trained, Bob had a very chastening remark he often used. It came about because I have always tended to cut corners in explanations. For myself I have always excused it on the grounds that, once one got to the specific point, the rest was obvious. But in mathematics what is obvious depends a lot on the beholder. And so when Rourke came across these neat passages that finessed big issues by finishing off essentially with "you know how it goes from here," he would pencil in the margin, "Ask your teacher." This was a devastating comment because we both knew that the teacher, leaning only on the text, didn't have a prayer of answering the next question on the subject going beyond the text.

When the Commission's main report was assembled in manuscript form, Bob was asked to take leave from Kent School and act as Executive Director. After a long leave, Albert Meder, who had served in this capacity, needed to return to his post at Rutgers University. Bob received an invitation to visit Russia and observe their schools, an opportunity he happily accepted. When he returned, he found galleys for much of the book on his desk. Imagine his surprise when he found that the technical mathematical terms "real and complex numbers" had been replaced throughout by "genuine and complicated numbers" by a well-meaning editor. Other changes of a similar sort produced much re-editing. He was still glad he went to Russia, but felt rather guilty that he had not been on hand to prevent this disaster.

Following the Commission's work, I thought Bob, George, and I might put together a statistics book, which indeed we did. It was used for Continental Classroom in 1961 on perhaps 195 commercial TV stations in the NBC network. Bob gave one of the 48 lectures, George declined. We published with George's publisher, Addison-Wesley, and I was involved with Addison-Wesley in various ways for many years.

At some stage in our relationship, Bob, along with others from Kent School, established a similar school for English-speaking children in Rome, Italy, and taught there until he retired. I think the intent was to make available an Episcopalian school for children of Americans abroad in an area generally served by Catholic schools.

George did not want to pursue the collaboration further than the first three books (and the two editions of the Commission's book on probability and statistics and its teaching manual), but Bob and I kept on and in 1973 put out *Sturdy Statistics*, a book on nonparametric methods, which we enjoyed preparing. Then we began a book we called BEST, for "Beginning Elementary Statistics." This was one of those labors of love. We were enjoying ourselves enormously, getting together frequently and voting on the effectiveness of the examples and homework problems, when Bob got sick—not once, but repeatedly. Strokes, heart attacks, etc. After that, Bob was never able to take up a full share of the effort and initiative. Meanwhile, Alice died in Switzerland, where they were vacationing. And so Stephen Fienberg and I finished much of the book with little help from Bob, though he took a great interest in it, and we talked a lot about it at his home just two weeks before he died.

★ ★ ★

Over the years, several group-writing efforts have helped me and others contribute to education in statistics, both elementary and advanced. For me,

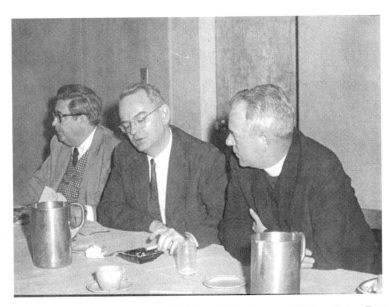

Fig. 18.1. Fred with Bob Rourke (left) and Headmaster Father John Patterson (right) at a meeting of the Commission on Mathematics, College Entrance Examination Board, at the Kent School, CT.

the first of these occurred when the Commission on Mathematics of the College Entrance Examination Board decided to produce a book on probability and statistics for secondary schools, mentioned above. Both the Commission and the working groups that prepared materials included secondary school teachers. Many people helped to prepare that book: Edwin C. Douglas, Frederick Mosteller, Richard S. Pieters, Donald E. Richmond, Robert E. K. Rourke, George B. Thomas Jr., and Samuel S. Wilks. In addition to the comments of the several authors, I was impressed by the value of the critiques that the teachers from secondary schools were able to contribute during the summer working sessions at Kent School. To give a notion of the effectiveness of these critiques, I wrote and revised a chapter I dearly wanted in the book nine times, but it never passed the review. All the other seriously prepared chapters were used in the final version.

When I was invited to speak at the Las Vegas meeting of the National Council of Teachers of Mathematics (NCTM) in April 1967 as President of the American Statistical Association, I thought it would be appropriate to propose a joint ASA-NCTM committee on statistical education. This invitation was accepted by Donovan A. Johnson, President of NCTM, and a committee was established,[3] initially under my chairmanship. The Sloan Foundation gave us a grant for the work of the committee.

The committee, after considerable exploration, decided that materials of two kinds were needed. First, although statistics books teach methods, they

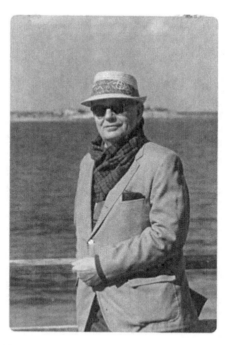

Fig. 18.2. Fred in Bermuda in 1970, while finishing *Sturdy Statistics* with Bob Rourke.

teach the methods in isolation. People, even those in statistics courses, usually do not get to experience the solution of whole real-life problems where statistics plays an important role. To fill this gap, the committee decided to create a book with many concrete examples of statistics in action leading to successful problem solutions. The committee picked areas where it thought good essays could be written, and it invited individual scholars to write short pieces, about 10 printed pages.

We had several ground rules. The story had to include a real example of a useful and successful statistical application. The paper had to be readable by a high school senior or a school superintendent. The exposition was not intended to teach how to do statistics but to illustrate the variety of applications and methods. We could not use mathematics that the reader would not have available.

Judith Tanur agreed to edit the volume. We started off with the notion that something like 50 examples would be a nice round number. As fast as drafts of the papers came in, several committee members criticized each one, as did the editor and I, and then the authors were supplied with the pooled suggestions. Authors were differentially able to use the critiques.

In spite of the most carefully worded instructions, authors tend to do as they please. A few thought that they could just make up illustrative data rather than provide genuine data. Others thought that high school seniors had surely mastered at least advanced calculus. The conflicts between these beliefs and the instructions wiped out a few of the planned examples.

We stuck to our guns. Some authors, though complying with the original mandate, could not seem to use the advice supplied by the readers, perhaps because they did not know what was meant. It took us a long while to solve this problem, but the ultimate device worked very well. Instead of supplying anew the critiques that an author had not properly used, we ourselves rewrote the author's piece according to the criticisms that the various readers had supplied. Then we wrote the author a note explaining that we had slightly revised the piece and that we hoped that the final draft was satisfactory—if not, please let us know. We never had any trouble about this. You might think that when a chapter is returned with many, many changes the author would have some corrections, but apparently not. Of course, many authors were able to take advantage of the original criticisms and produce excellent manuscripts. In all, we obtained 44 manuscripts for the first edition.

The book was published in 1972 by Holden-Day. It sold several tens of thousands of copies, and Frederick H. Murphy, President of Holden-Day, was kind enough to send a copy to two members of the editorial team, who brought it to Boston on the day I recovered from the anesthesia following surgery at Massachusetts General Hospital. The nurses set up a screen with an exhibit for the book. That may have been the fanciest first day for a book in my publishing career.

William Kruskal and I had worked hard on two problems, the illustrations and the title. The publisher's designer, Edward Millman, solved the problem of the illustrations by providing a small cartoon at the opening of each paper, and by arranging that graphs be done in a sort of hand-drawn fashion to make the book warmer and friendlier for the reader. He also helped us over the hump with the final title. I had wanted "A Guide to the Unknown," but Kruskal felt that the title had to have "Statistics" in it, and so it came out *Statistics: A Guide to the Unknown.*

In 1989, the book had its third edition, published by Wadsworth & Brooks/ Cole Advanced Books & Software. In the second edition (1978), we added a very few papers. In the third edition we produced new papers and eliminated many of the old ones. The third edition was carried out by the same group from the original committee and in the same manner as the other two editions; Erich Lehmann aided us in the revisions for the second and third editions.

The second activity of the ASA-NCTM committee was to produce material on statistics for several levels of students running from elementary through secondary school. This material was intended to provide engaging examples that would be used in teaching students basic ideas in statistical methods. Thus, it dealt with a different population of readers and had a how-to-do-it purpose rather than a cultural one. To get materials, we amplified the committee by adding members who had some experience in teaching statistics and probability in secondary school and by inviting some graduate students in statistics to participate. In all, we put together four slender volumes under the title *Statistics by Example*, and each volume had an associated guide for the teacher including answers to the problems. As with the first project, committee members read every piece, critiques were returned to the authors, and then the material was revised. Our losses in this effort were not so heavy, because each person who participated had very concrete material to present.

Addison-Wesley Publishing Company produced the volumes (in 1973). Again, tens of thousands of copies of the material have been distributed.

★ ★ ★

Among the consequences that have been especially rewarding is that examples produced both in *Statistics: A Guide to the Unknown* and in the four volumes of *Statistics by Example* have been extensively copied and used in statistics texts. From the beginning, we had hoped that such uses would be made, and that wish has been fulfilled. Now some new books similar to *Statistics: A Guide to the Unknown* have come out, and so these compliments have also been supportive.

The income from these publications has been used by the American Statistical Association to support the continuing work of the joint committee of the American Statistical Association and the National Council of Teachers of Mathmatics. The current committee, composed entirely of new members, has produced new materials and has new goals. The old committee reconvened only to revise *Statistics: A Guide to the Unknown*.

These two efforts have paid off a failure that I suffered when I had my first sabbatical in Chicago in 1954–55. For my project under the teaching organization supported by the Ford Foundation, I wanted to create statistical materials based upon great studies that had important statistical content, for example, Emile Durkheim's book *Suicide* or the Michelson-Morley experiment on the ether drift. This was part of my idea of having textual examples that had social or scientific importance. Although I worked hard on this idea in Chicago, I found that the great studies that I wanted to include usually required a level of analysis that the beginning student was totally unprepared to follow. And so after a good faith effort, I found myself defeated. Today it would be easier because we now have exploratory data analytic approaches, but then we were not so well prepared. Between the two sets of materials the ASA-NCTM committee prepared, I felt that I had finally paid off that debt, a little late—but it finished the job.

★ ★ ★

People sometimes ask me how I can handle so many items like this flowing by my desk. One answer is that editing seems to be something I can do good work at even with short snatches of time. Most of us find that some sorts of projects just cannot be started without an uninterrupted period of several hours available. I used to think this was true of editing manuscripts, but later I found that even a few minutes at a time can make a lot of progress through a manuscript, provided I write criticisms as I go instead of waiting until the end to organize them.

Since helping with these efforts, I have engaged with several others in joint works where multiple authors have participated. For example, several of us put together the book *Data for Decisions*, an exposition of statistics intended for people in the policy field who wanted to know what statistics is all about but not necessarily how to carry out specific methods of analysis. The book emphasizes data-gathering.

This book was written in a manner we have found to be especially effective. An author drafts a chapter, and then the other book authors act as critics and give the draft a thorough assessment. Then the paper or chapter is revised in light of the critiques.

★ ★ ★

At the same time that *Data for Decisions* was going on, David Hoaglin, John Tukey, and I were developing books on robust and exploratory techniques with the help of colleagues in the same manner. All these books have a definite plan, but the individual chapters are written by one, two, or three people and then subjected to heavy editorial criticism by the three editors. Our success in this kind of endeavor has continued because the papers turn out to have a mixture of original research and exposition that benefits the careers of the authors and their students. So far we have three books prepared along this line, and as I write, one and a half more are well along.

★ ★ ★

Two other efforts like this deserve inclusion. John C. Bailar III and I, together with Arnold Relman, wanted to produce a set of articles that would tell medical scholars what the state of the statistical art was as far as clinical research was concerned. With the support of the Rockefeller Foundation, the three of us developed a program of research to satisfy this need. Over a period of time with the help of visiting scholars and graduate students, we produced many articles and finally a book, *Medical Uses of Statistics*, that tells something of the state of the art of statistics for clinicians. Like *Statistics: A Guide to the Unknown*, the kind of writing required here was again very different from what our scholars were used to, and we had to be advised repeatedly by Dr. Relman, editor of the *New England Journal of Medicine*, just what he had in mind. After Bailar and I critiqued the articles, Relman pitched in. He wanted to tell physicians in the clinical research field what statistics of various kinds were being used for and what they should be paying attention to. But he did not want us to explain to the physicians how to carry out the analyses and designs that we mentioned.

Notes

1. Commission on Mathematics of the College Entrance Examination Board
   (Affiliations as of time of appointment)

Albert W. Tucker, Chairman	Princeton University
Carl B. Allendoerfer	University of Washington
Edwin C. Douglas	The Taft School, Watertown, Connecticut
Howard F. Fehr	Teachers College, Columbia University
Martha Hildebrandt	Proviso Township High School, Maywood, Illinois
Albert E. Meder, Jr.	Rutgers, the State University of New Jersey
Morris Meister	Bronx High School of Science, New York, New York
Frederick Mosteller	Harvard University
Eugene P. Northrop	University of Chicago
Ernest R. Ranucci	Weequahic High School, Newark, New Jersey
Robert E. K. Rourke	Kent School, Kent, Connecticut
George B. Thomas, Jr.	Massachusetts Institute of Technology
Henry Van Engen	Iowa State Teachers College
Samuel S. Wilks	Princeton University

2. The Canadian painters Tom Thomson, J. E. H. MacDonald, Arthur Lismer, Frederick Varley, Frank Johnston, and Franklin Carmichael, joined later by A. Y. Jackson, formed the Group of Seven in the early 1900s. Their work had a strong impact on the style and spirit of Canadian art (www.groupofsevenart.com/history.html).

3. ASA-NCTM Committee Members
   William Kruskal
   Richard Link
   Frederick Mosteller, Chairman
   Richard Pieters
   Gerald Rising

References

Bailar, J. C. III and Mosteller, F., editors (1986). *Medical Uses of Statistics.* Waltham, MA: NEJM Books. (Translated into Italian, *L'Uso Della Statistica in Medicina,* Rome: Il Pensiero Scientifico Editore, 1988.) 2nd edition, 1992.

Bowers, H., Miller, N. and Rourke, R. E. K. (1947). *Mathematics for Canadians: Book I.* Canada: J. M. Dent and Sons (Canada) and the Macmillan Company of Canada Ltd.

Durkheim, E. (1897). *Suicide: A Study in Sociology.* Glencoe, IL: The Free Press. Reprint, 1997.

Hoaglin, D. C., Light, R. J., McPeek, B., Mosteller, F., and Stoto, M. A. (1982, 2nd printing 1984). *Data for Decisions: Information Strategies for Policymakers.* Cambridge, MA: Abt Books; 2nd printing, Lanham, MD: University Press of America, Inc.

Hoaglin, D. C., Mosteller, F., and Tukey, J. W., editors (1983). *Understanding Robust and Exploratory Data.* New York: Wiley.

Hoaglin, D. C., Mosteller, F., and Tukey, J. W., editors (1985). *Exploring Data Tables, Trends, and Shapes.* New York: Wiley.

Hoaglin, D. C., Mosteller, F., and Tukey, J. W., editors (1991). *Fundamentals of Exploratory Analysis of Variance.* New York: Wiley.

Mosteller, F., Fienberg, S. E., and Rourke, R. E. K. (1983). *Beginning Statistics with Data Analysis.* Reading, MA: Addison-Wesley.

Mosteller, F. and Rourke, R. E. K. (1973). *Sturdy Statistics: Nonparametrics and Order Statistics.* Reading, MA: Addison-Wesley.

Mosteller, F., Rourke, R. E. K., and Thomas, G. B. Jr. (1961a). *Teachers' Manual for Probability: A First Course.* Reading, MA: Addison-Wesley.

Mosteller, F., Rourke, R. E. K., and Thomas, G. B. Jr. (1961b). *Probability: A First Course.* Reading, MA: Addison-Wesley. Derived from *Probability with Statistical Applications.*

Mosteller, F., Rourke, R. E. K., and Thomas, G. B. Jr. (1961c). *Probability and Statistics,* Official textbook for Continental Classroom. Reading, MA: Addison-Wesley. Derived from *Probability with Statistical Applications.*

Mosteller, F., Rourke, R. E. K., and Thomas, G. B. Jr. (1961d). *Probability with Statistical Applications.* Reading, MA: Addison-Wesley.

Mosteller, F., Kruskal, W. H., Link, R. F., Pieters, R. S., and Rising, G. R., editors. (1973). The Joint Committee on the Curriculum in Statistics and Probability of the American Statistical Association and the National Council of Teachers of Mathematics. *Statistics by Example* (four volumes). Reading, MA: Addison-Wesley.
- *Statistics by Example: Exploring Data* (with the assistance of Martha Zelinka).
- *Statistics by Example: Weighing Chances* (with the assistance of Roger Carlson and Martha Zelinka).

- *Statistics by Example: Detecting Patterns* (with the assistance of Roger Carlson and Martha Zelinka).
- *Statistics by Example: Finding Models* (with the assistance of Roger Carlson and Martha Zelinka).

Mosteller, F., with a group of the Commission on Mathematics of the College Entrance Examination Board (1957). *Introductory Probability and Statistical Inference for Secondary Schools.* New York: College Entrance Examination Board.

Mosteller, F., with a group of the Commission on Mathematics of the College Entrance Examination Board (1959). *Introductory Probability and Statistical Inference: An Experimental Course.* Revised preliminary edition. New York: College Entrance Examination Board.

Mosteller, F., with others (1959). *Program for College Preparatory Mathematics.* Report of the Commission on Mathematics. New York: College Entrance Examination Board.

Tanur, J. M., Mosteller, F., Kruskal, W. H., Link, R. F., Pieters, R. S., and Rising, G. R., editors (1972). The Joint Committee on the Curriculum in Statistics and Probability of the American Statistical Association and the National Council of Teachers of Mathematics. *Statistics: A Guide to the Unknown.* San Francisco: Holden-Day. (A 2nd edition with slight changes was published in 1979 with Erich Lehmann joining the editorial group; a much revised 3rd edition was published by Wadsworth & Brooks/Cole in 1989; a 4th edition was published in 2006 by a different editorial team: R. Peck, G. Casella, G. W. Cobb, R. Hoerl, D. Nolan, R. Starbuck, and H. Stern.) (Translated into Spanish and Chinese.)

19

The Cape

Among things that have facilitated my research, aside from people, summers on Cape Cod have been the most effective. About the time that Dave Wallace and I were working on *The Federalist* papers, Virginia and I rented a place in West Falmouth, and Dave and his family visited there for a while. Then we bought a place in Saconesset Hills, also in West Falmouth, and Dave rented a cottage right beside our place for part of the summer. This made it very easy to get together and discuss our work. My place has a garage made over into a small house that I use for research.

The main room is big enough to hold a conference of four or five people, though two is better, and it has a large table and chairs. As a further feature, the typewriter sits on a door laid flat over two two-drawer files.

The main living quarters are in a primitive house next door with only fireplaces for heat. It is not as convenient for cooking as at home, and Virginia has to put up with this lack of familiar equipment. The main house, while sparse on heat and equipment, has from the dining room table an excellent view of Cleveland Ledge Light, the southern entrance to the Cape Cod Canal. In addition, from a side window we look at a tidal marsh, often with egrets or herons. Finally, we have a deck, like a widow's walk, up one flight on a ladder. This deck gives a fine view of Buzzards Bay from the Elizabeth Islands on the south to Mattapoisett on the north. Then nearby, it has a complete view of Great Sippewissett Marsh. We can also see the back of Frank (in 1989 President of the National Academy of Sciences) and Billie Press's summer home in Sippewissett. I doubt that many summer homes, heated or not, have better views than we have.

The distance from the research office to the beach is perhaps 200 yards, and when it is swimming time as determined by the weather and the tides, we just change at once and go to the beach for most of an hour and then come back and get back to work. I don't enjoy lounging on the beach. A very small room in the ex-garage has bunk beds, and when Gale was young, she liked to sleep in the upper one. Bill was always wonderful about fixing up the houses. He learned to take windows apart and replace the ropes that hold the weights

F. Mosteller, *The Pleasures of Statistics: The Autobiography of Frederick Mosteller*,
DOI 10.1007/978-0-387-77956-0_19,
© Springer Science + Business Media, LLC 2010

that make it fairly easy to move a window up and down. He learned to replace the glass rectangles when they broke for some reason and to do the glazing properly. All the family finally learned to remake screens because the long winters gradually destroy them and taking them down was very inconvenient for us.

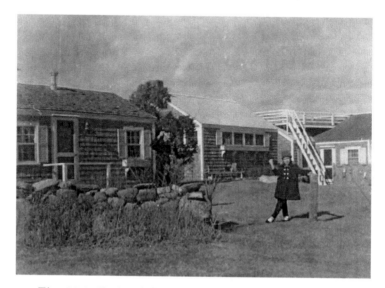

Fig. 19.1. Fred and Gale in front of the Cape house, 1963.

Decoration Day[1] weekend was our customary first visit to the Cape for three purposes: to check that utilities were in order, to cut the grass and trim the hedges, and to plant the window boxes. Over the years the window boxes gradually cracked, fell off their supports, and broke. One year Gale brought her power drill and built replacements that are holding up well after several years. Once the window boxes were planted, we hurried home because this is also a traditional time to plant tomatoes.

We tended to move to the Cape about the last week in June or the first week in July, the reasons being various—we couldn't break away earlier, the swimming was cold before the Fourth, and so on. We usually pulled out just before Labor Day. Nevertheless, those two months—July and August—produced a great deal of writing associated with research and exposition, to say nothing of committee work.

Many people have cute names for their summer homes, such as Wits End or Owl's Nest, and for a long time I thought The Bookmaker would be a nice name, but my neighbors might misunderstand. Recently I thought of The Bookery, which may not offend and still carry the message of production.

Both children learned to type and also to drive here on the Cape because of the Falmouth summer school. Both learned to sail, though Virginia and I never did. Gale even did some horseback riding.

Bill learned early to do computing and found himself having summer jobs, and so he usually was not available for participation in the summer work. Gale took courses that were especially helpful for my work, and she acted as the live-in computer, secretary, and mathematical assistant for several summers. When she was younger, she and I used to give the Mosteller Award of the Summer for Outstanding Contributions to American Literature. Gale and I would create a beautiful award diploma replete with stars, ribbons, and seals announcing who got the Award and then send it to the authors. We mounted the book itself against a sort of frame Gale made of red, white, and blue crepe paper and set it up in a prominent place. The first such award was given to Lincoln Moses and his coauthor Robert V. Oakford for their book *Tables of Random Permutations* of the integers.

Bill worked in computing for several organizations and wrote a book, *The System Programmer's Problem Solver*, on debugging systems programs. I believe he got the Mosteller Award of the Summer for that contribution. Virginia and I enjoyed reading it as he developed it, though we knew nothing about the subject, and did not speak debugging. I'm sure that we tried to send advice all the same.

We gave ourselves and our coauthors first priority when choosing a recipient. Having Gale as a steady secretary right on the premises, together with her experience with mathematics, speeded up a lot of the work for several years, but finally all good things must stop, and then Professor Gary Becker of the University of Chicago was the recipient of my excellent assistant. Gale went on to take a doctorate in Economics.

When at the Cape, although I had to return to Harvard every week or two, I did not stay long, just enough to meet various people who were working on our projects and make sure the work was on track, and then I returned to the Cape. These visits also gave me a chance to collect produce from our Belmont vegetable garden and to do a little weeding sometimes, though Virginia has always been the steady weeder.

Although swimming was a hobby at the Cape, we had one other—day lilies. The climate seems to be superb for day lilies on the Cape; as long as they get some sun, they thrive. Over the years we have added many kinds to the orange-yellow triples that were there in profusion when we arrived. The main problem is to beat back the advancing forces of nature.

Bird life here is fun to watch, and we have gradually purchased various kinds of feeders and swimming pools for birds. They come in profusion— cardinals, several finches, flickers, sparrows, chickadees, Carolina wrens, hummingbirds, green and blue herons, egrets, geese, catbirds, swallows, robins, brown thrashers, Baltimore orioles, grackles, red-winged blackbirds, terns, occasional hawks, toward the end of summer cormorants, and always sea gulls. One summer Gale captured a parakeet who seemed pleased to live the next few years with her. More accurately, to her delight, it captured her by suddenly perching on her outstretched finger. During the day Henry (or maybe Henrietta) flew freely through the house, landing on unexpected targets like a pencil or pen, or a head of hair.

Also we have some wild animal life, but that changes more from year to year than do the birds. We have a stable group of chipmunks and rabbits. Beyond that we have "the year of the...." The blank gets filled in according to the year. For example, the first time we noticed that we had an animal year was the year of the Groundhog—a great big grandfather groundhog that could be seen near the edge of the marsh, doing we did not know what. We have never seen him or another groundhog there since that year. The next important year was the year of the Toads. These stayed for two successive years. One year the toads lived underneath the automobiles. They would get out before we went anywhere in the morning. Another year, one lived on the deck, a rather large open porch. We couldn't understand where he went in the daytime because the deck was in full sun, but after many weeks we discovered that he would wedge himself between a little fence we had to protect children from falling down some steps and a brick chimney. He seemed to live vertically during the sunny part of the day. He grew very rapidly, and so he must have found it a good hunting place. Those were the two years of the toads.

Toads never threatened us, but the years of the Skunks were more harrowing. One year the skunks grew so numerous that the local highways were strewn with their bodies. At night as we tried to walk between the two houses, it was important to take a flashlight to spy out the route to make sure it was free of skunks. The large ones were very brave and yielded to no one. When we found one on the route, we just retreated and waited until they gave us back the front yard. This siege went on for two successive summers. Since then we've had no skunks.

The next year was the year of the Foxes. They did not seem well to me, though perhaps foxes always look a little thin and sick. Sometimes they would come and lie down and rest between the two houses. Dogs didn't seem to bother them, nor cats, although there were some of each around. I always assumed that they lived off the bunnies. I never saw many foxes.

After a year or two of no animals, we then had Raccoons. They would come in numbers and try to get at the garbage cans, and so we had to keep the garbage cans inside the houses. For the same reason, one couldn't put the garbage out for collection the night before the collectors came, because the raccoons would open up the can and spill garbage all over the neighborhood. Also they seemed to fight and snarl and squeal, at least I supposed that that was what they were doing.

In two separate years we had proud results from the Quail. Mama and Papa quail marched around, followed one year by a line of about 14 young. Sometimes they would come to our feeders and collect cracked corn from the ground beneath, where the other birds had thrown pieces they weren't pleased

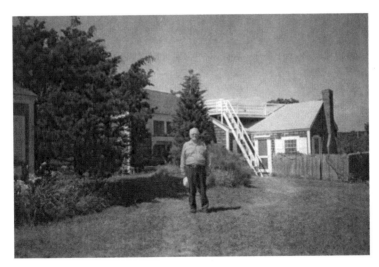

Fig. 19.2. Fred in front of the Cape house, 1985.

with. Another year we saw a dozen young. In 1989 we saw only Mama and Papa.

The main point about the Cape from the point of view of working is that it is easy to have a half-day of uninterrupted work on the same project. This is something that is hard to achieve anywhere. It is not that I can't work on a project with only a bit of time available, but large projects require substantial time to keep them moving, and so writing a chapter of a book or revising one requires lengthy attention.

I don't mind changing projects frequently if that is what the priority calls for, but books are helped greatly by long periods on one part, even when one knows just what is to be done.

The Cape provided uninterrupted time without losing the backup that goes with the help at the office. For example, in the late 1980s at the Department of Statistics, Cleo Youtz, and at the Technology Assessment Group, Marie McPherson and Elisabeth Burdick handled the summer. During the rest of the year the same group plus Marjorie Olson maintained our projects.

Then too the fun of looking out the window at a peaceable kingdom of birds and chipmunks seems most rewarding in itself, even if the mind does wander from the subject.

On reviewing this description, Gale said, "The Cape sounds positively idyllic. Apparently it does not have great plantings of poison ivy, a yearly ant invasion of the kitchen, tight-clinging ticks, house-raiding crickets with noisy chirps, the merry clatter of snapping mousetraps, week-long 'typhoons,' or summer weather requiring winter coats." Fortunately, these are not what I recall.

Note

1. The U.S. holiday now known as Memorial Day, the last Monday in May.

References

Moses, L. E. and Oakford, R. V. (1963). *Tables of Random Permutations.* Stanford, CA: Stanford University Press.

Mosteller, W. S. (1989). *The System Programmer's Problem Solver.* 2nd edition. Wellesley, MA: QED Information Sciences, Inc.

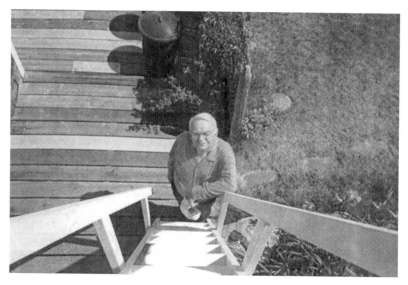

Fig. 19.3. At the Cape house, 1985.

20

Biostatistics

After our Faculty Seminar at the School of Public Health had continued for a few years, Dean Howard Hiatt decided to strengthen the quantitative side of his health services effort. Biostatistics had had a serious presence since the School was established in 1922. The founding chair of the department was E. B. Wilson, a mathematician who had earlier been chair of the Department of Physics at MIT. After he retired from Harvard, he was the project supervisor for Bill Cochran's research contract with the Office of Naval Research, and I got to know him more professionally than I had through the American Academy of Arts and Sciences, where he had been the Executive Officer. In the course of his visits with Cochran, he and I talked about a research problem in factor analysis whose results I still have not published. He checked over my approach and used it on a practical problem he was helping someone with.

Wilson was polite and formal, rather in the way people are sometimes portrayed as being at the turn of the century or earlier. In spite of this, I found him easy and enjoyable to talk with. In a 1927 paper in the *Journal of the American Statistical Association*, he had developed the idea of confidence limits for the binomial situation, possibly before others had done so. When I mentioned this to him, he made no claim to priority. He seemed unduly modest about it.

The Department of Biostatistics in Dean Hiatt's time was of modest size because it had not grown as the School had done. Between its teaching load and its consulting work for other departments, its faculty had little time for original research on its own methods, though consulting did breed new findings, as I have suggested elsewhere. Robert Reed had been chairing the department but had turned the chairmanship back to Jane Worcester, who had been one of Wilson's assistants at the founding of the School. Jane in turn was about to retire. After a good deal of searching for a new chair in 1974, Jane wrote Howard that he ought to make me the chair, and he in turn persuaded me. The major carrot was that Dean Hiatt wanted to enlarge the department. I continued with half-time teaching in Statistics at Arts and Sciences and devoted the other half to administrative and research work in Biostatis-

F. Mosteller, *The Pleasures of Statistics: The Autobiography of Frederick Mosteller*, DOI 10.1007/978-0-387-77956-0_20, © Springer Science + Business Media, LLC 2010

tics. When I came over to the medical area, the Harvard Medical School also gave me an appointment to help make me feel welcome.

In addition to Bob Reed and Jane Worcester, Biostatistics also had Nan Laird, who had been a research assistant and teaching fellow for me at Statistics, Margaret Drolette, who was a marvelous classroom teacher, and (part-time) Yvonne Bishop, who had written her thesis with me. I worked with the faculty to develop some new courses, which they were happy to do, and to bring in some new faculty. The personnel searches were very time-consuming and expensive because of modern hiring regulations. We also put our departmental colloquium on a more regular schedule, and we began to set up a consulting service that could ultimately support itself. Yvonne was especially good at developing the consulting service. Later she joined Lincoln Moses in the Department of Energy in Washington, D.C.

Somewhere along the line, we got the idea of using telecommunications to offer a course on both sides of the Charles River simultaneously (Statistics near Harvard Yard and Biostatistics in the medical area, about four miles apart). Nan Laird tried hard to make it work with a course in design of experiments. In theory, the lecture could be heard and seen in both places at the same time. As so often happens with technologies that are used occasionally, something often failed. Although NBC could do this daily with 195 stations, Harvard could not regularly connect two, probably because we were trying to do it only a few times a week and with few resources. Enough crying.

The point is that we were trying things new to us. Attempts at innovation proceeded on all sides. Milton Weinstein, an expert in policy analysis and decision theory who had attended classes I taught earlier at the Kennedy School, joined the department. Lawrence Thibodeau came to us from Minnesota, where he had studied with one of my former students, Stephen Fienberg. Together with Joseph Ingelfinger (son of Franz Ingelfinger, former editor of the *New England Journal of Medicine*), Thibodeau and I began to develop a quantitative course in biostatistics for physicians. It took several years, and we did not finish the book until James Ware came and helped. We attracted Thomas Louis from Boston University (he now heads a large department at the University of Minnesota). Christine Waternaux also joined us, coming from the University of Michigan.

Arnold Relman, editor of the *New England Journal of Medicine*, asked the department to review a collection of articles from the *Journal* to see how many needed quantitative refereeing. As I recall, it came to about 35 percent. In response, he purchased a large amount of Larry Thibodeau's time to help with the process. When Larry left Harvard, Relman got John Bailar III to take up the part-time post as statistical editor, a service he continued to perform in 1990 even though much of his work is now at McGill University.

A little earlier, Marvin Zelen, together with a substantial group of statisticians experienced in carrying out and analyzing clinical trials, especially in cancer, decided that they wanted to move from their base at another university. One possible new home was the Dana-Farber Cancer Institute at Harvard, and this would have served the cancer research side, but not the academic side of their needs. In such groups, the personnel have more promising futures if they can maintain a teaching appointment along with their research work.

Marvin and I had known each other through the American Statistical Association. Bringing a large experienced group to the department would break us out of the difficulty of never having enough faculty for our teaching and consulting tasks. It would also enable us to enlarge the small, ill-funded doctoral program.

All that remained was to figure out how to make the appointments. The School was managed mainly by faculty committees, and I could see that some-one planning to make 10 or 15 new faculty appointments was likely to step into a minefield. After a few fruitless starts, I recalled that I was new here. I went separately to Brian MacMahon, Chair of Epidemiology, and James Whitten-berger, Chair of the Department of Physiology, and explained my problem and asked what they would do if it were theirs. Although neither thought I had much chance, they separately outlined a program with many steps that they thought would be required.

Instead of looking for shortcuts, Ruth Werman (my senior administrator) and I set up the many meetings Brian and Jim had suggested, laid out the paperwork, and badgered Marvin for piles of documents. It turned out that, when department and committee chairs understood what we were trying to do and how it could be financed, the benefit for the School seemed obvious, though the story took a great deal of explaining and plowed through hills of skepticism. Fortunately, Marvin's group had an adequate number of strong publications, and so the question of extent of research did not arise. The group ultimately came in two waves, and that spread out the lumpiness of the move. In 1990, Biostatistics had about 34 faculty members, though not full-time on departmental work, and 58 graduate students.

References

Ingelfinger, J. A., Mosteller, F., Thibodeau, L. A., and Ware, J. H. (1983). *Biostatistics in Clinical Medicine.* New York: Macmillan Publishing Co. 2nd edition, 1987.

Wilson, E. B. (1927). Probable inference, the law of succession, and statistical inference. *Journal of the American Statistical Association*, 22:209–212.

21

Health Policy and Management

Among his innovations at the School of Public Health, Dean Hiatt created
a Department of Health Policy and Management (HP&M). Its existence responded to the reality that the health care system had become a complicated
structure with many players and tensions—regulation from government at
all levels, providers (physicians, hospitals, nursing homes, and other personnel), payors (insurers and government), and consumer interests. As the health
costs in the United States rose as a percentage of gross national product, using health resources wisely became ever more important. For example, some
hospitals were not well supplied with managerial staff who understood the
business side of the institution, and they could be helped by training in hospital management. The government should, of course, assess the impact of
its activities and regulations on the health care system because well-intended
regulations often create unintended bad outcomes—what economists call ex-
ternalities.

The department therefore included faculty with business training and special knowledge of health care, economists, evaluators, policy analysts, and
faculty concerned with the analysis of health care practices and with health
services research.

The administrative situation in the department in 1981 was in some ways
reminiscent of the Department of Social Relations in 1953. Instead of having
a chair, several faculty members formed a committee to run the department.
Although committees have their uses and I've had great success with them,
they do not shine at running day-to-day activities. If nothing else, communication becomes too slow for action in real time, and then people without
authority take initiatives that lead to trouble because "there wasn't time to
check, and decisions had to be made."

Never one to waste a helper, Hiatt thought that I should chair HP&M
because Marvin was chairing Biostatistics. My previous experience in statistics, evaluation, and policy at the John F. Kennedy School of Government
gave some support to that idea, but my lack of experience in economics and
management à la the business school did not.

F. Mosteller, *The Pleasures of Statistics: The Autobiography of Frederick Mosteller*,
DOI 10.1007/978-0-387-77956-0_21,
© Springer Science + Business Media, LLC 2010

Some alternatives to taking on this post would have been to resume heavier participation in the Kennedy School or to return to Statistics full-time. Under Graham Allison's leadership, the Kennedy School was making giant steps in growth, and being part of that group would have been very attractive, but I felt that they had so many strong senior people that one more person would make little difference to their future.

On the other hand, at the School of Public Health, with two or three exceptions, the HP&M faculty were young and were trying to organize a new field consisting of heterogeneous disciplines. Consequently, when I discussed my next step at this time with President Bok, I acknowledged that I would fit in well at the Kennedy School, but the need for my strengths—research experience, administration of departments, engagement in policy and evaluation—seemed greater at the School of Public Health. He seemed pleased with that view, and so I took the chair at HP&M.

To help me there, Nina Leech came from Biostatistics to be the department secretary. She had done much work with me at Biostatistics, and she continued to manage both correspondence and manuscripts at HP&M. Ruth Werman and her husband left Harvard and began spending much of their year in Boca Raton. Deborah Harris became the new senior administrator at HP&M, and Jaylyn Olivo was her assistant.

One difference between HP&M in 1981 and Social Relations in 1953 was that Social Relations was huge and thoroughly organized, whereas HP&M was of middling size—bigger than Statistics or Biostatistics, though, in students enrolled in the department—and was organized primarily at the level of courses with a large number of valuable faculty appointments as lecturers, not only from the Boston area, but from far and wide. Until I joined HP&M, it had been heavily committed to giving courses to people in the health care industry, such as hospital managers and heads of departments. These activities went on simultaneously with regular teaching of students seeking masters and doctoral degrees through full-time enrollment. The unique nature of HP&M meant that research of two kinds had to be maintained. For all the courses, but especially for the continuing education courses, new "cases" had to be created to illustrate real management problems, their consequences, and their treatment. Whereas in a statistics book the background to a problem might go on for half a page at most, in the case studies 50 or 60 pages of detail were common. The Business School and the Kennedy School use such cases very effectively in their teaching. Cases emphasize a whole problem with their many facets, including organization, finance, technology, science, marketing, and even personalities, rather than focusing on some key piece of the picture and trying to handle it. Preparing these cases is an expensive operation because one is writing the detailed history of an event. Through frequent changes in technologies and institutions, the older case studies became outmoded. Consequently, the demand for new cases has been very steady.

A second kind of research develops and applies theories and obtains data to prove points. Sometimes sample surveys or experiments are required. Usually such research has more disciplinary character than case studies, bringing to bear political science, planning, economics, law, public analysis, or whatever mixture seems appropriate. To progress in academia, professors must make a substantial contribution to this second kind of research.

When I joined HP&M, it was agreed that the heavy continuing education work would be developed outside the department by a schoolwide agency under the able direction of Dr. Dade Moeller. Happily, that effort has been successful in its own right. Department members still participate in such programs, but the organization, advertising, housing, and so on is removed from the academic department. This left more time to attend to the full-time students. It also made it possible for faculty to put more effort into their own research because they were less distracted by the daily crises of a business organization.

With the aid of Penny Feldman and Chester Douglass from the Dental School, we obtained some training grants to assist some students. We reviewed our course structure from the point of view of our masters degree program and our doctoral program. We decided to increase the numbers in the doctoral program.

The pace of research increased. William Hsiao reviewed the programs of reimbursement for physicians by getting panels of physicians to judge the features of a technology or treatment and how they should be weighed in deciding on payment. Inevitably, such a study, if it changes anything, will produce some dissent. We still do not know how this will all come out.

Several people prepared books based on their research. My own role in this part of the work was to encourage the authors to keep the work going and to advise them about some traps to avoid. Scholars often plan much larger books than their study can support, or that take longer than a scholar can afford in a competitive system. By recognizing that some problems can be put off to another book, to be written after this one is finished, writers can in good conscience complete a volume. I learned long ago in working with good doctoral students that they could be greatly helped by paring their theses down to just a few themes, and putting off some chapters for later papers. Book writers can use the same device, and they can be helped if someone will listen to their chapter plans and suggest matters that might be set aside in a first writing. Of course, the author has to make the decision, but the opportunity to talk about it is helpful, and I enjoyed doing it on a regular basis. Sometimes authors asked me to read and comment on chapters, and I did a great deal of such collegial work. The production of books and papers increased. Kenneth Thorpe developed projects with the health commission of the State of New York.

Harvey Fineberg, a professor in the department, was also a physician. He had been a student at the Kennedy School, but he had not yet completed his doctorate for them. When I was chairing Biostatistics, he wrote his thesis with me and thus completed his degree. When Dean Hiatt completed his term of office, Harvey was chosen to succeed him. With my own retirement in view,

I had rather expected Harvey to take over the HP&M chairmanship, but, by ascending to the deanship, he left us searching.

One important goal for me was to be sure I was replaced by a strong chair. If the person had some management background, that would help in HP&M. We were fortunate to get Robert Blendon, who had studied business administration and had foundation experience and substantial experience with technology assessment, to join the department as chair.

References

Hsiao, W. C., Braun, P., Dunn, D., Becker, E. R., DeNicola, M., and Ketcham, T. R. (1988). Results and policy implications of the resource-based relative-value study. *New England Journal of Medicine,* 319:881–888.

22

Health Science Policy

When David Hamburg came to Harvard to lead the Division of Health Policy Research and Education, he wanted to establish Working Groups somewhat comparable to the committees used by the Institute of Medicine (IOM) to guide its program. He and I had become acquainted when he was president of the IOM and I served on several of its committees. After several meetings, we developed the idea of a Health Science Policy Working Group that I would chair. To do this meant giving up the Surgery Group, which was still active in spite of the death of John Raker, who, with Benjamin Barnes, had advised us on surgery.

The new Division was an umbrella organization, university wide, but especially connected to the Medical School, the School of Public Health, and the Kennedy School of Government. Within the School of Public Health, the Center for the Analysis of Health Practices, directed by Howard Frazier, and the Department of Health Policy and Management, which I chaired, were units with special interests in the Division.

We formed the Health Science Policy Working Group from groups all over the university and beyond. The Andrew K. Mellon Foundation generously supported the Group, and we began meeting monthly in the fashion of the Faculty Seminar in Health and Medicine.

After the usual start-up problems, Michael Stoto, a statistician and demographer at the Kennedy School, became the Executive Officer, a task that Jay Winsten assumed when Stoto later went to Washington, D.C. to join the staff of an IOM committee, and that Jane Durch took on still later.

The members laid out three areas for initial study and over the years carried out several projects within each area. Subgroups met separately and regularly to do their work. And, of course, new areas emerged.

One policy area dealt with the distribution of resources for the Health Sciences both for the United States and for other countries. Michael Stoto initially led the subgroup, aided by Jane Durch. They found 85% of biomedical research concentrated in five countries—Japan, West Germany, France, the United Kingdom, and the United States, which alone carries out nearly half

F. Mosteller, *The Pleasures of Statistics: The Autobiography of Frederick Mosteller*,
DOI 10.1007/978-0-387-77956-0_22,
© Springer Science + Business Media, LLC 2010

of the world's total. Canada and Norway relied on universities for research; Denmark, France, and Sweden on public laboratories; and Switzerland and the United Kingdom on the private sector. Of the five major countries, only the United States does not have a ministry of education with responsibility to sponsor university research.

When Stoto became study director for a committee on the Organizational Structure of the National Institutes of Health, Donald Shepard chaired the subgroup and obtained a contract with the Fogarty International Center to study per capita expenditures for biomedical research in developed countries. They ranged from $1 or $2 in Portugal, Spain, and Ireland to $40 in Sweden, the U.S., and Switzerland.

Another policy area was the credibility of scientists and quality of research. This was a difficult topic because of the widespread distress about fraudulent work that had been revealed at several universities. One project was oriented to the media with the aim of improving communication to the public. Although we do much in professional scientific organizations to educate journalists and science writers about science, we do little to advise scientists how to work better with journalists. We had many meetings where outstanding journalists and science writers told us about their problems with their editors and with scientists. They told us too about their ethics and what various assurances with interviewed scientists meant. Within our group, the scientists found the information most instructive. For example, it is not insulting to ask a science writer how much he or she knows about a subject because it helps find the proper level for the interview. I had hoped that we would get a science writer to prepare a primer for scientists on dealing with the press. So far, no one has carried that out. (Neal Miller, a scientist, has written a helpful primer.)

Jay Winsten interviewed many journalists, science writers, and media professionals, and wrote a great article on the difficulties writers have in delivering their material. But I'm still waiting for the primer for scientists by a science writer.

Our interest in the media has encouraged the School of Public Health to seek funds to bring science writers to the School for a sabbatical year to learn more about science and policy in public health.

A related project was to encourage a science writer to write a primer on statistical methods for journalists. Victor Cohn of *The Washington Post* took this on after attending our meetings and a couple of six-week sessions at the School. He used the subgroup and the Department of Biostatistics as consultants for his book. Books take a while, and although the idea for the book began about 1983, Victor's book *News and Numbers* was published in 1989. The Russell Sage Foundation helped support this project. I enjoyed spending time with Cohn when he was writing it. Years before, when Wallace and I presented the results of our Federalist work at the Minneapolis meetings of the statistical societies, Cohn covered the meeting and after interviewing us wrote an extensive story. We were lucky to have had him as our first experience with a reporter.

As I dither on, you are saying, "Yes, yes, but what about fraud?" With the cooperation of other subgroup members, Penelope Greene, an anthropologist and statistician, and Jane Durch developed a plan to find out how well prepared academic institutions were to respond to allegations of fraud. To find out what sorts of policies research organizations had, they sent questionnaires to medical schools, teaching hospitals, doctorate-granting universities, and schools of public health in the United States. Their response, from two-thirds of the institutions, was very satisfactory for this sort of inquiry. Less than a quarter of the responding institutions had formal *written* policies. About a fifth said they had no plans to develop guidelines. (Although I shouldn't make light of a serious subject, I recall an unknown respondent saying that the quality of research was so bad at his institution that fraud would not matter.)

Penney, Jane, and coworkers Wendy Horwitz and Valwyn Hooper published the analysis of this survey, "Policies for responding to allegations of fraud in research."

The third area of our initial subgroups was led by David Blumenthal, who, in addition to being a physician, had experience as a staff person for Senator Edward Kennedy. Appropriately, he was teaching at the Kennedy School of Government. His subgroup's plan was to investigate the benefits and risks posed by university-industry relationships in research. Ultimately David and his colleagues sent out sample surveys to four groups: 1) administrators in universities and medical schools, 2) executives of companies with potential for such relations, 3) faculty members, and 4) graduate students and fellows. These surveys led to numerous publications at a time when contracts between universities and industries were increasing.

In addition to the surveys, Blumenthal and Shelley Epstein prepared a set of case studies of university-industry relations for universities that had made such arrangements with industries.

Obviously I cannot list all the projects the subgroups undertook, but these were important and very productive. Our speakers at the monthly meetings were usually people contributing to the work of one of the subgroups. The meetings contributed to the overall liveliness of the School of Public Health and the Kennedy School, and we usually met alternately on the two sides of the Charles River.

★ ★ ★

During 1984–85, Thomas Chalmers joined the Working Group, and a subgroup on meta-analysis was formed. Meta-analysis is a collection of methods for analyzing quantitatively a set of studies of similar nature to provide stronger answers to questions than the single studies did. Although the name comes from social science, in the field of medicine Chalmers had been the leader in applying and disseminating the method. You may recall, though, that Beecher actually carried out a meta-analysis when he found out how effective placebos were against a variety of ailments. I also reported some meta-analyses carried out by Gilbert, Light, and Mosteller as well as by Gilbert, McPeek, and Mosteller in Chapter 16. Chalmers was teaching a course in meta-analysis every year in my Department of Health Policy and Management, even when he was leading Mt. Sinai Hospital in New York. Later he retired from Mt. Sinai and moved back to his roots in Boston, and he and I planned to set up a Technology Assessment Group in the School of Public Health when I retired from active teaching.[1]

In 1986–87, several new groups developed. Alexia Antczak developed a very active subgroup on Dental Technology Assessment. With the support of the Working Group, John Graham, Bernard Guyer, and David Hemenway developed the New England Injury Prevention Research Center, bringing together faculty from the Harvard School of Public Health, Boston University, Tufts University, Massachusetts Department of Public Health, and Education Development Center, Inc.

* * *

What helps to make projects in the Health Science Policy Working Group and other such group efforts productive? Naturally, the people in the effort believe in it, or they would not be still contributing. Probably, devices that all organizations use to manage their affairs help. Each project has some definite goals before it begins. The regular meetings with public reports, capsule reports at every meeting from each project together with future timelines, plus featured full meeting reports whenever a project is far enough along, presented to a group of people who feel concerned about the product even when it is not their subgroup, give major support.

The full presentations scheduled well in advance set deadlines for progress of a type that projects create for their teams. And teams need the encouragement that these external stimuli offer. Most of us rise to deadlines. (Difficult labor negotiations rarely get anywhere until strike deadlines loom.)

As I've said elsewhere, whenever I was given a manuscript to criticize, I tried to respond quickly, and in my own work I have found suggestions helpful at hurrying me along toward a more complete and polished manuscript. The mixtures of advice on content, writing, figures, tables, and statistical methods all move the investigators along.

At regular intervals I do try to review the progress of each subgroup and each project with each leader to see whether something can help a lot to move the project along. Attention without nagging seems to be a facilitator.

I have one low-tech reminder system. On one sheet of paper I have a list of the projects we are working on—Harvard Yard on one side and Medical Area on the other. It's the only time I write on both sides of a sheet of paper. About once a week, I go over the list and make notes of what needs to be done or what is and has to be static. My impression is that reviewing the list and making the notes are helpful activities, but I don't seem to use the notes again. Probably the main merit is the poker up the spine that goes with being reminded of an activity that is both forgotten and not moving. Once in a while, we revise the list when papers get published or projects are completed. I once read advice from an efficiency expert that such a list shouldn't have more than 20 items. That is about what mine runs, maybe a few more, but my list includes several that other people have primary responsibility for.

Once in a while hang-ups occur that come from misunderstandings, and then sometimes a word from a senior person to another senior person can straighten things out. Or junior people working together fall out, and then sometimes a senior person can either reassemble them or separate them in such a way that projects can still go forward on new tracks.

Helping a totally stalled scholar restart research can contribute a good deal. Usually such a person is essentially down in a garbage dump staring at an overwhelming number of repellent tasks, all overdue. Although one could try to do a cost-benefit analysis to prioritize the tasks, as I've said elsewhere, a good rule to cut through that resistance, and the defeating count of obligations, is to choose one thing and do it. I advise choosing the thing that is nearest done. Elsewhere I've explained why, and because it has helped me through life, I think it helps others. For instance, do not start a three-volume work not yet outlined. It doesn't take more than a few minutes to decide which is the thing nearest done. Won't there be cheating because the stalled person will choose something less repellent? Well, the purpose of the rule is to get back into production; the advisor doesn't much care which project begins to move.

Occasionally, one finds that a project needs special support that no one anticipated, and then the leader has to try to figure out whether it can be obtained and afforded. Some reserve funds for such contingencies help a lot, but they are not always available. Solutions often are not monetary but organizational.

It is essential that someone be paying close attention to the expenditures of funds; otherwise people not used to handling money may get into trouble. It is important to review this regularly, just like the timelines for progress. In large organizations the project budget is often erroneously charged for items that were spent elsewhere, and someone has to be vigilant about these errors or they become permanent. I'm not good at keeping track of these matters myself, but I have been fortunate in working with people who can maintain pressure on these problems and who understand their importance. Pressure is required because organizations don't like to admit errors and like even less to fix them, as we have all found.

★ ★ ★

Most of us need encouragement or, even if we don't, we are cheered by it. All of us need to distribute more praise than we do, and most of us want more praise than we get. When a speaker has finished a talk, the one thing that person wants is for people to say, "That was just great, you've done it again!" Some other day you can send along the fundamental flaw underlying the whole presentation. Is that dishonest? No. Today praise the talk, tomorrow discuss the content. Of course, you will say that mature scholars do not need such support. Ha! Or as Tukey would say, "Haw-Haw!"

When I'm on trips, I enjoy sending postcards to people I work with and getting some from them when they travel.

Much of the strength of these group efforts comes because interdisciplinary work is fun. By its nature several collaborators are required, and groups seem to have more fun than individuals—fun may not be funny, but enjoyable and gratifying. When a management person like Nancy Kane or Alice Sapienza, or an economist like Kenneth Arrow or Richard Zeckhauser tells me how their discipline thinks about a problem, I find it exciting to see the way it upgrades the discussion. Each field has worked for centuries or decades to put iron into the reasoning, and so our tools become much more effective when they are adjoined. When we talk to people from our own discipline all the time, we do not realize that others have thought about nearly the same problems from very different points of view—some for efficiency, some for safety, some for distribution, and some for ethics. And so we are much broadened and sometimes chastened.

It may be easier to be original in interdisciplinary work than in one's own discipline, where everyone has been reworking and polishing the same key concepts. Interdisciplinary work forces consideration of combinations of things and thus increases the opportunities for original ideas and concepts. I was always impressed with how well interdisciplinary research seminars worked in Social Relations, as opposed to discussions of curriculum requirements, where the disciplines tended to oppose one another, fighting for more of the student's study time.

Editors' Postscript

Among the articles produced by the Health Science Policy Working Group, we note three related to AIDS: Hatziandreu et al. (1988), Stoto et al. (1988), and Siegel et al. (1990). The first two were written as background papers for the first IOM report on AIDS, Confronting AIDS: Directions for Public Health, Health Care, and Research *(National Academy Press, 1986).*

Note

1. Chapter 23 describes several activities of the Technology Assessment Group.

References

Beecher, H. K. (1955). The powerful placebo. *Journal of the American Medical Association*, 159(17):1602–1606.

Blumenthal, D., Gluck, M. E., Louis, K. S., Stoto, M. A., and Wise, D. (1986). University industry relationships and biotechnology: Implications for the university. *Science*, 232:1361–1366.

Cohn, V. (1989). *News and Numbers*. Ames, IA: Iowa State University Press.

Gilbert, J. P., Light, R. J., and Mosteller, F. (1975a). Assessing social innovations: An empirical base for policy. In R. Zeckhauser, A. Harberger, R. Haveman, L. Lynn, Jr., W. Niskanen, and A. Williams, editors, *Benefit-Cost and Policy Analysis 1974: An Aldine Annual on Forecasting, Decision-making, and Evaluation*. Chicago: Aldine Publishing Company. 3–65.

Gilbert, J. P., Light, R. J., and Mosteller, F. (1975b). Assessing social innovations: An empirical base for policy. In C. A. Bennett and A. A. Lumsdaine, editors, *Evaluation and Experiment: Some Critical Issues in Assessing Social Programs*. New York: Academic Press. 39–193.

Gluck, M. E., Blumenthal, D., and Stoto, M. A. (1987). University industry relationships in the life sciences: Implications for students and post-doctoral fellows. *Research Policy*, 16:327–336.

Greene, P. J., Durch, J. S., Horwitz, W., and Hooper, V. S. (1985). Policies for responding to allegations of fraud in research. *Minerva*, 23:203–215.

Greene, P. J., Durch, J. S., Horwitz, W., and Hooper, V. S. (1986). Institutional policies for responding to allegations of research fraud. *IRB*, 8(4):1–7.

Hatziandreu, E., Graham, J. D., and Stoto, M. A. (1988). AIDS and biomedical research funding: A comparative analysis. *Reviews of Infectious Diseases*, 10:159–167.

Louis, K. S., Blumenthal, D., Gluck, M. E., and Stoto, M. A. (1989). Entrepreneurs in academe: An exploration of behaviors among life scientists. *Administrative Science Quarterly*, 34:110–131.

McPeek, B., Gilbert, J. P., and Mosteller, F. (1977). The end result: Quality of life. Chapter 10 in J. P. Bunker, B. A. Barnes, and F. Mosteller, editors, *Costs, Risks, and Benefits of Surgery*. New York: Oxford University Press. 170–175.

Miller, N. E. (1979). The scientist's responsibility for public information: A guide to effective communication with the media. Bethesda, MD: Society for Neuroscience.

Miller, N. E. (1986). The scientist's responsibility for public information: A guide to effective communication with the media. In S. M. Friedman, S. Dunwoody, and C. Rogers, editors, *Scientists and Journalists*. New York: Macmillan Free Press. 239–253.

Siegel, J. E., Graham, J. D., and Stoto, M. A. (1990). Allocating resources among AIDS research strategies. *Policy Sciences*, 23:1–23.

Stoto, M. A., Blumenthal, D., Durch, J. S., and Feldman, P. H. (1988). Federal funding for AIDS: Decision process and results in fiscal year 1986. *Reviews of Infectious Diseases*, 10:406–419.

Winsten, J. A. (1985). Science and the media: The boundaries of truth. *Health Affairs* (Millwood), 4(1):5–23.

23

Editors' Epilogue

The manuscript that we inherited went only to around 1990—just before Fred "officially retired" from teaching and administration in 1992. Virginia Mosteller became seriously ill after he completed that draft; she died in 2001. Fred maintained an office in the Department of Statistics at Harvard, and he remained active, even tackling important new projects. He continued to live in the house in Belmont, though he suffered a serious fall in 2002. In January 2004 he moved to Arlington, Virginia, to be near his children and grandson, but he continued to work on multiple projects. Many of his friends and colleagues had occasion to visit with Fred after his move. He died, after an extended illness, on July 23, 2006.

Without Fred's perspective from the center of his web of activities, we cannot hope to cover the years after 1990 in substantial detail. We are fortunate, however, that in response to our request for help, a number of people who worked closely with Fred have given us written accounts of selected projects and accomplishments from that period and earlier years. We gratefully acknowledge these contributions from John C. Bailar III, Graham A. Colditz, John D. Emerson, John Hedley-Whyte, Howard H. Hiatt, and James H. Ware. We have built on their material, without quotation marks, to assemble this epilogue, which meshes with Fred's chapters on Education, Teaching, Group Writing, Biostatistics, Health Policy & Management, and Health Science Policy.

★ ★ ★

When Howard Hiatt was appointed dean of the Harvard School of Public Health in 1972, he learned that the department of biostatistics was small and minimally visible in the world of statistical scholarship. This was troubling because biostatistics and its sister discipline, epidemiology, are considered to be the pillars of research on populations. Hiatt soon began to consult with Fred about strategies for statistical science at the school. He persuaded Fred to lead a faculty seminar at the school on statistical problems in health, building

F. Mosteller, *The Pleasures of Statistics: The Autobiography of Frederick Mosteller*,
DOI 10.1007/978-0-387-77956-0_23,
© Springer Science + Business Media, LLC 2010

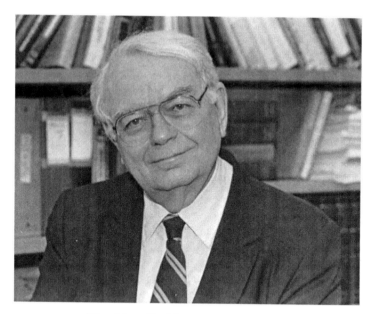

Fig. 23.1. Fred Mosteller, circa 1990.

on his long and productive history of collaborative work on important issues in medicine and public health. The Faculty Seminar on Health and Medicine became very popular, sometimes attracting more than 100 participants to its meetings. The participants met over dinner, often had a guest speaker, and then separated into their chosen working groups. Fred was an active member of the Surgery Group, which focused on costs and benefits of surgery. Using his unequaled ability to convene scholars, he brought together surgeons, anesthesiologists, statisticians, and students in all of these fields to complete a groundbreaking study, *Costs, Risks, and Benefits of Surgery*, which set a new standard for the assessment of surgical procedures and for research on surgical practices. Fred and Hiatt continued to collaborate on a variety of projects for the ensuing decades.

In Chapter 20 Fred mentioned the project that reviewed quantitative aspects of articles from the *New England Journal of Medicine*. As Fred described briefly at the end of Chapter 18, the effort grew into a broader project (with support from the Rockefeller Foundation) to write usable papers on various aspects of statistics in the *NEJM*. Twelve of these were published in that journal, and a few more appeared elsewhere. The project as a whole resulted in *Medical Uses of Statistics*, edited by John Bailar and Fred and published by NEJM Books in 1986. The volume was highly successful, and further work led to a second edition in 1992. Before Fred moved to Virginia, he and Bailar laid the groundwork for a third edition and recruited David Hoaglin to help. After his move, Fred remained interested in the project. He was eager to know how the revisions were going, and he sometimes offered very helpful suggestions. That edition, with Bailar and Hoaglin as editors, appeared in 2009.

When Harvard created its Division of Health Policy Research and Education, Fred chaired the Health Science Policy Working Group. In 1986, its subgroups included Resource Allocation, Media, Meta-Analysis, Regulation, Technology Assessment in Dentistry, and University-Industry Relations. By

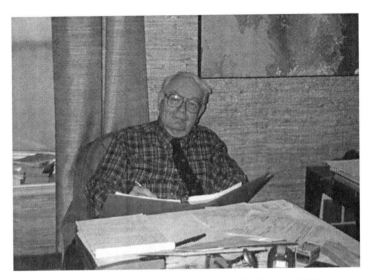

Fig. 23.2. Fred working at home in Belmont, 1989.

1987, project groups on Case Severity Adjustment and on Registries and Datasets had formed under an umbrella subgroup for assessment of medical technologies. The results from the work of the Registries and Datasets Subgroup were published as a special issue of the *International Journal of Technology Assessment in Health Care* in 1991, and in later issues of that journal. One major focus during the period 1988–90 was to examine the use of medical registries and data sets in the assessment of medical technologies. These data constituted an increasingly important resource for technology assessment in health care. Fred presided over monthly early breakfast meetings where participants critiqued methods and results and interrupted guest speakers with predictable regularity.

The Technology Assessment Subgroup evolved into the Technology Assessment Group (TAG—in the Department of Health Policy and Management) under Fred's directorship, with Thomas C. Chalmers as Associate Director. The work was supported primarily by a grant from the Agency for Health Care Policy and Research. The TAG occupied a windowless area in the base-

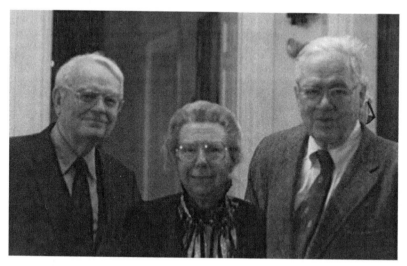

Fig. 23.3. Fred, Virginia, and John Tukey at Fred's "retirement" party in 1987.

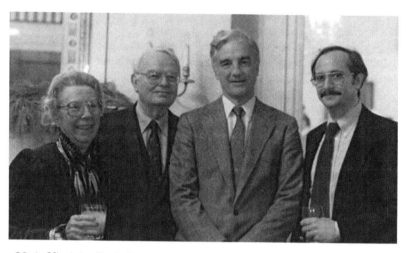

Fig. 23.4. Virginia, Fred, Harvard President Derek Bok, and chair of the Harvard Statistics Department, Don Rubin, at Fred's "retirement" party in 1987.

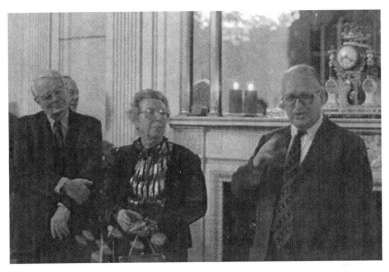

Fig. 23.5. Fred, Virginia, and Henry Rosovsky (Harvard Dean of the Faculty of Arts and Sciences) at Fred's "retirement" party in 1987.

ment of the Kresge Building, but the work environment was stimulating, lively, and fun. As he did in so many other projects, Fred attracted a large group of scholars, including young graduate students and postdocs, to engage the challenges of evaluating medical technologies. Their work contributed to the complex processes by which advances in medical technology lead to new policies and practices that serve the public good. Fred's earlier contributions included chairing the Institute of Medicine's Committee for Evaluating Medical Technologies in Clinical Use, which produced the landmark 1985 volume *Assessing Medical Technologies.*

A primary emphasis in the work of the TAG was meta-analysis, a collection of statistical methods that formally aggregate quantitative scientific findings from multiple primary research reports. Members of the TAG used these tools almost routinely to evaluate new therapies—for example, by combining odds ratios from randomized controlled clinical trials. Their work identified methodological challenges, and members of Fred's team worked on these problems too. One such problem was that of combining risk differences when random-effects models were deemed appropriate. A related effort focused on heterogeneity, an issue that had historically been ignored in the epidemiology literature but is actually one of the richer features of a meta-analytic project. In another earlier study, Fred worked with Graham Colditz on assessing the effect of study design on gain in evaluations of new treatments in medicine and surgery. Jim Miller, then a student at the Kennedy School, was a co-conspirator on this substantial project. They applied several of the methods developed in the *Cost, Risks, and Benefits of Surgery* project to translate the verbal summary of a finding about gain into a 6-point scale. Among the challenges in this work

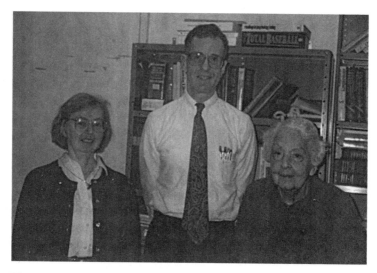

Fig. 23.6. Marge Olson, Dave Hoaglin, and Cleo Youtz, early 1990s.

was the approach to summarizing data across many designs and measures, and Fred developed an application of the Mann-Whitney statistic to summarize measures across many studies. Thus, this empirical study not only produced an evaluation of the potential impact of study design on the evaluation of new technologies but also yielded a methodologic contribution. In keeping with an interest throughout much of his career, Fred also tackled statistical questions of robustness—for example, in trying to ensure that meta-analytic tools were not unduly influenced by a small number of anomalous studies or even by errors in the data. However, the driving focus of Fred's work at TAG was to make good sense out of multiple research findings in order to bring benefit to public policy and to medical practice.

In 1990, Fred turned the efforts of the Registries and Datasets Subgroup to a more general assessment of the contributions contemporary medicine makes to health. The prospect of health care "rationing" and the complex socioeconomic incentives underlying the growth of managed care provided additional impetus to a project on "The Benefits of Contemporary Medicine." Howard S. Frazier served as co-chairman and co-editor of this effort. A diverse group of co-authors met regularly to refine the scope of the investigation, for dialogue with guest speakers, and to review and critique the book chapters that evolved. *Medicine Worth Paying For: Assessing Medical Innovations*, edited by Howard S. Frazier and Frederick Mosteller, was published by the Harvard University Press in 1995. This group continued to meet as the Technology Assessment Group's Seminar on Effective and Affordable Health Care, which later became the Seminar on Technology Assessment in Health Care. Its monthly breakfast meetings have continued, under the leadership of John Hedley-Whyte since 2003 (with Debra Milamed as secretary), addressing such diverse areas as the increasing role of complementary and alternative medicine; the design and analysis of clinical trials; costs, risks, and benefits of health care modalities; and the safety and performance of medical equipment. A Divinity School Fellow with an interest in biomedical research ethics was among the Seminar's more recent attendees. Upon completing his program, he expressed gratitude for "The Technology Assessment in Health Care Seminar ... as a procedural model of collegiality that is very impressive." As of 2009, the Seminar continues on Fred's foundation of critical dialogue, to address issues of statistical methodology, research ethics, data collection, analysis, and communication in a broad spectrum of areas.

In 1991, the Centers for Disease Control and Prevention called for an independent evaluation of the efficacy of BCG vaccine for prevention of tuberculosis. The emergence of drug-resistant TB raised important policy questions for the CDC. This project fit nicely into Fred's larger vision of bringing data to bear on policy. The team of experts consisted of Harvey Fineberg, Mary Wilson, Cathy Berkey, Graham Colditz, and later, Tim Brewer, who had completed infectious disease training at Massachusetts General Hospital. Fred linked the project to a series of methodologic issues that aided in quantifying the efficacy of BCG. He mentored Cathy Berkey on this project, linking her with Carl Morris to develop and apply a random-effects regression approach to the data. This development and application of methods has become the standard teaching piece for software such as STATA, which uses the BCG data set as its demonstration of the application of this method. The project, bringing together expertise in policy, infectious disease, and statis-

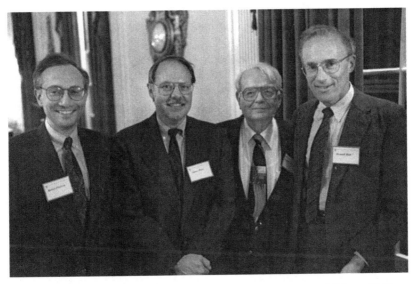

Fig. 23.7. Harvey Fineberg, Jim Ware, Fred, and Howard Hiatt, 1992.

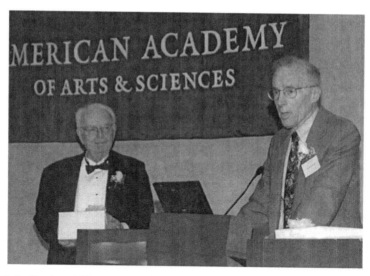

Fig. 23.8. Fred and Howard Hiatt being honored for their work together on the Initiatives for Children project in 2002.

tical methodology, exemplified the interdisciplinary work that Fred fostered and cherished so dearly.

In 1990, Howard Hiatt began a project entitled "Initiatives for Children" at the American Academy of Arts and Sciences (located in Cambridge, near Harvard). He was eager that programs affecting children, particularly teaching programs, be subjected to the kind of rigorous evaluation that Fred, his colleagues, and their successors had applied to medical procedures. Fred agreed to oversee such a process, providing that he not be charged with finding grant support for its activities. Fortunately, Harriet Zuckerman, one of Fred's many great admirers and Professor of Sociology at Columbia University, had recently become vice president of the Andrew W. Mellon Foundation. When Howard told her that Fred had agreed to evaluate programs in the education field, she was delighted. She said that she was confident that the Mellon Foundation would provide Fred with whatever resources he needed to carry out such work, and it did. Again he began with a seminar series on educational issues that was extremely productive and led to a number of studies and several publications. The scope of the project was broader than its name suggested: it addressed issues of health, education, discipline, law, and public policy that pertained to human subjects ranging from newborns through college students. Fred's choice of specific topics always reflected his desire to produce work that could help make a better world.

One example of his influence on the field of education: at an early conference on the issue of optimal class size, Fred mentioned that not many careful studies could be found in the literature, but indicated that the Tennessee experiment on class size was an exception. It was a great surprise that many of the educators present had not heard of it! But it led several people present to suggest that it be used as a model for further research.

As in much of his work, for Initiatives for Children Fred assembled small teams of researchers who identified a societal need and then systematically located a related body of research and tried to make sense of the aggregated findings. For example, Edward Miech, Bill Nave, and Fred carried out a massive search for research literature that examined the use of computer-assisted instruction (CAI) in the teaching of foreign languages. Another project by John Emerson, Cleo Youtz, and Fred addressed the validity of student ratings of college teaching by synthesizing findings from primary studies that worked with multiple sections of the same college courses. Fred and John Emerson also worked with Lisa Boes to assess the current state of knowledge about the teaching of critical thinking at the college level. Fred's other projects also used systematic literature searches and the synthesis of primary research findings to provide reports on the current status of important research agendas that related to the well-being of children. Even after Fred moved to Virginia, his participation on projects that grew out of this work continued, largely via telephone conference calls and letters.

One unifying theme of Fred's work in public health and medical technology, and his research in education, was his commitment to the use of experimental research in prospective studies. Meta-analyses of medical technologies carried out by the Technology Assessment Group often limited their inclusion to primary studies of randomized controlled clinical trials. In his work with the Initiatives for Children project, Fred stressed the need for randomized trials to evaluate educational interventions. Fred and Robert Boruch edited a book

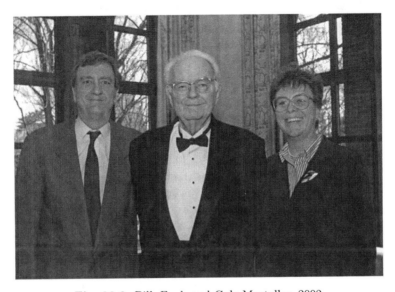

Fig. 23.9. Bill, Fred, and Gale Mosteller, 2002.

of conference proceedings entitled *Evidence Matters: Randomized Trials in Education Research*. Fred clearly believed that some of the triumphs for using rigorous research methods in medicine could be, and should be, replicated with rigorous research on important questions in the field of education. When the Initiatives for Children program ended in 2002, both Hiatt and Fred were honored by the American Academy "for their successful efforts to place the health and welfare of children on the Academy's agenda," and in 2005 Fred received the Rossi Award from the Association for Public Policy Analysis and Management partially in recognition of this work.

★ ★ ★

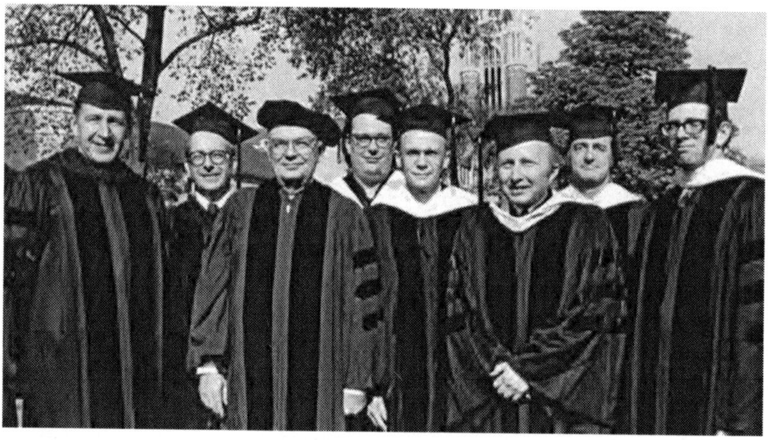

Fig. 23.10. *From left to right,* Leo Goodman, Paul Meier, Fred, Mike Wichura, David Wallace, Bill Kruskal, Pat Billingsley, and Shelby Haberman on the occasion of Fred's receipt of an honorary degree from the University of Chicago, 1973.

Fred was a master at leading a team of investigators in carrying out large-scale projects whose ultimate scholarly production was substantial and impressive. His success in doing this can be attributed in part to the ways in which he organized and carried out these projects:

- He assembled people with diverse areas of expertise and interest, and thus brought a variety of perspectives to bear on any given challenge. This diversity of people tended to make the work more interesting and exciting for all.
- He organized regular meetings of the team at which each participant reported on progress and sought the advice of others. This approach tended to be motivating for all, because the participants knew that others cared about, and even depended on, the work they were doing.

- He guided the team in subdividing a project into manageable chunks that could be tackled without a sense of being overwhelmed.
- He insisted that write-ups of findings and results begin very early and be shared with others in the group for commentary and for exploring possible next steps. He used the notion of a "zeroth draft," and often such drafts were quite informal and handwritten. These benefited the author by stimulating thoughtful and serious discussions of ideas that were still at a formative stage.
- Fred called these various drafts "memos," and each one typically had a title, number, and date, and was cataloged. This system yielded a highly organized and visible record of progress. The completion of a particular memo, often by a pair of collaborators, became a short-term and immediate goal; this almost always proved motivating.
- Project participants felt obliged to read and provide comments right on the drafts in preparation for the next meeting of the team. Fred expected this feedback to be honest and constructive, to challenge the ideas and the work that was presented, and sometimes to suggest different directions for that component of the project. Often the group considered and discussed the commentary of individual participants, and the end result was that the authors of the original memo got many ideas for improving and extending their work.
- Collections of memos eventually became more polished drafts of papers or chapters, and these received lots of "editorial" attention from the group. Fred had some pet peeves, which most of his collaborators came to share;

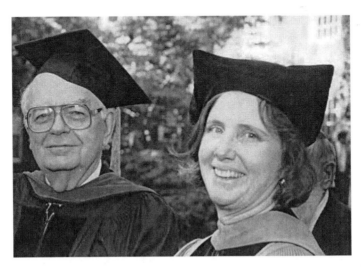

Fig. 23.11. Fred with faculty escort Nan Laird, his former student and now professor of biostatistics, at the Harvard University commencement ceremony, 1991.

he disliked the passive voice and excessive use of the verb "to be." His goal was clarity of exposition and ready access to the material by the reader, even in articles for highly technical journals. Sometimes Fred would encourage an author to ask for a critique of a draft by one or two of Fred's collaborators who were not part of the current project team.

- After a thorough but not overly lengthy revision process, Fred's goal was to "get the paper out the door"; that is, to submit the work for review and potential publication. He discouraged procrastination. Perhaps the only event more uplifting to Fred than seeing a manuscript finished and submitted was the arrival of the reprints or published book.

Over the years, recognition of Fred's accomplishments came in many forms. He received honorary degrees from the University of Chicago (1973), Carnegie Mellon University (1974), Yale University (1981), and Wesleyan University (1983). He was also an honorary fellow of the Royal Statistical Society, an honorary member of the International Statistical Institute, and an elected member/fellow of the American Academy of Arts and Sciences, the American Philosophical Society, and the Institute of Medicine. One of his proudest moments came in 1991, when Harvard University gave him an honorary doctorate after his retirement.

At the celebration of the 50th anniversary of the Department of Statistics (in 2007), Judith D. Singer, professor in the School of Education at Harvard and one of Fred's last Ph.D. students, surprised the audience when she announced that she had tracked down the films of Fred's Continental Classroom course, and that the American Statistical Association had converted them to electronic form. Since August 2008 they have been available from the ASA Archives.[1]

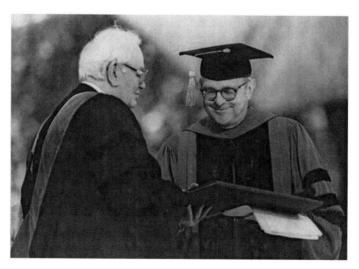

Fig. 23.12. Fred receiving an honorary degree from Harvard University, 1991.

★ ★ ★

Editing this book has given us yet another opportunity to appreciate the breadth, depth, and benefits of Fred's many contributions. We are grateful for the ways in which, as teacher, mentor, collaborator, and friend, he enriched our lives and helped to advance statistics, science, and society.

Fred with the editors

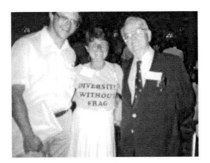

Fig. 23.13. Steve Stigler, Judy Tanur, and Fred, circa 1982.

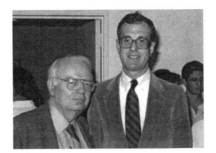

Fig. 23.14. Fred and Dave Hoaglin, 1987.

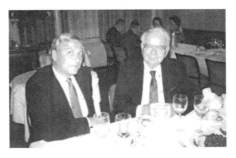

Fig. 23.15. Steve Fienberg and Fred at the International Statistical Institute meeting in Paris, 1989.

Note

1. A nearly complete set of Fred's Continental Classroom series (46 tapes in all) can be viewed at the American Statistical Association Archives Collection at Iowa State University:

Special Collections Department
403 Parks Library
Iowa State University
Ames, IA 50011-2140

http://www.lib.iastate.edu/spcl/manuscripts/MS349.html

Unfortunately, the videos cannot be loaned out or sold because they are still under copyright by the Ford Foundation. They are, however, available on location for viewing.

References

Antczak-Boukoms, A., Burdick, E., Klawansky, S., and Mosteller, F. (1991). Medical registries and data sets in technology assessment. *International Journal of Technology Assessment in Health Care*, 7(2):123–126.

Antczak-Boukoms, A., Tulloch, J. F. C., and Klawansky, S. (1991). Technology assessment in the Normative Aging Study. *International Journal of Technology Assessment in Health Care*, 7(2):143–149.

Bailar, J. C. III and Mosteller, F., editors (1986, 1992). *Medical Uses of Statistics*. Waltham, MA: NEJM Books. 2nd edition; Boston: NEJM Books.

Bailar, J. C. III and Hoaglin, D. C., editors (2009). *Medical Uses of Statistics*. 3rd edition. Hoboken, NJ: Wiley.

Bunker, J. P., Barnes, B. A., and Mosteller, F., editors (1977). *Costs, Risks, and Benefits of Surgery*. New York: Oxford University Press.

Burdick, E. and McPherson, M. A. and Mosteller, F., guest editors (1991). Special Section. The contribution of medical registries to technology assessment. *International Journal of Technology Assessment in Health Care*, 7:122–199.

Colditz, G. A., Berkey, C. S., Mosteller, F., Brewer, T. F., Wilson, M. E., Burdick, E., and Fineberg, H. V. (1995). The efficacy of Bacillus Clamette-Guérin vaccination of newborns and infants in the prevention of tuberculosis: Meta-analysis of the published literature. *Pediatrics*, 96:29–35.

Colditz, G. A., Brewer, T. F., Berkey, C. S., Wilson, M. E., Burdick, E., Fineberg, H. V., and Mosteller, F. (1994). Efficacy of BCG vaccine in prevention of tuberculosis: Meta-analysis of the published literature. *Journal of the American Medical Association*, 271:698–702.

Colditz, G. A., Burdick, E., and Mosteller, F. (1995). Heterogeneity in meta-analysis of data from epidemiologic studies: A commentary. *American Journal of Epidemiology*, 142:371–382.

Colditz, G. A., Miller, J. N., and Mosteller, F. (1988a). The effect of study design on gain in evaluations of new treatments in medicine and surgery. *Drug Information Journal*, 22:343–352.

Colditz, G. A., Miller, J. N., and Mosteller, F. (1988b). Measuring gain in the evaluation of medical technology. *International Journal of Technology Assessment in Health Care*, 4:637–642.

Colditz, G. A., Miller, J. N., and Mosteller, F. (1989). How study design affects outcomes in comparisons of therapy. I: Medical. *Statistics in Medicine*, 8:441–454.

Committee for Evaluating Medical Technologies in Clinical Use, Division of Health Promotion and Disease Prevention, Institute of Medicine (1985). *Assessing Medical Technologies*. Washington, D.C.: National Academy Press.

Emerson, J. D., Boes, L., and Mosteller, F. (2002). Critical thinking in college students: Critical issues in empirical research. In M. A. Fitzgerald, M. Orey, and R. M. Branch, editors, *Educational Media and Technology Yearbook, 2002 volume 27*. Englewood, CO: Libraries Unlimited, Inc. 27:52–71.

Emerson, J. D. and Mosteller, F. (1998a). Interactive multimedia in college teaching. Part I: A ten-year review of reviews. In R. M. Branch and M. A. Fitzgerald, editors, *Educational Media and Technology Yearbook, 1998 volume 23*. Englewood, CO: Libraries Unlimited, Inc. 23:43–58.

Emerson, J. D. and Mosteller, F. (1998b). Interactive multimedia in college teaching. Part II: Lessons from research in the sciences. In R. M. Branch and M. A. Fitzgerald, editors, *Educational Media and Technology Yearbook, 1998 volume 23*. Englewood, CO: Libraries Unlimited, Inc. 23:59–75.

Emerson, J. D. and Mosteller, F. (2000). Development programs for college faculty: Preparing for the twenty-first century. In R. M. Branch and M. A. Fitzgerald, editors, *Educational Media and Technology Yearbook, 2000 volume 25*. Englewood, CO: Libraries Unlimited, Inc. 25:26–42.

Emerson, J. D., Mosteller, F., and Youtz, C. (2000). Students can help improve college teaching: A review for an agenda for the statistics profession. In C. R. Rao and G. Szekely, editors, *Statistics for the 21st Century*. New York: Marcel Dekker. 145–172.

Emerson, J. D. and Mosteller, F. (2004a). Cooperative learning in schools and colleges: I. Teamwork in college mathematics. In M. Orey, M. A. Fitzgerald, and R. M. Branch, editors, *Educational Media and Technology Yearbook, 2004 volume 29*. Westport, CT: Libraries Unlimited, Inc. 29:132–147.

Emerson, J. D. and Mosteller, F. (2004b). Cooperative learning in schools and colleges: II. A review of reviews. In M. Orey, M. A. Fitzgerald, and R. M. Branch, editors, *Educational Media and Technology Yearbook, 2004 volume 29*. Westport, CT: Libraries Unlimited, Inc. 29:148–162.

Frazier, H. S. and Mosteller, F., editors (1995). *Medicine Worth Paying For: Assessing Medical Innovations*. Cambridge, MA: Harvard University Press.

Klawansky, S., Antczak-Boukoms, A., Barr, J., Burdick, E., Roberts, M. S., Wyshak, G., and Mosteller, F. (1991). Using medical registries and data sets for technology assessment: An overview of seven case studies. *International Journal of Technology Assessment in Health Care*, 7(2):194–199.

Klawansky, S., Burdick, E., Adams, M., Bollini, P., Falotico-Taylor, J., and Orza, M. (1991). Use of the SEER cancer registry for technology assessment. *International Journal of Technology Assessment in Health Care*, 7(2):134–142.

Miech, E. J., Nave, B., and Mosteller, F. (1997). On CALL: A review of computer-assisted language learning in U.S. colleges and universities. In R. M. Branch and B. B. Minor, editors, *Educational Media and Technology Yearbook, 1997 volume 22*. Englewood, CO: Libraries Unlimited, Inc. 22:61–84.

Miech, E. J., Nave, B., and Mosteller, F. (2001). Large-scale professional development for schoolteachers: Cases from Pittsburgh, New York City, and the National School Reform Faculty. Chapter 7 in R. J. Light, editor, *Evaluation Findings That Surprise, New Directions in Evaluation*, No. 90. San Francisco: Jossey-Bass. 83–99.

Miller, J. N., Colditz, G. A., and Mosteller, F. (1989). How study design affects outcomes in comparisons of therapy. II: Surgical. *Statistics in Medicine*, 8:455–466.

Mosteller, F. (1995). The Tennessee study of class size in the early school grades. *The Future of Children*, 5:113–127.

Mosteller, F. (1997a). Project report: The Tennessee study of class size in the early school grades. *Bulletin of the American Academy of Arts and Sciences*, L(7):14–25.

Mosteller, F. (1997b). Smaller classes do make a difference in the early grades. *The Harvard Education Letter*. July/August:5–7.

Mosteller, F. (1997c). The Tennessee study of class size in the early school grades. In D. R. Brillinger, L. T. Fernholz, and S. Morgenthaler, editors, *The Practice of Data Analysis: Essays in Honor of John W. Tukey*. Princeton, NJ: Princeton University Press. 261–277.

Mosteller, F. (1999a). The case for smaller classes and for evaluating what works in the schoolroom. *Harvard Magazine*, 101:34–35.

Mosteller, F. (1999b). How does class size relate to achievement in schools? Chapter 6 in S. E. Mayer and P. E. Peterson, editors, *Earning and Learning*. Washington, D.C.: Brookings Institute Press and Russell Sage Foundation. 117–129.

Mosteller, F. and Boruch, R., editors (2002). *Evidence Matters: Randomized Trials in Education Research*. Washington, D.C.: Brookings Institute Press.

Mosteller, F., Light, R. J., and Sachs, J. A. (1996). Sustained inquiry in education: Lessons from skill grouping and class size. *Harvard Educational Review*, 66:797–842.

Nave, B., Miech, E. J., and Mosteller, F. (2000a). A lapse in standards: Linking standards-based reform with student achievement. *Phi Delta Kappan*, 82:128–133.

Nave, B., Miech, E. J., and Mosteller, F. (2000b). The role of field trials in evaluating school practices: A rare design. In D. L. Stufflebean, G. F. Madaus, and T. Kellington, editors, *Evaluation Models: Viewpoints on Educational and Human Services Evaluation*. 2nd edition. Boston: Kluwer Academic Publishers. 145–161.

Sharp, S. (1998). sbe23: Meta-analysis regression. *Stata Technical Bulletin 42*, 16–22. `www.stata.com/stb/stb42`.

Name Index

Page numbers in *italics* refer to figures.

Subject Index

Breinigsville, PA USA
01 April 2010
235343BV00002B/74/P